ALL
IN MY
HEAD

ALSO BY PAULA KAMEN

o o o o o o o o o

Her Way: Young Women Remake the Sexual Revolution

*Feminist Fatale: Voices from the Twentysomething
Generation Explore the Future of the Women's Movement*

PAULA KAMEN

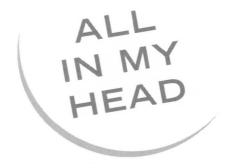

ALL
IN MY
HEAD

An Epic Quest to Cure an Unrelenting,

Totally Unreasonable, and Only

Slightly Enlightening

Headache

Da Capo
LIFE
LONG

A Member of the Perseus Books Group

For My Parents
and
Dedicated to the Memory of
My Friend Iris

Designed by c. cairl design
Set in 10.5-point Fairfield Light by The Perseus Books Group

Cataloging-in-Publication data for this book is available from the Library of Congress.

First printing, 2005
ISBN 0-7382-0903-1

Published by Da Capo Press
A Member of the Perseus Books Group
http://www.dacapopress.com

Da Capo Press books are available at special discounts for bulk purchases in the U.S. by corporations, institutions, and other organizations. For more information, please contact the Special Markets Department at the Perseus Books Group, 11 Cambridge Center, Cambridge, MA 02142, or call (800) 255-1514 or (617) 252-5298, or email special.markets@perseusbooks.com.

1 2 3 4 5 6 7 8 9—08 07 06 05

CONTENTS

○ ○ ○ ○ ○ ○ ○ ○ ○

PART FOUR: THE VERDICT

PART FIVE: CLOSING REMARKS

PREFACE

○ ○ ○ ○ ○ ○ ○ ○ ○

A Burning Bush in Gary, Indiana
(1979)

I could interpret the strange fact that the title of my sixth-grade science project was "The Control of Chronic Pain," and that I later developed years of constant pain (felt primarily as a dagger of criminal nerves behind the left eye), in one of two ways:

1. It's just a coincidence. No connection. There is no real system of meaning in the universe. After all, I'm hardly unique. More than a quarter of all Americans experience some form of chronic pain each year, and about 20 percent of women have migraines or some type of persistent headache, a term I have used as shorthand to name my particular mystery affliction. For God's sake, the headache is the most common medical condition plaguing human beings! And there you have it.

OR

2. You see, the New Agers, much of the alternative medicine and self-help industry, and all those psychoanalysts are right. All pain has some meaning. Everything in life happens for a reason, so we can *grow*. There are no accidents. The sixth-grade science project was a clear sign from God or Spirit or the Higher Power of Your Understanding that all along I was meant to experience these headaches, learn from them, and then teach others to relieve their suffering.

More specifically, as I interpret this second popular philosophy, we are each basically nothing more than ageless, continually reincarnating souls on an eternal mission for enlightenment, seeking to learn the vital and often painful lessons that our previous selves neglected. Just before we are born, our invisible spirits, just released from dead people, hover in the twilight—somewhere between the clouds and heaven—waiting for the next baby, which will represent their next and most effective learning opportunity. Then, at the proper moment, like synchronized swimmers lined up on a long series of diving boards by the pool's edge in a 1930s Busby Berkeley musical, they each seamlessly dive sideways and gracefully in cascading sequence into their individually designated earthly human containers.

So, from this perspective, what evidently happened to me was that on the day I was born, April 9, 1967, my particular soul looked down and had the foresight, as souls often do, to choose my unassuming bourgeois South Suburban Chicago human life-form. It knew that, through a series of hapless errors in judgment and general misfortune, this bipedal hominid would offer the soul the perfect opportunity to fulfill its particular mission: having a really, really bad headache.

In its infinite wisdom, the soul recognized that I would grow up with an anesthesiologist uncle who started one of the earlier chronic pain clinics in America, in Gary, Indiana—a land mass which is comparable in its cosmic power significance only to the sacred continental energy-vortex center underlying the Great Pyramid of Giza, or to that freaky thing in Sedona that attracts all those tourists. At the age of twelve, a traditional age of initiation into the world, my uncle would suggest as a topic for my sixth-grade science project "chronic pain," offering valuable foreshadowing. That science project would serve as my own personal burning bush, as a platform on which the Divine could manifest itself on earth and alert me to my purpose.

The soul knew that despite the initially apparent dry nature of this topic of chronic pain, its mysteries would soon powerfully capture my imagination. After all, it posed so many more haunting and mesmerizing questions than the garden variety projects of my classmates, what with their pedestrian baking-soda volcanoes and hamster-perplexing mazes.

I was drawn to the topic of pain the same way I was to the riveting made-for-TV John Travolta movie *The Boy in the Plastic Bubble* of that era, about the freakishness that results when the body goes awry. It had the same pull as the horrible, terrorizing historical accounts of Jewish girls my age hiding from the Nazis, such as in the Scholastic book *Marta and the Nazis*, which was most likely ordered from the back of a *Weekly Reader*, about a German girl stashing the family diamonds in the head of a doll she carried away in the train going over the border. And then there was the story of the more famous real-life Dutch girl hiding in an attic covered in movie posters, in a story still too dark for me to fully comprehend. Probably Catholic kids feel the same weird connection to tales of martyred saints riddled with arrows, sleeping on piles of bricks, wearing gloves filled with nettles, and/or willingly starving themselves to death. They just eat that stuff up.

Indeed, the subject of chronic pain—full of mysteries and unimaginably endless suffering—would fascinate with its stories of people with phantom pain in limbs that had been cut off years before. Sometimes they would even feel the sensation of nails digging into palms that no longer existed. The topic would capture my imagination with the accounts of the rare children born without the ability to feel pain, which isn't as fortunate of a thing as you would at first suppose, as pain can actually give you useful warnings. Such children would almost always die early in life, after years of tearing up their bodies by doing something as simple as jumping off a swing too hard. Just as too little pain was bad, I learned, so was too much of it. I would think about what it must be like to go on with pain that was not "acute" (temporary), but "chronic" (from the Greek word *chronos*: "concerning time, constant, continuous"), meaning that despite having no apparent medical purpose at all, it wouldn't go away.

My resulting science project—a report and a thick three-paneled poster board display, which I recently dug out of my parents' attic—reveals that I really got the drama of it all. On the middle board is the title, with the words "Chronic Pain" spelled out in twisting white wire garbage bag ties colored with a red marker. "Most of us well know what pain is and experience it quite often," reads the carefully printed explanation below, which was laid out on four strips of white construction paper pasted onto a red square, "but in the United States alone, for 40,000,000 people constant pain is a way of life. Here are some of the main ways people use to cope with their agony." I illustrated the intricacies of the nervous system with a diagram of nerves made of dried spaghetti noodles and a spinal cord of Styrofoam vertebrae, probably cut out of a disposable cooler, connected by a spine of blue drinking straws.

On the surrounding white poster board I had illustrated different remedies. One was "drugs," signified by a bulbous jar labeled "opium" and surrounded by a smattering of road-safety signs—"do not enter," "caution," "yield"—cut out of my mother's driver's ed book. I knew this was the most basic tool, as scientists had found traces of morphine in mummies unearthed from thousands of years ago. I also displayed another ancient method, acupuncture, using a photocopied line drawing of a hefty goateed warrior standing resolutely, his body dotted with acupuncture points. On display below was a vial of real acupuncture needles. But I had more license to play with the biofeedback machine on the table, which literally provided audio and visual feedback to a patient about the effectiveness of certain tension-reducing techniques. Demonstrating the machine required the use of an electricity-conducting pad from my limited stash. I would peel away a tab to expose the pad's side of sticky gel, which gave off a bitter odor of alcohol and petroleum combined. Then I would affix the pad to my forehead, plug the biofeedback machine's arm into the pad, and then contort the forehead at will. The machine, which resembled a professional version of a transistor radio, with its tiny bulbs and dials and handsome black carrying case, beeped in proportion to the tension levels I was creating.

But the pièce de résistance was an "interactive" board game, "The Control of Chronic Pain." The game's mission was serious, the players taking the perspective of someone trying to achieve pain relief; but the format was whimsical, ripped off from Candyland. The players, using a cardboard playing piece of a human figure, the kind that you see on public men's room doors, advanced along the steps of an upwardly curving path of blue footprints, with the ultimate destination point designated by the label "Pain Is Under Control." The players were escaping the villain, Pain, who was personified by three cardboard thieves who were pasted to the game board and who wore masks and stood in suspicious, hunched-over, lurking poses. A sign on the board explained the premise: "Wanted: PAIN. Charge: Hurting Millions of People. Reward: Relief." After rolling the dice, the players moved forward to spaces that gave further instructions, all soberly realistic, such as "Try to stop villain by surgically taking him out of nerve. It works. But there is numbness. Stay where you are." Another: "Advise a helpful drug to the victim. The victim gets addicted. Move back two spaces." The moral was illustrated by another sign on the board: "Pain Doesn't Pay!"

And not to toot my own horn, but this display was also quite adept at illustrating basic neurological concepts in the treatment of pain. Fundamental was the gate theory, first formulated in 1965, which demonstrates how counterirritant pain blockers (Ben Gay, electrical stimulators, acupuncture needles) work, by blocking pain signals from the spinal cord. On the right lower panel of my poster board display, this process was illustrated by two parallel spaghetti noodles, representing the C nerve, the source of the pain, and then the friendlier A delta nerve. At the point where they reached the spinal cord, the A delta branched downward to overlap the C and impede its signals with a little "gate." In another diagram, I illustrated another relatively new scientific concept of that time: endorphins, "pain-fighting chemicals which are made in the pituitary gland in the brain." I explained that we try to activate these natural opiates in a variety of ways, such as placebos (fake pills that the patient thinks are the real thing) or acupuncture.

The result: I got a B on it.

Indeed, in the end, with so many possible interpretations, the really awful part of having a really bad headache that won't go away is the *confusion of it all*. What does it all mean?

How we conceptualize and treat real physical pain is indeed rooted in our culture, and our culture today gives us more mixed and extreme messages than ever before. On the one hand, everything I know from growing up in an educated, doctor-worshiping Jewish home in the Midwest pulls me to the first answer, that basically "shit happens" in life, and that Western doctors are the answer. But then, the whirlwind of popular alternative medicine philosophies of the past several years—not to mention, my own natural internal quest for meaning—alert me to a second universe of other possibilities.

But I do know for sure that I'm not alone in asking such difficult questions about the experience of chronic pain in the United States, in one form or another. In our culture, experiencing chronic pain or any long-term illness can be a complicated, isolating, self-blaming, guilt-ridden process. Millions of chronic pain sufferers in the United States like me have silently suffered their own individual and profoundly strange battles. In the process, we've questioned and overturned basic concepts of ourselves, of the medical system, of the world, and of illness and its metaphors. We need to share our journeys through this strange terrain for the benefit of those just beginning their struggles. More than a decade ago, when I embarked on my search for a cure for an American headache, I was painfully ignorant about the real, often hidden limits of many common treatments, from both Western and alternative medicine. I wish I had been armed with such essential, hard-won, critical information.

Needless to say, this book, my second major lifetime report on chronic pain in the United States, has been much more complicated to research than the one I did in 1979. When I wasn't a patient with actual pain, understanding how to control it seemed so much easier, so much more straightforward. In my sixth-grade report and display, I was just giving the obvious facts, which had been mapped out for me in the clinical literature and were translatable to a two-dimensional cardboard display.

In this book, in addition to developing and expanding on some of that information, I try to fill in some gaps, examining many popular and culturally rooted myths denying the physical realities of chronic pain. Most basically, I describe the experience and ask questions from the perspective of the *patient*. And as in my other writing as a journalist, I hope to give the "bigger picture," so that my story doesn't start and end just with me personally. As well as eventually telling about other patients I have met, I also report some findings about chronic pain, culled from texts, interviews, and medical meetings.

I hope also to reveal some complexities of the experience. Most popular health books, including those on headaches, are of the self-help variety, written by a doctor or New Ager with a single limited agenda or practice to promote. They typically sell a one-size-fits-most perspective of pain relief, a variation of *Ten EZ Steps to Total Health and Enlightenment*. And many of the health stories that do exist from a patient's perspective, such as in articles in women's magazines, follow a preordained formula to recount the valor, and ultimate triumph, of rich and famous celebrities. According to these media narratives, we are all supposed to be like Ronald Reagan, riding away on a horse days after his surgery. Or Christopher Reeve, directing a film right after becoming paralyzed. Or Lance Armstrong, winning six consecutive Tour de Frances, after battling a very advanced case of testicular cancer. In contrast, patients with more invisible, yet still often disabling, chronic illnesses, which characteristically hit young women, from chronic migraines to fibromyalgia to rheumatoid arthritis to vulvodynia (vaginal pain), see their less dramatic problems hardly covered at all.

But telling more realistic and sobering stories such as mine can be just as powerful and, ultimately, hopeful. This telling raises the social awareness of chronic pain as a major unresolved public health issue and gives both doctors and patients a more effective and down-to-earth grip on this problem. The fact that our culture often glosses over the complexities and difficulties of chronic pain only compounds the suffering, self-blame, and isolation of patients like me. We believe the uniquely American work ethic, as applied by alternative medicine, that if you just work hard enough, you will get better. When we don't, we think it's our own fault. Perhaps there is a psychological issue we aren't dealing with appropriately, perhaps we aren't listening to our soul's code, or perhaps we are suffering a waxy yellow buildup of the chakras. We also believe the credo that doctors actually know everything about stopping pain, and that if they can't cure you, the problem must be yours. As a physical therapist friend has told me, this is the only culture on earth that fails to accept chronic pain as a fact of life.

Sharing patients' real stories also sheds light on chronic pain as a women's issue, the focus of my past writing. Chronic pain mainly affects women, both in overall numbers and in accounting for those primarily affected by most types of pain disorders, including chronic migraine and head pain. Many studies show that women's chronic pain is seriously undertreated medically by not enough painkillers being prescribed, compared to the treatment of men with chronic pain. Instead of responding adequately, many doctors, therapists, and cultural critics dismiss it, using the catchall psychosomatic diagnosis of "hysteria," and overstating the influences of any contributing mental, emotional, and political factors. Many academics, even feminists, are in the business of talking about how our culture "creates" certain illnesses (such as chronic fatigue syndrome, a common target), but not about how strongly that same culture often *denies* them. This is a legacy that continues in full force a hundred years after Freud, denying major scientific discoveries of the past several decades, such as information gained through advanced types of brain imaging.

In our society, illness as a metaphor is an especially potent and pervasive force when that illness is "invisible," when it is experienced mainly by women, and when the causes are largely unknown. These forces all combine to form a recipe for the accusation: "It's all in your head." Ironically, feminists in the women's health movement, a separate branch of feminism that emerged fully in the 1970s, have not yet fought back significantly. In fact, they have largely avoided addressing the topic of women and pain, fearing that such attention will lend credence to the age-old disparagement of women as "the weaker sex," an attitude that has justified terrible discrimination.

Telling our stories can also raise awareness of how far we—both men and women—*haven't* come in actually treating chronic pain, especially the most severe and frequent forms, despite significant strides in understanding its neurochemistry and triggers. Popular media reports on pain, often in the form of news-magazine cover stories, are often devoted to overpraising the latest so-called wonder drug (read: "It's so new that we don't know its side effects yet") as pain patients' savior of the day. Providing testimonials are a carefully selected group of patients, very often fed to journalists by pharmaceutical companies and the doctors interviewed. As a result, pain patients who aren't cured by the latest "miracle discovery" or who can't solve their pain through sheer gumption and force of will feel their already debilitating sense of isolation and self-doubt compounded.

In 1979, in that poster board display, I summarized the major treatments of pain of that era: acupuncture, drugs, and biofeedback. Today, more than twenty-five years later, despite some notable gains, this is still the case. Although modern medicine allows us to replace severed limbs and excise the most precariously placed brain tumors, our effectiveness in treating chronic pain and many other disabling invisible illnesses has not significantly advanced. In fact, in reality, we are hardly better off than in 1979 B.C.—when the people whom we know today as the leather-faced mummies in museums walked the earth, all too conscious of their humanity because of their crushing toothaches, their shingles, their labor pains, their cluster headaches.

When I was twelve and unburdened by chronic pain, I couldn't yet describe the full experience, neither physically, emotionally, nor spiritually. This wasn't possible until years later, when I was twice that age and one continuous headache gradually started to define itself and then take nonstop residence behind my left eye and in my left temple, like a bad, inconsiderate roommate who never leaves the apartment to give you peace. I then found myself starting a trial, as well as *going on* trial, as a chronic pain patient. I was in the odd position of playing for real that board game that I had devised so many years ago, following another circuitous, unpredictable, and ultimately (somewhat) enlightening path.

Part One:

TRIAL AND PUNISHMENT

1

Big Pharma (1991)

○ ○ ○ ○ ○ ○ ○ ○ ○

MORE THAN A DECADE AGO, at the age of twenty-four, in a single moment, I found myself going from "girl, emerging author" to "girl, interrupted."
I was doing something quite mundane at the time, putting in my contact
lenses in the bathroom of the downtown Chicago Hyatt Hotel at a journalism
conference. Somehow, inserting the left lens set off a chain reaction to ignite
a constellation of nerves, which radiated backward from behind the surface
of my eye. The pain was deeper and more piercing, and generally more unreasonable, than any other headache I had ever experienced, and I instantly
realized I was dealing with an entirely new and different species.

Although this process was instantaneous, the new connections seemed to
be made in slow motion, in several discrete consecutive stages, much as
when they light up the huge White House Christmas tree on television. You
see the bottom level and then the middle and then the top turn on in sequence, one immediately after the other. Click, click, click.

As I later realized, nearly everyone with a chronic health issue has a distinct story of the moment she or he was stricken, although the symptoms
had probably been creeping up all the time, often for years and years. A man

describes the beginning of his depression as taking place on the first morning he couldn't get out of bed. A woman pinpoints her multiple sclerosis as starting when she reached for change in her purse in line at the grocery store and couldn't feel the coins. Such moments are probably defined by the feeling that we shouldn't be struggling this much to do this simple a thing.

Still, at that moment at the Hyatt Regency, I knew never to underestimate the power of repression and compartmentalization, exalted skills of journalists everywhere. I looked in the mirror, and although the surface of the eye felt like broken glass was lodged in it, I saw no sign of irritation. It wasn't even red. I went back to business and tracked down the appropriate meeting room, whatever it was called, probably one of those hotel-conference-room-type names like the Venice Room, or the Sequoia, or something evoking the majesty of one of the Great Lakes.

I was interested in meeting one of the panelists, a noted writer on urban poverty, who was deeply committed to the issue of poverty in the inner city and, as far as I could tell, was neither married nor homosexual. I sat through the panel without fully comprehending the words and then made the journey up to speak to the man, who was surrounded by admirers. I lacked the stamina to push through the crowd and instead waited for them to leave, one by one. Finally, we were left alone in the room. He looked up at me, confused. "Do you know where the next session is?" he asked. "I don't see it in the program."

"Sorry," I said, shaking my head. I knew that it was up the escalator outside and to the right, and I probably should just walk with him there. But I didn't have the energy. My eye was on fire.

Then he walked away.

I ran to the bathroom, popped out the contacts, and continued to feel the cutting pain at full force. I rushed out of the conference area and into the guts of the adjoining underground Illinois Center complex, concentrating on retracing my steps to find my way back to South Water Street and the Metra train. I staggered through the low-ceilinged maze of narrow, uniform tunnels, whose sides resembled single floors of Chicago's modernist skyscrapers, made of uniform sheets of frosted and then clear glass, bordered by sleek black steel beams. I kept running, trying to find my way out.

A few months before that, in March 1991, I had just come out of the closet, in the literal sense. I had spent that winter writing a book on young women and their views of feminism, under deadline, while hunched over a beady little Apple Macintosh screen in a walk-in closet in Kenosha, Wisconsin. As I had predicted, I had confronted very few, if any, distractions in that small city, where I had just left a job as city reporter and had months of rental time left to go in the apartment behind the Pick 'N Save on Highway 50.

My editor, at a small independent publisher, had wanted the book out as soon as possible, as *Time* had just done a cover story on this new mysterious generation, Generation X, featuring a multicultural cluster of twenty-some-things staring ahead plaintively into the future. And she had a feeling that further discussion of just what they were thinking about would be in the media soon. So I did what I had always done under pressure: worked like hell and planned to recover later.

One day after finishing my book, I moved out of the writing closet and the apartment. That day was marked by the worst headache of my life, up to that point, a searing yet diffuse sensation in the forehead. I was sure that this was merely the result of withdrawal from Eight O'Clock Bean. And so I clutched my head without panic during the ride back to my parents' split-level house in the Chicago suburbs, where I arrived with a handful of change, what had been left in my Kenosha checking account.

When the caffeine-type headaches continued, I went to a nearby general practitioner. I took his advice to lay off the caffeine altogether, but then a greater variety of pains started taking temporary tours of various durations and intensities in different parts of my head and eyes. I also noticed a trend—which had very gradually emerged over the years and was now accelerating—of both of my eyes becoming more and more sensitive and inhospitable to contact lenses. Over the years, I had had to put the lenses in later and later in the day, waiting until just before the start of the event at which I wanted to look good. The process became still more painful when I got less sleep the night before. This was even the case with the new onionskin-thin high-tech daily-wear ones, which I hadn't bothered to wear at all during my four months' hermitage in the closet. And increasingly, as with that most jolting May episode at the Hyatt, when I put them in, the left lens would trigger a severe day-long pain that shot from the back of my eye toward the core of my head, without ever seeming to stop.

Like many who experience migraines and other types of chronic headaches, I assumed all these things were part of a problem originating in the eye. I was suspicious that it was the result of an accident a few years before when I had been using a phone in my parents' house and felt an electrical shock leap from the receiver to the back of the socket of my left eye. The pain at that time wasn't bad, just a little pinch. I went to see an ophthalmologist, who gave it a good look and said no apparent damage had been done.

I took his advice and stopped wearing contacts for a while, but the pain, as usual, was smarter than I was. By the time I moved into Chicago that summer, right after the Hyatt episode, the headaches started self-generating, without any apparent external trigger. And then, by October of that year, the release date of my book, the pain behind the left eye and in the left temple was constant.

To cope, I greedily shoveled aspirin and Advils down my throat. But usually, the only effect was a hollow gnawing feeling in my stomach. Excedrin worked at first and then suddenly stopped, leaving me wired and sleep-deprived because of its high caffeine content and, as a result, with even more pain. Like many headache sufferers, I had a love-hate affair with caffeine, a blood-vessel-tightening chemical used for more than a century as an ingredient in migraine medications. Caffeine is truly a double-edged remedy: It can both trigger and relieve headaches.

I was also beginning to realize that painkillers of all types—whether over-the-counter or stronger—were effective to use once in a while, but not every damned day. Used constantly, they could wear the body down. And I even later learned that if taken too often, over-the-counter pain medications can worsen the pain, by suppressing natural pain-relieving endorphins and making the nervous system more sensitive to pain. Such overuse can result in "rebound" headaches. (In fact, doctors think that many people who suffer frequent headaches are primarily victims of this rebound effect.)

The next logical step was to call my uncle, whose opinion our family always trusted above all others. A former head of intensive care at Northwestern University Hospital in Chicago, my uncle started his first pain clinic in the 1960s in Gary, his home base. The clinic was his response to the needs of his great diversity of patients, many of whom were facing work-related injuries, the most common being herniated disks. They also included U.S. Steel and Inland Steel workers who had had parts of their arms and hands ripped away in confrontations with large moving rows of raw metal. We knew he was good at seeing the bigger picture of things, such as in campaigning against the rampant pollution of the steel mills, which was aggravating his patients' health problems. He took note of the serious pain and discomfort that many patients were suffering with the rigid plastic breathing tubes that had been planted in their throats and often caused ripping, scarring, and infection. With another doctor, he devised a new type of cuffed tube (formerly known as the Kamen-Wilkinson tube) made of polyurethane foam that expands to fit each patient individually, which is still in use today worldwide. Of course, we were all quite proud.

My 1991 visit to his pain clinic office was my first one to him as a patient. At that time, I remembered my earlier, more lighthearted research trip from sixth grade, when I had had my picture taken with his life-sized plastic skeleton on wheels, a fixture of the place. On the wall had hung a large sledgehammer and a sign, "Other People's Pains Are the Easiest to Bear."

But this trip involved less levity. When I got to his present office in Merrillville, Indiana, he took out a very large needle, which was filled with cortisone and some kind of pain-killing drug. He gave me a nerve block, which was an especially common procedure with his back pain patients. To ease the tension, he pretended to be confused, asking himself, "OK, just give me a minute to remember where this goes." He then swiftly injected it into selected tender points at the base of my skull and on the sides of my head. I felt a crunching as the needle went in and then swirls of numbness filled the nerves encircling my head. That was from the painkiller. That first time, it seemed to work. But only for a day.

I returned a half dozen times more and had less success every time. Each visit, I walked in hopeful and left surprised that my uncle couldn't help me more. Through his long career he had resuscitated countless people from the brink of death—and had even devised a better mousetrap for their breathing comfort and ease. But now, with this seemingly simple problem, he was stumped.

On the way back from what was to be our last visit to the clinic in Indiana, my parents and I stopped at an Arby's for lunch, and I realized that the caffeine from the cardboard-cup-flavored iced tea there was more effective in relieving my pain than occipital nerve blocks. For about an hour, the headache went almost completely away. Later that day I called my uncle, who agreed there was no point in continuing the nerve blocks. But he didn't have any alternatives.

"Don't worry," he said. "These things always burn themselves out."

"What do you mean?"

"Chronic pain burns itself out, eventually."

"What do you mean by 'eventually'?"

"Eventually."

"Months?

"I don't know."

"Years?"

"It's hard to say."

"Decades?"

He didn't know.

I knew I couldn't wait for "eventually." It was time for a force bigger than us all, Big Pharma, to step in. I needed a preventive prescription medication, something to take on a daily basis that would raise my threshold to pain and make all these other weak, and even eventually harmful, stopgap treatments unnecessary.

As many new patients are surprised to learn, visiting a neurologist is a different experience from visits to other types of doctors from one's past. Here, because of the "invisible" nature of neurology—and this is not a complaint—the patient typically has no physical contact with the doctor. Business is conducted with the same level of human intimacy that you would expect from a bank clerk in opening a new Roth IRA. The nurses do the preliminary grunt work, such as taking blood pressure.

And then you go in to see the doctor, who sits opposite you behind a large desk, which in my opinion and in my case, resembles a judge's bench. This first exam, often costing several hundred dollars more than the others, is known as the "consultation visit," or the one visit where the neurologist actually displays an interest in talking to you.

Like other doctors to come, this first one I met, a general neurologist at a South Suburban hospital, was attentive, optimistic, and spry—in the beginning. The questions he asked were typical, revealing many common concepts behind the understanding of headaches in our culture.

First: "How old are you? What year is it? Who is the president? How many fingers am I holding up?"

Despite my assumption that my answers to him were correct, I answered nervously, afraid I would space out, perhaps fixate on one of those mundane matters that floats through the brain from minute to minute, such as a phone call I had to return or "What's the deal with that 'Priority Mail' thing at the post office? Is it really the same as regular first class, but they're making you pay more for it? They guarantee delivery in two to three days for 'Priority Mail,' but isn't that the same time that first-class mail takes? I just saw them dump the last package I mailed earlier today into the same bin as the first-class mail. Oh, wait a minute, who are these young fellows in the white coats, and why are they taking me away?"

But luckily, I remained focused and passed that hurdle. Then he asked about past head injuries; I had had a concussion in second grade, after falling backward on the ice from the insanely high Timbertown jungle gym, which was later razed after a spate of such injuries occurred at my school (a casualty of a less-protective era, along with punishing dodgeball games, the humiliating exercise of picking teams, and asbestos-lined classrooms). I'd been unlucky that it was winter; my blow had not been cushioned by the scattering of "protective" wood chips on the ground, which were well covered by a layer of ice. I ticked off past surgeries: adenoid and tonsil excavations in grade school. He checked my reflexes and asked me to accomplish challenges like touching my index finger to my nose and walking in a straight line.

Then there was the task of describing the pain, which is famously difficult to do, even with something that has been a constant companion for months. One of the toughest parts, which many writers have mused about, is simply to pinpoint when it began. In perhaps some of the most noted lines of verse describing pain, headache sufferer Emily Dickinson wrote:

> Pain has an element of blank
> It cannot recollect
> When it began—or if there were
> A day when it was not.

Another often-repeated quote by another famous headache patient, Virginia Woolf, in her classic 1930 essay *On Being Ill*, relates the odd difficulty of describing the ever-changing headache—its intensity, when it began, how it feels. "The merest school girl when she falls in love, has her Shakespeare or Keats to speak her mind for her," she wrote, "but let a sufferer describe a pain in his head to a doctor and language at once runs dry."

That challenge is true, but the task of accurately describing what a headache feels like is possible, if you stop to examine its overall character. For this reason, headache experts strongly recommend keeping a daily headache diary and then analyzing it with the doctor. Although a headache may change often, it also exhibits particular general patterns over time. It's comparable to a particular climate in a particular region in a particular season, which may seem unpredictable day by day. But when viewed in general retrospectively, one can see that it is basically sunny and humid in the summer, averaging 80–90 degrees, cooler near the lake.

Describing a headache is also a matter of the doctor's asking the right questions and offering the patient some useful choices of descriptions. At my exam, I answered that, yes, mine definitely resembled a clamp pinching the nerve at various levels of tightness or a dagger piercing through the eye or temple. But through the years, I have kept other, more eccentric descriptions to myself. I privately have conceptualized the headache pain as caused by a fishhook, pulling backward on the nerves behind the eye, with varying intensities through the day. A more accurate analogy came to me more recently during housecleaning, while I was soaking a showerhead in vinegar, to release the little bits of foreign gravel that accumulate there over the months and impede the flow of water. I thought that my eye pain has always felt as if those same little irritants were traveling upward from some unknown source in the brain through the nerves, trying to make their way out through the frustratingly impermeable eye-membrane nozzle.

The doctor's more clinical diagnosis was migraine, an atypical one, because the pain was constant. Usually migraines are episodic; they come and go. To him, a major clue was that the pain was only on one side of my head and behind the eye, characteristic of migraines. That was true although I had no nausea, or light or sound sensitivity, or auras of spots or pinwheels, or the other accoutrements that often go along with classically defined migraines. I just had the pain.

"This is just the way you're wired," he said. "It's not your fault. It's based in the personality. You're a Type A."

"Then I'll change," I said. "I'll learn to be different."

"You can't change your personality. That's the way it's going to be."

This was the beginning of a long dialogue that I would engage in over the years about "the migraine personality," also which is considered one of repressed anger and hostility. About twenty-five years before my experience, in her well-known 1968 essay about her chronic migraines, "In Bed," writer Joan Didion was already questioning one specific idea of the "migraine personality," defined as "ambitious, inward, intolerant of error, rather rigidly organized, perfectionist." She recalled, "'You don't look like a migraine personality,' a doctor once said to me. 'Your hair's messy. But I suppose you're a compulsive housekeeper.' 'Actually my house is kept even more negligently than my hair'" (170).

Yielding to reality, and the doctor's assessment, I took his prescription for the drug amitriptyline (under the brand name Elavil), which was actually one of the most well-used and effective chronic headache "preventives" at that time and continues to be today. As I found out only while researching this book years later, this was a tricyclic antidepressant (an older type affecting the neurotransmitters serotonin and dopamine). As many patients do not realize, antidepressants are common treatments for chronic pain. This is not because doctors are blaming the pain on depression, but because these drugs actually treat the same neurotransmitters involved in the pain cycle. Neurotransmitters, a term with which I would become very familiar in studying chronic headaches, are basically signal messengers between brain cells that can help determine levels of pain (and depression), among many other conditions.

Blessedly, this drug worked, for a month or so. It seemed to stop after I had an unusually heavy night of drinking, while sitting in a bar distracted with playing cards for a long time in a group of friends who kept refilling my glass. I still don't know if there was any connection, as alcohol was "contraindicated" for this drug. At that time, with the pain under control, I had almost forgotten about it.

At some point, as a typical course of action for a headache patient, I got my first MRI, a milestone in any young woman's coming-of-age story. I had it done just over the border in northwest Indiana, where brain scans are cheaper than in Chicago, just like gas and cigarettes. The suspense was great, but with the hope that they would indeed find something. As I waited for the results, I longed for the announcement of a very small, benign, and easygoing brain tumor, something that would be taken care of with one swipe of the scalpel, before the doctor's afternoon round of golf. I would take a week or two to recover, perhaps stopping to relearn a bit of hand-eye coordination and what had happened to me in the 1980s, as perhaps those parts of my lobes would have been sacrificed during surgery. A tumor, I rationalized, would offer concrete and irrefutable proof to the entire world—and to me—that something was really wrong. I wanted to believe that the problem was indeed all in my head, but not in my mind.

But to my dismay, the results showed that there was nothing visibly wrong. Although this pain was as real to me as anything I had ever experienced, I was being told that there was no evidence of it. Although I have to admit that I was happy I had no brain tumor, this nonfinding was a mixed blessing (as it is for others with "invisible" illnesses). Only fewer than 1 percent of headaches in the general population are caused by a dangerous underlying disorder.

The neurologist was disappointed about the drug pooping out. He was also miffed that my mother, not I, had subsequently called him with a few questions. She had asked me about my progress, and I said I wasn't sure about the next step and would call later after some deadlines were met and I finished traveling. She then offered to call the doctor herself to find out. I hadn't seen the harm in it; after all, she had offered, she was good at that kind of thing, and, as I reasoned to myself, she was the stereotypical Jewish mother with no sense of boundaries.

On the heels of her involvement and with a new weariness, the neurologist asked me if I had ever considered counseling. I decided to try another doctor, perhaps a headache specialist, instead of a general-practice neurologist.

Although my mother had annoyed this doctor, I knew I was lucky to have her on my side. A former medical social worker, my mother was relentless in doing research of all types, especially in seeking health care information. Although she had stopped working outside the home, like others of her generation, when she had kids in the late 1960s, she still had a strong "can-do" attitude. Years before, she had suffered severe back pain, which immobilized her for a few weeks. The doctors had told her that surgery was the only way out. Instead, she had talked to dozens of other back pain patients, some total strangers she had met in the grocery line, and sifted through the great detritus of random advice to find the few relevant nuggets. With great discipline, she followed their best hints, most of which involved different ways to hold and retrain the body. She scattered old blue Compton's Encyclopedia volumes on the floor of our house, in places like at the bases of all the sinks, to use as a supportive step when she stood still. And then she got better. We were sure that type of resourceful thinking would work for me.

When sleuthing for my immediate health matters, my mother found the name of a headache specialist neurologist at the cutting-edge University of Chicago Hospital, a few blocks from where I then lived in Chicago's Hyde Park neighborhood. The office was just beyond the large gray-and-bronze-colored brushed-metal statue on Ellis Avenue. Hollowed out in different points on the bottom with a bulbous top, it resembles both a mushroom cloud and a human skull. The monument marks the spot of the first "self-sustaining controlled nuclear chain reaction" set off by scientist Enrico Fermi in December 1942. That experiment laid the groundwork for the atomic bomb. This monument also reminded me of the university's historic role in developing new technology, for better and for worse.

I had plenty of time to reflect on such matters. The wait for the renowned headache expert was two months long. In the meantime, I stumbled through as best I could. I wasn't in the frame of mind to do anything more high-powered and challenging than write the occasional short freelance story and serve at temp jobs.

My tactic to get treated sooner, on the advice of the new doctor's nurse, was to go to the emergency room, which sounded like a good idea at the time, as it does at one time or another to the majority of chronic headache patients.[1] I went on a day when the pain was particularly piercing and I couldn't work anyway. They gave me a CT scan, which again, unfortunately, turned out normal, and an injection of Compazine (prochlorperazine), a typical one-size-drugs-all tool in the ER to treat migraineurs (meaning *all* people who suffer migraines, not just the French ones). It is also a close relative of Thorazine, the old tranquilizing antipsychotic. Compazine is commonly given for migraine partly because of its antinausea qualities, without the fact of its common lack of pain control effectiveness and extremely impairing side effects as an impediment to its widespread use. The ER staff also wasn't deterred by the consideration that there are many types of headaches, and mine did not include any nausea. Another added "benefit" of Compazine to medical staff is discouragement of "drug seekers." Unlike with narcotics, they don't have to worry about devious ploys to get a hit of it. After all, no one in their right mind is going to lie, cheat, steal, and/or whore themselves on the street for some Compazine.

The Compazine did work in one way; it shut me up from complaining about the headache, which had only been muted a bit. My parents took me back to their home, as I was too drugged out to function on my own. While I was lying down, trying to figure out where things had gone wrong, the phone rang, and I stared at it, very confused, unsure of how to go about the task of picking it up and bringing it to my ear. About a day later, the Compazine finally wore off.

I returned home and tried the bright red Midrin, an old-time migraine-abortive drug that the ER doctor had prescribed, again without much explanation. The drugged stupor returned—as I later found out that Midrin contains a sedative—and I struggled not to fall asleep at the desk of my temp job downtown. I left early, staggering to the bus, scared of feeling this unexpected loss of my faculties.

Finally, the day of my appointment with the University of Chicago doctor arrived. He confidently explained that he saw this type of headache frequently after a person had some kind of trauma, such as divorce. The pressure of quitting my job and writing that book in a very short time had probably triggered it, and this would be temporary. He gave me another mysterious drug, desipramine (Norpramin), another tricyclic antidepressant. As with many drugs to come, I never knew if these little red tablets were working because of the normal daily fluctuations of pain, which in my case I would rank as from a 2 to a 6 out of 10 each day. When I called the doctor with questions, he would just tell me to wait awhile, as these drugs typically took a very long time to kick in. Then he would instruct me to double the dose I was on, which I did repeatedly for the next five months. Finally, he told me to stop and did not go on to offer any alternatives. Besides, he was leaving soon for another job, on the East Coast.

I thought to myself that these drugs should have worked by now on my so-called migraine. Why wasn't I closing the little spaghetti pain gate, like the one that had worked so well on my sixth-grade poster board display, and why couldn't I get those little endorphins going?

This was a simple problem, to the point of being ridiculous: It was too invisible to inspire sympathy, too strangely embarrassing to talk about, and too common to be a disability.

A headache, after all, especially one proven *not* to be caused by a tumor, was the most unserious thing you could have. And as far as I knew, unlike with a majority of migraine sufferers, no one in my immediate family (parents) had headaches, which would have pointed to a genetic connection. (Years later, I found out about many aunts and cousins with migraine, but I'm not sure if that even counts.)

Judging by the apparent initial confidence of my doctors in the drugs I had been taking and their subsequent loss of interest in me, I was sure I was the only one with such an absurd ongoing struggle. Besides, I figured I was alone in having a constant headache. Most people I knew who suffered "migraines" only got them once in a while, like right before their periods or after eating a particular kind of aged cheese. I didn't even think like them, in terms of identifying "triggers," as the pain was constant.

Worst of all, I didn't know of any celebrities with it, Oprah had never done a show on it; I had never seen it written about in the Tuesday "Science Times" section of the *New York Times*. Therefore, how real could it be?

Next, I went to another doctor, a very well-regarded and much more folksy osteopath (who has a degree called a doctorate of osteopathy, or D.O., not a medical doctorate, or M.D., and goes to a different type of medical school, which is still mysterious to me) in the suburbs of Chicago, who had helped a friend of a friend of my mom's. He diagnosed me with tension headaches, because that was one type that was considered to have constant pain involved. Although a tension headache was then considered to be different from migraine, a result of muscles that contracted too tightly, researchers today tend to see all these types of headache in the same spectrum.

First, he tried physical manipulations, such as cracking the neck and rotating the shoulders (which osteopaths specialize in) and then hypnotism.

"Your eyes are getting heavy," he told me.

"They are?" I answered, totally awake.

And then he turned to the drugs.

That summer, we tried a battery of typical drugs used for chronic headaches—Inderal (a blood-pressure medication, surprisingly), Cafergot (an ergotamine), Anaprox (an anti-inflammatory)—which, unexpectedly to me, gave no or temporary relief, while typically making me feel hazy and/or lethargic. This was a very different experience from my relatively simple and easy use of drugs in the past, such as to treat allergies.

From the start, this process seemed random and inefficient and experimental—mainly because, as I later found out while researching this book, it indeed was.

In reality, as patients rarely realize from the beginning, neurological problems, especially those involving chronic pain, are often complicated to treat. Patients usually don't understand the biological fact that every person has a unique type of pain, responds differently to medication, experiences different side effects, and requires a different dose. Also often unexplained is that "preventive" drugs, if they do ever work on headaches, typically take awhile to kick in, often more than a month. And so, the typically long and circuitous journey of finding the correct headache medication is very similar to that described by patients suffering psychiatric illnesses, such as depression or bipolarity. These patients are also dealing with a complex problem involving highly individualized brain chemistry, which you can't see or objectively measure, with an X-ray or blood pressure meter.

Also befuddling patients is that the majority of drugs they are given for prevention of headaches were never specifically approved for this purpose. In reality, most preventive "headache drugs" are drugs that the Food and Drug Administration (FDA) had approved for other problems, like high blood pressure. Somewhere along the way, lo and behold, doctors discovered they helped patients' headaches. As a result, as well as for chronic pain disorders in general, they are prescribed "off label," or without FDA approval for that specific use.

In fact, as of this writing, the FDA has approved only four drugs that are available in the United States for *migraine* prevention: the anticonvulsants Topamax and Depakote, and the blood pressure medications Inderal and Blocadren.

One strike against better regulation is that the medical guidelines for chronic daily or near-daily headaches as a class of its own are just being established, after years of being overshadowed by episodic migraines. And the pharmaceutical companies don't comprehensively test these drugs for these other uses because, well, they don't have to. Legally, these companies are

OK, as long as they don't directly advertise these products to doctors for off-label uses. In this way, they avoid the cost of the rigorous and expensive research required for FDA approval for these added purposes. And despite the lack of research behind them, doctors are still willing to prescribe drugs for off-label uses.

Actually, a great number of "headache drugs" of all types were primarily devised for and used to treat depression in particular, which shares with chronic headaches similar imbalances of both neurotransmitters and aggravating hormones. In fact, almost every drug used for psychiatric treatment has at one point or another been used for headache prevention.[2] Indeed, drugs for daily headaches are usually the bridesmaid to the bride of depression (or maybe epilepsy or bipolar disorder; all four of these have similar overactive brain neurochemistry). To use another metaphor, with less status and attention in their own right, chronic headaches are like the second-class free-loading relative of depression, crashing on depression's couch.

But doctors in the trenches often fail to communicate the reasoning behind giving an antidepressant off-label to a headache patient. As a result, the patient often just recognizes the drug as one given for psychiatric purposes and then might get angry with the doctor, seeing him or her as "judging" the patient's problems as purely psychosomatic or even ignoring them, like others in the patient's life.

Adding to the confusion is lack of specific medical study and recognition of chronic daily headaches (at least in the past one hundred years, since other doctors have written about it through the centuries). Like others with this ailment, I lacked proper medical terminology to classify it, and this affected both my treatment and my ability to convey the experience to others. No existing official diagnosis really explained what I had—as I seemed to fit somewhere between tension headache and migraine, two of the main categories (besides cluster headaches, which are much rarer). The only type of constant headache classified at that time was chronic tension-type headache, which mainly involves a bandlike pressure around the whole head, not a migrainelike stabbing on one side, like I had. As shorthand, I just called what I had "migraines," a word that people were familiar with and that carried a certain gravitas, one that *tension headache* just can't muster.

But there is a real and important medical distinction between *chronic daily headache* (which became a standard term in the 1990s) and *migraine*, about which most people are not aware. Doctors are now more careful to call what has been perceived as migraine as *episodic migraine*, which, by definition, typically only happens once in a while. But I learned recently that the separate concept of *chronic daily headache* (CDH) is newer. The latest revision of International Headache Society classifications, made only as recently as 2004, describes it as distinct in treatment, neurology, and symptoms.[3] Instead of just one type of CDH, which it had in its first edition in 1988, it now defines ten different types, the most common being *chronic migraine*, classified in the migraine category.

Although this term *chronic daily headache* may seem very contrived and noncommittally generic—seemingly hatched by a crafty marketing staff somewhere trying to push more drugs—it is very useful in making an important distinction with the three words of its name. It is defined as a headache that happens at least fifteen days a year and for at least four hours a day. Although CDH accounts for a minority of headache sufferers, such patients comprise the great majority of patients in headache clinics, a factor adding to doctors' very recent growing awareness of them. They are the ones who keep coming back, the dreaded and traditionally suspect "thick folder" patients, which I was becoming.

But episodic migraine has overshadowed this other category in treatment and research for many reasons. After all, migraine affects an amazingly high number of people across all populations and cultures (not just high-maintenance white middle-class women), about one in five women and one in twenty men. Yet, as more recent studies have shown, CDH actually affects

The Art and Science of Classification: It's Enough to Give One a Headache!

Revealing the evolving and also complex challenge of diagnosing a headache, the list of those that have been officially classified goes on and on and on. The revised International Headache Society (IHS) classifications for 2004 total 151 pages and are more detailed than ever. In an effort to reduce the chaos of each doctor using different terminology, the first IHS criteria came out in 1988 (with twelve different categories) and was partly modeled after the third edition of the American Psychiatric Association's *Diagnostic and Statistical Manual of Mental Disorders* (DSM-III), used to diagnose psychiatric disorders.

The classifications now include a total of fourteen headache categories, the first two listed being the most familiar and common:

- Migraine headaches (with twenty types listed, mainly defined by whether they are accompanied by a visual aura).
- Tension-type headaches (totaling about nine).   *(continues)*

(continued)

After that are the even more intense—known as the most severe head pain syndrome known to humankind:

- Cluster headaches (with 8 types, including a renamed type of short-lived chronic daily headache, "chronic cluster headache).

Following that is a miscellaneous primary category with eight types, with the most evocative names of all, including

- Primary stabbing headache.
- Orgasmic headache (see Chapter 6).
- Hypnic headache (a new addition, meaning a dull, short-lived form of chronic daily headache that wakes one up, previously known as alarm clock headache).
- Primary thunderclap headache (also new; defined as a "high-intensity headache of abrupt onset mimicking that of ruptured aneurysm").

These listed here are all "primary types" of headaches, that is, pain that is not a result of another underlying problem. The rest of those classified in ten categories are the rarer secondary types; that is, they stem from other issues, such as a tumor, drug withdrawal, or head or neck trauma.

only 4–5 percent of the population, with 0.5 percent, or one in two hundred people experiencing the pain nonstop, 24/7, as I was.

Numbers aside, migraine is also still more established in the medical and public psyche as "real" because of the numerous drugs that have been approved for it over the past century. These two classes involve ergotamines, first introduced as effective drugs in the 1920s, and the much more streamlined and modern triptans first rolled out in the 1990s, such as Imitrex, Relpax, and Zomig. These drugs' resulting effect on public opinion reveals their secondary use in society as a sort of diagnostic test. If it can be treated effectively with drugs, then a malady is "real." If not, the patient is making it up (usually on a subconscious level, allegedly).

In my adult years, I have witnessed this process in the use of Prozac to validate depression. If someone takes a chemical (Prozac) that successfully treats depression, then that depression is considered chemical in nature (not imaginary or a moral failing). Today, patients with chronic daily headache are in the same position as many of those who had depression in the pre-Prozac era, relying on a motley assortment of drugs, such as lithium and anticonvulsants, many taken off-label, that sometimes work (a bit) and sometimes don't.

In contrast to chronic daily headache patients, episodic migraine sufferers have more choices and hence more legitimization. (See the sidebar on page 18.) In the early 1960s, they were widely validated by the ergot-derived Sansert. As a "serotonin antagonist," it was created directly as the result of chemical studies of the basic mechanisms of migraine. Sansert was touted as getting to the neurological root of the problem, instead of simply constricting blood vessels, as other migraine drugs in that class had been perceived to do in the past. As a result, Sansert made a dramatic difference in changing the view of migraine as a neurological disorder, instead of as primarily a psychiatric problem. In public opinion and to doctors, this view of serotonin as central seemed more legitimate and "less neurotic" than just the old view of dilated blood vessels as the culprit.

Then, the triptans, first introduced with Imitrex in 1993, further distinguished themselves from past episodic migraine drugs by selectively targeting receptors of the neurostransmitter serotonin, preventing dilation of arteries in the head (an action that causes pain). Ironically, as ergotamines, the drugs of the past, were discovered to be serotonin antagonists (reducing its effects), these modern triptans were serotonin agonists, enhancing its action.

In its unprecedented level of effectiveness, Imitrex was like the Prozac for episodic migraine sufferers, changing lives with its highly targeted smart-bomb effect, instead of just the multiple-neurotransmitter carpet bombing of the past, as with the cruder ergotamines. At that time, as a result of Imitrex's effectiveness, doctors started describing headaches more generally as being the result of a neurochemical problem, and not as being primarily a blood vessel or vascular disorder, which was what had been visibly observed to cause pain in the past.

But alas, just like the ergotamines, these triptans, which are meant to be taken as needed to stop migraines as they emerge, often do not work for poor schmendricks with constant head pain. They are also expensive, a cost of twenty dollars per pill being common, and have time limits on how often they can be taken. And like analgesics, they can cause "rebound" headaches if taken too often.

Perhaps doctors who are aware of the challenges and nuances involved in diagnosing and treating CDH have some good reasons not to communicate them to patients. They may want to raise patients' expectations and preserve some kind of "placebo effect"; after all, if the patient is positive, perhaps a drug will work better. (Encouraging the patient is fine, but the ethics behind this practice of downright nondisclosure are still questionable, with a shady history involving women, as well as minorities. In fact, as feminist author

A Short History of Migraine Drugs: From LSD to Imitrex

The most basic (if flawed) class of migraine drugs, with a very storied past, is the ergots. This means that they were derived from ergot, or *Claviceps purpuria*, purple fungus of rye and other types of grains. Ergot is a multipurpose agent of mythical proportions, used for centuries for everything from relieving hemorrhaging after childbirth and inducing abortion in Europe (hence a German name for it, *Mutterkorn*) to serving as a hallucinogenic for Aztec ritual practices. Doctors had made note of its crude and intense blood-vessel-constricting powers centuries ago, in the Middle Ages, as causing gangrene. (Today, doctors would refer to this problem as a side effect.) At that time, black bread contaminated with ergot fungus was found to be the root cause of epidemics in which people's limbs rotted off, giving them the appearance of being badly burned. This malady, killing tens of thousands in Europe, was called St. Anthony's fire, after the saint at whose shrine relief was sought. (Some people believe that relief was really caused by the lack of contaminated bread ingested through the pilgrimage there.)[4]

From the late nineteenth century on, noting its blood-constricting effects, researchers worked to refine ergot for migraine treatment—without such unseemly limb-rotting effects. Their results were mixed. As early as 1868, a crude and only marginally effective extract of ergot was used for migraine. Then it became more widely used and standardized for migraines in the 1920s after an improved pure alkaloid of ergot had finally been extracted, as "ergotamine titrate," in 1918. However, afterward, the "father of headache research," Dr. Harold Wolff, made note of the possible resulting disease of "ergotism," which could happen with drug overuse. This could involve violent vomiting, hallucinations, seizures, and gangrene.

One attempt at a better migraine remedy by Sandoz Pharmaceuticals in Switzerland in 1938 synthesized lysergic acid, which failed as a painkiller, but nevertheless emerged in popular consciousness, both literally and figuratively, by its other name, LSD (lysergic acid diethylamide). During a lab experiment in 1943, the scientist Albert Hofmann accidentally went on the first acid trip in recorded history when the substance seeped through his fingers. He reported seeing for two hours "an uninterrupted stream of fantastic pictures, extraordinary shapes with intense, kaleidoscopic play of colors."[5]

In the early 1960s, the pharmaceutical industry finally got it right and released a highly selective derivative of lysergic acid, methysergide, under the brand name Sansert (called Deseril in Great Britain). This was heralded as a wonder drug for migraine prevention, its makers estimating that it could relieve 90 percent of all cases of severe migraine—as its notable side effects were not yet well known. (The manufacturer, Novartis, stopped making Sansert in 2002. A reason may be concern over the side effect of fibrosis, or scarring of heart tissues. Sansert also has been known to cause terrifying hallucinations.[6])

And then, in the early 1990s, the heavens parted and a more refined and effective solution was rolled out to stop migraines in their tracks. Out came the triptans, for which many with episodic headache had been specifically praying for decades. These drugs had been in the pipeline for development since 1972, when a pharmaceutical company executive launched a search for an effective migraine treatment for his daughter. This class includes the first triptan, Imitrex (sumatriptan), and then, as of 2004, six more, including Amerge, Zomig, and Relpax. Triptans do pose possible side effects to an organ widely considered important; for example, they constrict the heart's blood vessels. But they generally have been effective in aborting episodic migraines for many at the first sign of symptoms.

Barbara Seaman (1995) has written, it was common in the 1960s not to inform women of the typically high instances of side effects of the then-much-more-potent birth control pill. "If you tell a woman she'll get a headache, she'll get a headache" was the rationale.) Or maybe doctors don't want to admit a "weakness" in their own or their field's expertise, maintaining the omniscient and omnipotent veneer that they and their patients have come to expect.

But of course, a result of this lack of knowledge is that such patients often suffer tremendous self-blame, feeling that they are the only ones who are not responsive to these drugs. And like me, they also may resent the doctors for seeming incompetent, random, and insensitive. When treatments fail again and again, doses are constantly over- and underestimated, and totally unexpected, debilitating side effects emerge—such as prolonged dizziness and insomnia—we often get the feeling that the doctor has absolutely no idea what he or she is doing.

Starting to sense that *every* drug was fair game to be used off-label for headaches, I began to fear that doctors were blindly reaching for anything, as if they were playing a game of darts with the open *Physicians' Desk Reference* as a target. I imagined them thinking, "Well, her name is Kamen. Kamen— that sounds like Calan, the calcium channel blocker. How about some Calan? Here's a prescription. See you in six months. Bye!"

It was like with the grab bags we had at holiday time in grade school in the 1970s. But here, instead of getting a toy troll with green hair or a book of Lifesavers, I got a tricyclic antidepressant.

Finally, after I had gained ten pounds as a side effect and the pain showed no sign of budging, the osteopath told me to abandon the standard preventive drugs I was taking. He admitted that if he went on, he would just be guessing about which drugs to try.

I looked at the calendar and realized that I had been in nearly constant pain for more than a year. And I had so much I wanted to do. An ego-caressing highbrow publisher approached me about doing a book. The total advance, about fifteen thousand dollars, was almost enough to live on for the year I estimated it would take me to research and complete the book. This seemed like a luxurious amount of time, as it was twice what I had had for the book before it. And I was fascinated by the topic, current female sexual attitudes, which had always confounded me because of the mixed messages of empowerment and double standards I had observed. At the same time, on college campuses I had visited while lecturing on my first book, I was impressed by the boldness and sense of entitlement of many vocal women students. They stood out, even from my slightly older peers, in their openness and lack of shame about gay and lesbian and even bisexual issues, safer sex, acquaintance rape, dating abuse, and other tough issues that were not a part of widespread popular awareness in "my day." Their activism for control—and their obviously high rates of casual sex—defied the popular wisdom at the time that the fear of AIDS was ruining sex for young people.

But my energy, spent from constantly pushing through the pain, was diminishing, and my front was crumbling. Ironically, the old "not tonight, dear" excuse was alive and well, with a headache threatening to stop a sex book.

The pain, which averaged a moderate level, was usually mild enough not to stop me from doing routine things, but strong enough to make everything more difficult, to introduce an underlying layer of resistance. It was as if I was driving with the parking brake on. I was constantly battling to break through an invisible barrier between the world and me, which only I could see.

The osteopath then asked me if I had ever considered "something else," and I braced myself for the recommendation of counseling (which seemed to imply that this was not a real medical condition and only insulted me). Instead, he referred me to the Chicago Headache Clinic (not the real name, but close),[7] a nationally famous operation, mentioned in nearly every major national media article at the time, and continuing today, about headaches. Founded in 1964, it was the first such private clinic in the country, later spawning the at least fifty that now exist in the United States and abroad. Its well-known founder had been reacting to an increased medical interest in headaches, which had accelerated twenty years before with World War II veterans returning home with head injuries. This center had followed the first-ever headache clinic, established in 1945 at the Montefiore Medical Center in the Bronx, New York.

The interesting part was that's all they did there at the Chicago Headache Clinic: treat headaches. And they took them very seriously (at least as long as you weren't on Medicaid). The doctor stressed that I was lucky that it was based in Chicago, as people from all over the world had made pilgrimages to the Chicago Clinic as their ultimate hope for relief. It looked like I had a chance to get some well-planned, scientifically based, personalized care, with some more innovative thinking. I immediately called to make an appointment.

2

Mecca

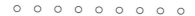

THE CHICAGO HEADACHE CLINIC was on the far North Side of Chicago, in a two-story plain red-brick building, across from a Shell station and a Korean strip mall. It was just south of the old Jewish neighborhood of West Rogers Park, Chicago's equivalent to parts of Brooklyn or Queens. When I was little, my elderly Yiddish-speaking grandmother had lived about a mile away from this place, in that type of squat yellow courtyard apartment that Yiddish grandmothers lived in, with couches hermetically sealed in brittle plastic covers.

My always-irreverent father was very skeptical of this plan to go to a so-called headache clinic, as he was about most doctors. Not helping was that my uncle, the one doctor whom he trusts, told him that this place had a better reputation among the public, exposed to the constant uncritical media coverage of its accomplishments, than among some practicing physicians, such as himself. But I saw this clinic as a great hope and eagerly counted down the days until the appointment.

Besides, my private, flexible, non-HMO insurance, which my business professor dad had wisely researched and advised me to get earlier, after leaving my job, would cover most of it. So I didn't worry about the high cost, which was immediately foreshadowed in the waiting room. For reading material, both the Sotheby's and the Christie's catalogs were displayed.

But I still felt more at home there than with past doctors. Many patients were visibly in pain, hunched over and shielding their eyes from light. At one point, the elevator opened, and the man inside was vomiting and pounding his head on the wall. This is a common reaction to one of the most painful types of headaches, clusters (mainly experienced by men, by a five-to-one ratio). The pain is so severe that the sensation of hitting one's head violently is a pleasant distraction from the pain. According to the first recorded description of such a headache, dating from the 1700s, the sufferer felt "as if his eye were slowly being forced out of its orbit with so much pain that he nearly went mad."[1] Nurses quickly ran to the elevator to help.

Here, with the problem taken so seriously, I first learned to define what I had as "headache," that is, without the *a* before it, which sounded eminently more legitimate.

At some point, I saw the doctor assigned to me, another osteopath (which, it turns out, is basically a mix of an M.D. and a chiropractor), who was friendly and optimistic. The doctor asked me what I wrote about, which I usually declined to mention to doctors, for fear that he (and up to this point, they were all "he") would see me as a hostile, man-hating feminist. But I revealed myself, and he won my trust by answering that he was a board member of the National Organization for Women.

I described my symptoms. Like other doctors, he discounted the shock-in-the-eye and concussion incidents from years earlier as irrelevant. Before I was even finished talking about them, he almost cut me off, confidently stating a diagnosis. He had seen this a lot. I did not have migraine but was unofficially classified then as a "mixed" headache, meaning both migraine and muscle-contraction tension headache. This was the common term for a constant headache, before *chronic daily headache* became better known soon after.

I was relieved that this doctor was experienced with this problem and had a plan. I was not alone, after all. He told me he would prescribe a series of aggressive preventive medications, along with an IV treatment of Dihydroergotamine (DHE), an old-time ergot alkaloid, to stop the headache cycle. That sounded good to me, I said, anticipating that I would get a few shots and the whole nightmare would soon be over, at last. He said he would send a nurse in to take care of the details.

He left and a nurse entered the room.

"I'm ready to check you into the hospital," she said.

I was startled. So she explained that these medications were too strong to just give to me, that the doctor had to monitor me while I was an inpatient, and that they had to be administered over a period of days. The typical stay was about a week. I asked if I could delay this a day, to give me time to get "my affairs" in order. She grudgingly said that was fine, as long as I took just one day.

Charged with the doctor's sense of urgency and optimism, I checked myself into the Chicago Clinic's decade-old inpatient unit at Weiss Hospital, just off Lake Shore Drive, early the next morning, as directed.

They gave me an IV, to which I reacted by swiftly and dramatically passing out. Aggravating matters, they probably had to dig around for a vein, which is common in many women, who often have dainty little blood vessels that are deep and hard to locate. When I came to consciousness, the needle seemed uncomfortable, like it wasn't in just right, but the nurse assured me it was fine. They fitted me with a medical bracelet, which I wasn't to remove, even after leaving the hospital, and that stated I was on an "MAO inhibitor." I signed a "treatment contract," in which I promised to attend all classes and biofeedback sessions, on time; not take previously prescribed medications; and, of course, not smoke.

Everyone on my floor wore his or her regular summertime street clothes, giving a casual summer-camp-at-Bellevue vibe. I observed the others, who like me, were acting in reversal of common stereotype, to enter a hospital to get *on* drugs, not to get *off* them. There was one woman, actually, who was there to get off drugs, headache drugs, as I was told she wanted to safely have a baby. I also met an accomplished and understated college professor and was astonished that she could teach and write with her constant headaches. I had not attempted any major mental project since I had been struck, and not being able to do so in the future was my greatest fear. She shrugged, saying she just had to make herself do it. At least a few others were also teachers, who were there on their summer breaks. Without any small talk first, another woman, a puffy-faced blond woman in her early twenties, complained to me very sadly that she had gained twenty pounds, as a medication side effect. I was almost starstruck meeting a young man who told me, after hearing I had lived in southeast Wisconsin, that he was a relative of the owners of Mars Cheese Castle, a famous landmark to Illinoisans traveling over the border.

Many people were either too fat or too skinny, reflecting the biological fact that the appetite centers in the brain overlap those that deal with migraine and the common weird weight-affecting consequences of headache drugs. I met my first roommate, an emaciated middle-aged rural Minnesota woman, who told me she had been in too much pain to eat for many months. When she got up, I saw her legs were almost pure bone covered with skin, with about nothing in between.

She was optimistic about the Chicago Clinic, explaining that she had been treated successfully there years earlier, and that the drugs they had given her had changed her life. But like many other patients there, she was a repeat visitor. Over the years, the wonder drugs had worn off, so she was in for a new round. She actually seemed to enjoy herself, complimenting the food and recommending to me Salisbury steak on the night's menu. If I wanted it, she told me, I could have vanilla ice cream for dessert, which was available in tubs in the refrigerator down the hall. Her sister visited, and they eagerly described their future visit to the Mall of America, just outside Minneapolis, which was opening that month. The mother of all malls, it was the largest such structure in the world, with a multiride theme park featuring a roller coaster in the middle. I was intrigued.

Every eight hours or so, a nurse would come in with a small paper cup, like the kind that would hold a minimuffin, filled with four colors of pills. The centerpiece of the collection, the orange pellets, were Nardil (phenelzine), known as a monoamine oxidase inhibitor (MAOI). She also gave me injections of a painkiller, while also monitoring the IV, which also was filled with drugs (and which was by now turning my left hand purple).

After one such visit, I finally turned to the worksheet in the blue folder they had given me and looked for the first time at what the nurse had written under the heading of "New Prescribed Medication and Warnings." The list went on for quite a while:

- IV DHE 45 (ergotamine abortive) will be given every 8 hours for a total of 9 doses. You will receive an injection of Tigan $1/2$ hour before DHE to control nausea. Any coldness, numbness, tingling of extremities, chest, flank or back pain—call nurse.

- Calan SR 240 mg. every day (calcium channel blocker). Do not stop abruptly. May cause nausea, constipation.

- Nardil, 15 mg., 3X/day, MAO Inhibitor tab 3X/day. Side effects: possible weight gain, leg cramps, insomnia.

- Toradol 60 mg. Im PRN (anti-inflammatory) will be given every 8 hours as needed. May ca [sic, it stops there]

- Sparine 100 mg. every 6 hours as indicated for 48 hours (anti-anxiolytic) will be given and may cause drowsiness.

- DHL, DHI Non narcotic analgesic, may take every 3–4 hours as needed.

The spectacular inventory of drugs blended together in my brain, literally and figuratively, and as the hours went on, I felt myself getting more and more hazy. But I still dragged myself to the workshops on drug and pain management, as I had promised. A required one was a lecture by the clinic's founder, a general practitioner (not a neurologist) then already getting up there in years. It was about "tyramine-free" foods to avoid while on an MAOI. To my surprise, almost everyone on the floor was attending that session and was taking a drug cocktail similar to mine.

The doctor explained that MAOIs deactivate the enzymes needed to metabolize the amino acid tyramine (a building block of serotonin and adrenaline), and too much of it was not desirable. Then he painstakingly outlined page after page of prohibited foods, including those that were well-known migraine triggers, such as cheese, caffeine, chocolate, and alcohol. But this list, which went on to fill several pages, also included anything fermented, pickled, or marinated, in every food group, even in food groups that I hadn't even known about before as existing. These included "hot, fresh homemade yeast breads," doughnuts, nuts and seeds, pole or broad beans, lima or Italian beans, snow peas, fava beans, navy beans, pinto beans, pea pods, sauerkraut, garbanzo beans, "onions except for flavoring," garlic, olives, pickles, and MSG. The only cheese allowed was farmer's cheese and the only alcohol was vodka. Yogurt was allowed, but in no more than a half-cup serving. He even cautioned us not to have certain types of over-the-counter drugs, such as antihistamines. If we had a cold, we could only use decongestants.

After at least a half hour of this, the audience's mood shifted from polite interest to stunned silence. At the back of the room, I raised my hand, cleared my throat a few times, and in a purposely light and casual tone asked, "So, I . . . uh, what happens to us if we *don't* follow this?"

After all, I was only human. What if I had a drink at New Year's? What if an errant fava bean somehow found its way onto my plate? What if I got attacked by a giant three-bean salad at my next potluck dinner?

His answer was vague: It was best just to follow these directions. I decided to comply, especially after my mother told me that someone she knew on these drugs ended up in the emergency room after eating some chopped liver. A few years later, I saw an episode of *Chicago Hope* that further informed me. It featured a boy going into a near coma after the doctors mistakenly gave him a sedative. "Oh my God, he's on Nardil!" the attendants cried, discovering his medical bracelet under his coat. But I found out the real risks only very recently while researching this book. "Ingestion of tyramine-containing foods, in the presence of medication that blocks monoaminime oxidase, can result in hypertension and even cerebral hemorrhage," wrote Dr. Stewart Tepper in his 2004 guide *Understanding Migraine and Other Headaches* (92).

Apparently, as I also found out more than a decade later, Nardil is an even older antidepressant than the first drugs I had been on. It was actually an antique, from the 1950s, a holdout from the era immortalized in literature of when tragic confessional writers like Janet Frame, Sylvia Plath, and Robert Lowell were institutionalized—and used MAOIs as a chaser to their regimens of electroshock therapy, lithium, and Freudian psychoanalysis. This old-fashioned drug apparently affected numerous neurotransmitters, implicated in both headaches and depression. And this is precisely the reason it has been found so effective for headache patients, even more than Prozac, because it affects more of the complex chemistry involved in headache pain. Serotonin is actually just one piece of the puzzle.[2]

In other words, even more than any other drug I had been on, this Nardil was basically a neurochemical whore. Totally undiscriminating. It would brazenly interact with almost any old neurotransmitter that moved—inhibiting the breakdown of serotonin, dopamine, and norepinephrine—without caring a bit about what the others thought of it. In contrast, Prozac, which came out later, was "cleaner," indeed a *selective* serotonin reuptake inhibitor (SSRI), meaning that it worked only to balance one neurotransmitter, serotonin. The tricyclic Elavil, which I had taken on the advice of my first doctor, was somewhere in between these two categories in selectiveness, working on two neurotransmitters.

And thus, the potent MAOIs have gained quite a reputation as being very complex and difficult to monitor. For this reason, doctors have had serious reservations about giving them out to severely depressed patients. People who are emotionally unstable have had trouble maintaining the clarity needed to avoid the numerous feared interactions. Patients also have resourcefully recognized MAOIs as a suicide drug of choice, made all the more effective, and pleasant, by being downed with a few cocktails.

But, as I mentioned, I didn't know anything about medications then. I'm only adequately informed now because of research I have done to understand my experiences. Indeed, I'm only just now for the first time reading many of the handouts from the Chicago Headache Clinic that were in that blue folder. I'm not sure whom to blame. The early 1990s were pre-Internet, so information wasn't as easy to come by. And I had a strong basic faith in doctors and very limited energy, which I used just to get the essentials done. So much of my life was gobbled up already by the headaches that I had little interest in giving my remaining energy to researching medications. And this problem of a headache seemed so simple that reading about it seemed as useless as reading about how doctors fix broken arms before getting a cast on. At some point, anyway, I figured you just have to follow what the doctors say.

I went to other workshops on more enjoyable things we couldn't do, all of which triggered headaches. People with headaches, we were told, had exquisitely sensitive nervous systems, which were aggravated by the slightest provocation, and we needed as much routine and order and blandness as possible. We had to keep the same sleep schedule every day, not sleeping in. We had to eat at the same time every day. We couldn't take too much stress.

I also worried if sex was out of the question, if it also somehow had headache consequences, like everything else that threatened the puritanical nervous system. I was thinking about that woman—the one I had seen only from a distance as a shadowy figure lying in her partially enclosed room, the one whom my roommate had described as getting off the drugs, presumably so as not to scramble the brains of her future baby. I gingerly took aside one of the doctors, and he very briefly answered me that if I used birth control and was "careful," sex should be fine. I was almost as embarrassed as he was but reassured myself that I was about to write a book on sex and had to get over such prudery.

As a needed distraction, friends came to visit, bringing increasingly inappropriate gifts. My brand-new boyfriend, Lance (whom I'll name after Lance Armstrong, whose autobiography I just read) gave me a copy of Ken Kesey's *One Flew over the Cuckoo's Nest* and inquired about conjugal visits. Some friends brought chocolate, which I had to dump into the garbage immediately after waving them good-bye and watching the elevator doors close. A college friend brought me a novel he had enjoyed, *Black Water*, by Joyce Carol Oates, a harrowing first-person account of a young woman losing control of her life.

At one point, I attended an art therapy session, which was apparently designed not to tax our increasingly enfeebled minds. One project was to make "stained-glass" birds. They gave us simple clear-plastic birds that were divided on the surface by little raised grids. They were like hard-plastic cookie cutters. But instead of filling them in with little pieces of glass, we just colored them in with markers, which made faint stains, like spilled fruit juice. And then, as I showed my sister, to her amusement, we had a macaroni and glue project. Nothing too elaborate either. They just had us glue macaroni on a plain piece of paper, in no particular order.

In the monotony and haze, I had one memorable bright moment. At some point, I finally managed to convince a nurse that my IV was indeed put in wrong, presenting my increasingly swollen and purple hand as primary evidence. She changed it, and it was then painless.

Yet, surprisingly, the pain in my head was not diminishing at all. After a few more days, I decided to find out more from my doctor. I queried him during

morning rounds, and he assured me that things would change soon. Not entirely convinced, I had my parents give the list of drugs to my uncle, who immediately became concerned. He asked me if he could call the doctor to
discuss the regimen with him, as these drugs were extremely powerful. I assumed that the Chicago Headache Clinic doctor would be open to such a
conversation with a colleague.

The next morning, my doctor was brusque and angry, no longer looking me
in the eye. He told me that he was the doctor, and that I should not have my
family interfere in my treatment. I needed to have patience, he explained,
and I might have to be there a few more weeks.

I had overlooked similar recent incidents as just my being too sensitive,
but now I was angry. Now too extreme to ignore, this treatment was a new
concept to me, of doctor as dictator, not partner. I realized that this doctor
was used to the old ways of doing things.

But I decided to tough it out and make the best of the experience. I had to
remain hopeful. After all, I had no choice. The Chicago Headache Clinic was
supposed to be the end of the line.

Feeling dejected and more and more groggy, I found it more difficult to get
to the educational sessions. I barely made it to one with a handful of others
to learn biofeedback. After a few minutes of lecture, the instructor realized I
had been staring straight ahead without any reaction. She quizzed me:

"Did you hear what I just said?"

I couldn't answer.

"OK, I'll explain again."

"Hmma," I answered.

Then, for the first time since I could remember, I started to cry, and she
told me I should go back to my room. I'd learn it another day.

"Hmma, hmma," I agreed.

Later, noticing that my shorts were tightening, I tried to work out in the
exercise room. I was surprised this was happening already, since I had just
bought new clothes after going up a size in the months before because of
drug side effects. But I soon saw a workout was not possible. I was so weak
and dizzy from the drugs that I only lasted for a few minutes on the exercise
bike, although it was dialed way down to the easiest level of resistance.

I gave up on trying any type of physical activity. I went back to bed, feeling
both the familiar drill behind the eye and the heavy meds filtering my senses.
How did I get into this spot, I wondered. Whose fault was it? In true "migraine personality" form, I thought that they were right, that I was indeed
angry and hostile—that is, at doctors.

But I was most mad at myself. This whole mess was entirely my fault, I thought. Me and my migraine personality. I fit the description exactly—hard-driving, sensitive, Type A, and OK, well, not really a perfectionist, and not really rigid. After all, I did identify with what we had discussed earlier as being a common personality trait of migraine sufferers, having an "inner locus of control," or being driven by inner forces instead of outer ones. I was always too tense. Although depression had never been a major issue in my life, I had to admit that I had always been high-strung. I thought back to all the anxiety I had experienced trying to finish that first book over the months of 1991 within a very short three-month deadline that had preceded the onset of this pain. That had probably caused the whole problem. As with every writing assignment I ever had, I never really knew if I'd be able to do it, until it was done. And now I was learning the hard way that nothing was worth this worry. Nothing. "It's not worth it," I said to myself, out loud, to reinforce this message: not to ever let anything like this happen again and never again to take anything too seriously.

Perhaps this was the greatest proof of my inner locus of control, that I was mostly blaming my problems on my inner locus of control. (In reality, recent studies show that this distinction is not true, that people with an "inner locus of control" don't have more migraines. In fact, they are better at managing the pain they have, more likely to take an active part in their treatment.[3])

After about ten days in the inpatient unit, I felt the pain shift. It didn't go away, but it fell to a lesser level, in a slightly different part of my head. My doctor was encouraged and said I could probably go home soon. I became more hopeful. On one of the final days, after two weeks there, I was even feeling strapping enough to go on the organized daily afternoon walk, which culminated in a visit to the Walgreen's drugstore across the street. We first strolled for about fifteen minutes through the slums of the surrounding area of the Uptown neighborhood, a leading inpatient release center of Chicago. We seamlessly mixed with the roaming hordes of the methadone-seeking, demented, and just plain down-and-out, an oddly high number wearing winter coats and hats in the middle of August. Like us headache patients, these other zombies were in a state of limbo, not totally a part of the mainstream world, hovering on the margins, not totally well and not totally sick. Well, look on the bright side, I thought. I can walk around talking to myself in this neighborhood as much as I want, and no one will ever notice.

The nonurban patients from out of state, which seemed to comprise the majority, were stunned, never having witnessed such scenes of urban decay and blight so close. When we finally got to Walgreen's, the only candy we were allowed to buy was Gummy Bears, and we walked out with bags of them under our arms.

We returned to the Chicago Headache Clinic floor of Weiss Hospital. My old roommate had checked out. I had a new one, a thirty-something mother from somewhere in northern Wisconsin. I expertly explained to her the rituals of the floor and the expected content of the dining menu. That night, I pointed out, we would have spaghetti, and you could have all the vanilla ice cream you wanted, but don't even bother asking for chocolate.

I stopped my monologue, suddenly realizing a new worry. Sometime in the past few days, I had started to like the place. It was safe. They were keeping me on a regular sleep schedule, which I had never experienced through my adulthood, feeding me carefully balanced meals, and shielding me from the stresses of the outside world, all triggers for pain. All this safety had me worried. Feeling as drugged up as I did, I feared that I wouldn't have the lucidity and energy to plan my life so well when I was sprung. (A week later, at a temp job at the University of Chicago, the avuncular tweedy head of the sociology department, for whom I worked part time, asked me about the stay and explained this phenomenon. I was oddly open, saying it was almost hard to leave the hospital. He looked up, intellectually intrigued, saying, ah yes, that there was a whole body of literature about that socialization process.)

But of course, despite some mixed feelings, I really wanted to go home. On the last day, my dad and sister came to pick me up. I left with a bill, as I recall, of thirteen thousand dollars, which my premium-level insurance would almost entirely cover, and a paper grocery bag filled to the top with drugs. It was a beautiful sunny day, and we walked on the long Montrose Street pier that spiraled out onto the lake and looked at the hospital across the street safely in the distance.

We went back to my apartment and saw that the past two weeks had been as hard on my car also. The silver 1982 Olds Cutlass had been broken into and the inside dashboard gutted. My dad hotwired it and drove it to a junkyard, where he picked up a new steering wheel, heater, and radio, all from different models and in different colors. We hoped for a full recovery.

The next morning, Lance and I didn't waste any time going on a long-awaited and delayed trip to Michigan, to enjoy the last remaining beach days of the year. We were already starting to feel a slight chill in the air. Before we left, he opened his trunk, which was half empty. He said he had made room for my drugs. He wasn't kidding.

The first night, I couldn't sleep, caught in a growing state of fear, confused about how to deal with the drugged-out feeling, how to function with all the waves of dizziness coming at me. I hardly knew what I was doing, able to focus only on resisting the swirling cloud. It was about 4:30 A.M. and Lance was awake, too. We were both hungry, so we walked across the parking lot of the Red Roof Inn to a corporate country diner. Lance faced me in the booth and gave me some basic directions about the art of drug taking.

"You have to give up control. You're trying to take charge of your mental state, and you can't. You have to just go with it until you get used to it. Don't fight it."

That was a new and highly useful concept. I appreciated that, in great contrast to me, Lance had been a bit of a stoner in high school and had such expert advice to impart.

We went back to the room and went to sleep until the early afternoon. The trip got better after that. My most vivid memory from the next day was my painstaking effort to peel the waxy chocolate coating from the ice-cream bar I bought at the beach concession stand when we finally arrived at 4 P.M. And at night, in the privacy of our room, we reached a new level of intimacy. Before going to sleep, I clutched my now-favorite part of his body, the one that some women secretly envy in men, the bulging blue veins wrapping conspicuously and with great virility around his forearm. With veins like that, giving blood would always be uncomplicated and sure.

3

The Revenge of the
Ortho Tri-Cyclen Girl

o o o o o o o o o

IT WAS ABOUT THIS TIME when I started dreaming of the Ortho Tri-Cyclen girl.

Perhaps you have seen her, this fictional spokeswoman for the Pill, in many different yet amazingly similar incarnations over the past decade. The one I remember best, from around the mid-1990s on TV, was a pixielike, fresh-scrubbed all-American woman in crisp Capri pants showing off a framed photo of her and her husband vacationing in France, standing before the Eiffel Tower. A 2004 print ad campaign for Ortho Tri-Cyclen Lo pictures a similar diminutive woman poised alone on top of a giant flower, just like a sexless little Tinkerbell or a hummingbird–she-mutant. "A girl who finds the right birth control pill finds bliss," reads the copy.

During this difficult time in my life, I looked to this Ortho Tri-Cyclen spokesfigure as my ultimate role model, as the person whom I would most like to be. It's not because I considered taking the Pill, as it has been largely contraindicated for women with migraines (because of an added risk of stroke, and it can make headaches worse).[1] This had nothing to do with sex. More than anything, the Ortho Tri-Cyclen sprite symbolized those coveted consumers who found instant and complete fulfillment through prescription drugs.

After I had pondered her further, her other meaning dawned on me. As I continued to interact with doctors, I realized that her innocent yet attractive brand of sex appeal is so much a part of our culture that it is actually a driving engine of the pharmaceutical industry itself.

You see, the Ortho Tri-Cyclen woman has close cousins, women I came to dub the Sirens. They are significant as comprising the living, breathing foot soldiers of corporate drug promotion. About every time I sat in a doctor's waiting room, I observed these sultry yet perky twenty-something sales reps making their rounds of doctors' offices. They always stood out as beaming with health, dressed in close-fitting Ann Taylor coordinates, and pulling their little carts filled with pillars of drug samples and coveted orange Zocor Post-it Notes. They really had the whole thing down. In fact, in their effectiveness, I thought they imitated the actions of some of the most successful drugs they promoted, such as Prozac. They were like the neurotransmitters of the pharmaceutical industry, facilitating selective transmission and reuptake of industry data from company to doctor.

I also realized that because of the tireless and persuasive efforts of this corps of motivated young women, I was now very heavily medicated. The good news is that the stew of drugs marinating in my brain did indeed start harmonizing my own nerve synapses. As the months went on, I did feel the most powerful of them all, the Nardil, gradually kick in and really decrease the pain. The relief was so gradual that I didn't notice it until my doctor at the Chicago Headache Clinic, on a follow-up visit in early fall, asked me about the pain's intensity and duration, and I realized they both had lessened. Not completely, but enough so that this was no longer a major handicap in my daily life. And so I signed my new book contract with confidence, certain that I would meet the fall 1994 deadline, one year away, and that this whole silly and embarrassing business was at last behind me.

The bad news: I had to keep going out to buy new pairs of pants.

A few months after my hospital release, I noticed a strange web of reddish iridescent stretch marks lining my stomach and darting downward from my armpits. I consulted the doctor, who said that it was normal to expect a ten- to fifteen-pound weight gain from an MAOI.

Then the weight gain quickened, from the socially normative 130s, past the still-reasonable-for-my-height 140s, past the still-average-for-the-Midwest 150s, past the now-I'm-wearing-Lane-Bryant 160s, and way past the thank-goodness-my-boyfriend-is-from-a-working-class-Italian-background 170s. It seemed—or actually, it was the case—that every time I stood on a scale, I had gained 5 more pounds. I was outgrowing clothes so fast that I thought maybe I should start buying them in three different sizes, like Liberace, who allegedly found that practice useful to make up for his weight fluctuations. Always lacking something to wear, I anxiously sorted through the items in my closet that I had worn just a few months before; each time, they seemed as tiny as doll clothes.

Finally, a mere four months after my institutionalization, my weight went up to almost two hundred, the critical point at which comedians unofficially make fun of people for being fat, and when you can accurately say that you weigh "hundreds of pounds." And I looked even heavier because the drugs also had water-retaining effects, puffing up the cheeks. I asked the doctor about it, and he shrugged, replying that the drugs must have erased my "set point," or the natural internal body-weight-stabilizing mechanism. His reaction—and my own sense of what was really important—made me feel vain to even worry about it. As my headache was naturally a bigger concern, I dropped the subject, but I never forgot about it.

As I learned later, doctors really don't know why so many drugs used for daily headaches, as well as for depression, among other neurological problems, cause weight gain. They could change the metabolism, and they could also increase appetite, which I was definitely experiencing. In my case, the constant companion of headache was supplanted by the nagging fury of hunger. Indeed, I was beset by a sharper, louder, and more painful type of hunger, which seemed to make my body into one large screaming hunger gland. If I didn't obey it, the gland would wake me up in the middle of the night, sometimes more than once, bidding me to go and get some toast to feed it.

To resist, I tried to motivate myself to go against all instinct and go hungry by trying to think like an anorexic or bulimic. But this was difficult, as I had the misfortune of growing up in a family where no one had eating disorders and all maintained a healthy attitude toward food. Sadly for me, my parents, who grew up in poverty with immigrant families, weren't "high-class" enough to promote an eating disorder; they considered someone who left good food on the plate morally bereft. So, reversing years of conditioning to eat when hungry, I tried to make myself an "antiaffirmation" tape in my head. In particular, I imagined that I was that one superskinny girl I would see at every gym to which I had ever belonged, joylessly trying to hoist a tiny weight over her head in the corner. Is this how she thought?

"Oh, my self-esteem is based on my size," I dictated to myself. "I must be in total control of my body. For if I am in control of my body, I am in control of my life. Small = virtue. Virtue = small. Fat is so ugly and icky. It is so horrid to think of anyone judging me, thinking negatively of me. That means I would lose control. I must be spare, understated, like good prose. God knows the most attractive thing in a woman is a well-defined waistline, and a well-defined clavicle, and a well-defined tailbone.

"Oh, look at that delicious dinner of Yankee pot roast, mashed potatoes and gravy, and green beans. Wouldn't it just be fun to cough it up in a half-digested state?"

And if that didn't work, I brought in the motivational big guns: "Oh, and even worse, there is my career to think about. How could I ever be allowed, as a woman under forty, to write a memoir about myself without being an erotically appealing, mentally disturbed waif with an eating disorder, only interrupted by periods of reckless and compulsive promiscuity? It's just not done."

Although I couldn't quite buy this on any level, I was still stuck in an odd quagmire. Despite my years of feminist reading and writing and my lack of prior history of really thinking about weight that much (at least compared to a lot of other women), I was now obsessed with it. This lack of control over appearance only heightened that same disorienting feeling that had resulted from the pain. I didn't know who I was anymore. I didn't have a realistic concept of even what I looked like, since it clashed so much with my previous conceptions. I didn't know if I looked a little heavier than normal or like pre-gastric-bypass Carnie Wilson in the old Wilson Phillips video in which the producers hide her behind a rock.

In other words, to use the previous generation's related pop music metaphor, I was somewhere between Michelle Philips and Mama Cass (of the earlier Mamas and the Papas), and I never knew quite where I fit. To get some concept of what I really looked like, I hung out by the scale at Women's Workout World to see what women of my weight looked like.

"Hmm," I thought, "she's 185 and she doesn't look too bad. Passable."

I also feared that this weight gain would not stop, ever. I would be one of those obese people featured on *Geraldo* who had to carve out the front seat of the car in order to drive. I didn't know how much longer I'd be able to fly coach. When they asked me if I wanted an aisle or window seat, I thought I would have to reply, "Both."

Although I knew I was not to "blame," I still felt guilty, as if my weight gain were a moral failure. (Ironically, at least one study has shown that patients with no prior history of weight problems experience the greatest initial weight increase with such drugs.[2]) This is the other side of the coin of how skinny people are viewed with moral praise, such as my sister, who is naturally about 110 pounds, without any effort to diet. (At that time, I started calling her my "half sister," because she was literally half my weight.) At a family wedding, I was irritated walking around with her and hearing relatives' constant cries of adulation, as I stood by her, trying to maintain my frozen smile.

"Don't praise her," I thought, "praise her irritable bowel syndrome."

Yes, I hate to admit it, but knowing how others thought, I was worried how others would judge me. This was especially the case with people I had known from my past, from high school or college, whom I occasionally ran into. Would they imagine that I let myself go, that I was depressed, that I was sitting alone at home all night in a corner gorging on Little Debbie's snack cakes and cookie dough? That was if they even recognized me. Many times, I waved at a distance to people I had known, just to see their confused stares. Then, after introducing myself, I just kept a stiff upper lip and kept talking to them as if nothing had changed. After all, I wasn't willing to just hide out in my apartment in a large muumuu. Life had to go on.

Although I didn't feel comfortable going into detail with most people about why I had gained the weight, I did tell my close friends. They were witnessing my ordeal step by step, pound by pound, and they knew something of my struggle with the headache. As a surprise to me, this weight gain ended up being the greatest source of sympathy, and even pity, I have ever had. This, and not constant pain, was something that they could personally identify with. Yes, I could tell them about a year of headache and get barely a shrug of a shoulder in response. But when I mentioned gaining at least fifty pounds, I've seen women break down and get on their knees, almost sobbing: "The horror! How does God let such things happen? Indeed, that is one of the true riddles of humankind."

Of course, besides the social stigma, there are the additional health risks of excess poundage. We've all heard the doctors' and the nutritionists' warnings, as they tick off the numerous health problems correlated with obesity: type 2 diabetes, hypertension, gallbladder disease, and coronary heart disease, among others.

But most health care professionals usually fail to just cut to the chase and discuss overweight women's most urgent concern: It's going to be really tough for a heterosexual female to get laid by an upwardly mobile white man.

At that time, I very clearly noticed others' negative reactions. This was especially true of hipster white males in my social group, who seemed to consider listlessness from anemia a sexy concept. In contrast, I was now the absolute robust ideal of groups of young black men I passed on the street. "Hey, there's the mama of my baby," I recall one young lad shouting to me. "There's the mama of my baby right there!"

In addition, the biostatisticians usually neglect to mention another very tangible risk for women gaining weight: getting any decent clothes. Now that the 1980s, with their characteristically oversized styles, had come and gone, "regular-sized" departments were now especially out of the question for me. What had passed for a medium size in the 1980s was now an XXL. To make matters worse, at that time, in the early 1990s, the plus-size stores and sections in department stores expressed a strange fondness for stirrup pants and sweatshirts decorated with teddy bears and/or sequins. I thought to myself, "I just gained some weight. I didn't have a lobotomy." Apparently, as sizes went up, plus-size clothiers felt that IQs plummeted. I described this problem to a friend, and she was also dumbfounded, guessing that perhaps plus-size clothing makers didn't think that women who bought them ever left their homes.

I dreamed of finding something actually understated and hip, like singer Natalie Merchant's understated shiftlike dress in an admirably drab olive color, which Lance had pointed out to me on her CD cover as desirable. But I soon gave up hope. The best I could do was find something as plain and basic as possible, such as the rare unadorned T-shirt, and get it in black. Otherwise, the colors were not suitable for a night of going to storefront theater or hearing alternative folk music. If the clothes weren't pastel, they were too bright, with all the subtlety of the color scheme of a pack of Skittles. I tried "one size fits all" outfits in "normal" stores, but I realized that label was a matter of opinion.

Whereas the largest sizes in the "normal" clothes section were mostly too snug, when I could find them, these plus sizes were actually too big in most places, except maybe the waist. These designers had not yet grasped the concept of tailoring, thinking instead that arms and legs suddenly doubled in width when you hit a size 16. The offerings all looked like the cover of a beanbag chair, with holes punched in it for the arms and head. It was as if clothing designers had given up, and said, "Hell, after a size 12, these women are just fat. That's their size: Size Fat. Just increase the waistband and shoulder width a few inches for each size and just shove as much material in there as you can, and that should do the job. Yeah, good enough."

Ironically, some of the names used to refer to this group of clothes are not demeaning and are actually positive. They seem to describe what is normative and healthy, calling bigger clothes *women's* sizes. Sometimes these words for bigger clothes are even downright compliments, such as the *plus* size, which suggests that these women have something greater to offer. Meanwhile, stores seem also to belittle other women, calling their sizes *pe-*

tites, misses, or *juniors.* The signs seem to marvel, "Aren't they just darling?" while reaching over with a giant hand to pinch their cheeks.

But between the lines, the actions of department stores communicate a different message than this upbeat sizespeak. I remember going to try to find the "women's department" in the Marshall Field's in suburban Oak Brook with a friend who lived nearby. We finally found it at the back of a very high floor, past the toddler wear and cutlery and sewing notions. We got off the elevator and wandered around this gulag. I almost expected water to be dripping from the ceiling into buckets, bulbs flickering. The curtain on the dressing room was thin and tattered, barely covering the entrance. Inside, castoff parts of mannequins—legs, arms, heads, torsos, chests—from other departments in the store were piled up in the corner. We were all in the same boat, the mannequins and I, casualties of fashion.

I tried to accept these indignities and concentrate on being grateful for the diminishment in pain. As with many strong drugs, I was trading in one malady for another, like the Little Mermaid trading her voice for legs, so she could go to land and court the prince. In my case, I assumed the best, that weight gain was definitely not as bad as a constant headache. If only all this had happened with a thing health care activists call informed consent; I would have liked to be clearly warned about the extent of the side effects. From the start, I would have had to expect that this level of change was a possibility and not find out about it only as it was happening, as had been the case with the Nardil.

As much as I certainly cared about the weight gain, a part of me was blithely indifferent. On one level, it was a stupid thing to worry about. I thought, "Who cares what the shallow people around me think?" After all, I was a writer and didn't have to look good (as long as I didn't have any aspirations to be on TV). I cheered myself up by reminding myself that I wasn't, for example, someone like a trophy wife, who would be thrown out on the street to eat out of a dumpster with such a transgression. Besides, despite the dogma of my antiaffirmation track, I didn't think I looked that bad. I didn't equate thinness with beauty; people naturally come in all sizes. I was never the kind of person who gets "offended" by fat people. This was something that I would just accept.

Side effects and public ridicule were not the worst thing, I knew. Headaches were the worst thing. While I was in severe pain, little else in life seemed possible.

I learned I was not alone in this conflict. Weight gain is a side effect that has greatly preoccupied writers who have taken drugs to combat invisible illnesses. People suffering from mood disorders, such as Lizzie Simon, in *Detour: My Bipolar Road Trip in 4-D*, have complained about weight gain from drugs like Depakote and lithium. Early in her memoir, *Prozac Nation*, Elizabeth Wurtzel explains that she didn't want to go on lithium for depression because of fears of weight gain and other physical symptoms "that I think would make me more depressed than I am without lithium" (4). Andrew Solomon, in *Noonday Demon: An Atlas of Depression*, mentions his struggle with increased appetite on the mood stabilizer Zyprexa: "Nowadays I can eat a perfectly normal meal and still be famished, and that hunger can be so extreme as to drive me out of my house in the middle of the night to get food. I sit with my hunger and think about how ugly a paunch can be; I remember hours of exercise that only burned a few calories. Then I feel that if I don't eat, I'll die, and I go and stuff myself" (242).

For many experiencing invisible illnesses, this weight gain, and other "beauty" issues, may be the only outward sign of the health problems. Another common cosmetic complaint about drug side effects is the loss of hair where you are supposed to have it or its growth in new places. For those with more stigmatized illnesses, such as bipolarity, these changes may go entirely unexplained to others because the person is afraid to "come out" about the root problem.

For me, there were other more privately felt side effects to tolerate, many involving sleeping. Occasionally, I would wake up with my entire body paralyzed, unable to move for what seemed like a few seconds, while my mind was fully alert. I had nightmares that were so vivid and so like my daily life that they seemed like hallucinations. One time, I lay down on the bed in the dark and soon noticed the figure of a strange man at the foot of my bed; he then crawled under the covers to grab me. I'll never forget that image: It was as vivid and as real as the office I'm sitting in right now. I woke up screaming and completely terrorized, not realizing that I had fallen asleep and it was all a dream. When I went back to the Chicago Headache Clinic for a follow-up appointment, I met a heavyset woman in the waiting room who told me she had woken up and, while still panicked, given her husband two black eyes. She had been on Nardil.

One challenge of all these side effects was having to wait weeks until my next appointment at the Chicago Headache Clinic to ask questions about them. For the time period before our next visit, we were given a sheet listing three to five half-hour to forty-five-minute intervals during the week when we were allowed to call our doctor. And even those allowances were limited. If there were too many people ahead of you, you typically had to wait days to try again. And there was a ten-dollar charge for each call. "We at the Chicago Headache Clinic have always endeavored to keep our costs down," reads the handout. "However, we too are victims of inflation."

(Since then, the Chicago Headache Clinic has started a practice of allowing open calling to physician assistants, who answer the questions directly or call you back after consulting a doctor—sometimes without charge. This is a common practice of headache clinics, which typically experience very large volumes of calls from patients trying a long series of very complex drugs.)

The pattern became predictable: Complain of a symptom and take home another prescription. I started taking more drugs to combat the side effects, such as a diuretic to control water gain. I also became increasingly concerned about my strong dependence on Nardil. Once, when I traveled, I forgot to pack enough Nardil with me for the entire trip and felt myself becoming very weak and sluggish, as if my batteries were running out. I cut the trip short and came home early, running into my home to take the pills.

Good lord, I thought. Instead of the Ortho Tri-Cyclen gal, I resembled Elvis, bloated in his later years. In fact, as I read years later, I was indeed a lot like Elvis in reality. One theory is that his fatal drug overdose was due to the interaction of a variety of off-label medications used to treat his intractable migraines. In fact, an investigator from the National Migraine Association (MAGNUM) explained his 1975 hospital stay for vision problems as his trying to cope with a migraine aura, which distorted his eyesight. After he died, the drugs found in his system were common ones that I had also taken for head pain: painkillers (like Demerol), antiemetics (antinausea drugs like Compazine, the blood-pressure medication sometimes useful with migraine), propranolol, and the ergot-derived DHE (which was mistaken for LSD because of its similar chemical properties). This news was not reported until 1999, by sleuths at the National Migraine Association in Alexandria, Virginia.[3]

Although I did not know about Elvis's chronic migraines at the time, I remember watching a video of him in his later years with which I did identify. He was clearly struggling to concentrate through a fog of drugs, as I had done so many times.

Suddenly, I knew that the stakes were too great with this combination of such powerful drugs. I couldn't risk also dying in middle age on the toilet of an accidental overdose. So I checked myself into the poor man's Betty Ford Clinic, my parents' house, for a few weeks and stopped taking the Nardil. Before that, the doctor had assured me that this drug was nonaddictive, and I shouldn't have any problem just stopping it. But then I started to feel burning in my arms and legs, along with a strange shaking.

Disturbed by that reaction, I started taking the drug again and went back home to Chicago. I would have to make friends with the Nardil and go against my natural urge to resist it. I'd have to go with the flow, as Lance had suggested. At least I had learned that Nardil was having a real physical effect on me, that it was a real tool, not just a placebo.

However, I did realize at that time that I did have a placebo boyfriend. As time passed, he was there in name only. Just as with real placebo medications, I had seen what I had wanted to see. Everything had fallen apart very slowly in the six months after our glorious trip over New Year's to the Mall of America in Minnesota, when everything seemed to be fine. But when we returned to Chicago, our real roller-coaster ride with each other began.

"I have never met anyone who was more of an Aries in my life," he said, explaining himself as an exasperated borderline Cancer. I didn't know what all that meant, but judging by his tone, it couldn't be good. Besides, if he was bringing up something as silly as astrology, then he was losing all credibility with me anyway.

About a month after the inevitable breakup, making matters worse, the companion that I had figured would be much more lasting, the Nardil, also pooped out. It just stopped working. And the pain returned with a vengeance, like that guy with the mask coming back to terrorize Jamie Lee Curtis in the *Halloween* movies after she thought she had certainly killed him. As doctors have found out by observing patient reports (and not through laboratory studies), this is a very common experience with MAOIs, along with many other types of drugs affecting mood. Again, as with weight gain, doctors are stunningly casual about this effect, although it often tears apart one's world and grinds everything to a sudden, unexpected halt.

When I think about this common problem, the character that comes to mind most is Charlie from the classic Daniel Keyes story (which was later adapted into a film and novel), *Flowers for Algernon* (1975). This story, which many people I talk to remember from their middle-school English classes in the 1970s and 1980s, is a powerful and poignant metaphor for the roller-coaster-like experiences that many patients experience with a temporary pharmaceutical boost. *Flowers for Algernon* is about a young developmentally disabled man who undergoes a surgery that results in his intelligence slowly developing from a very low IQ to genius levels. The only catch, which doctors fail to mention to Charlie, is that the effects of the surgery will run out, and they don't know when. He finds this out almost by accident at a presentation at a medical meeting in Chicago, when his doctors very coldly reveal that a mouse, Algernon, who had previously had this same surgery, is starting to fade. Hearing this news, Charlie feels more like an experiment than a person. "Like Algernon, I found myself behind the mesh of the cage they had built for me," Charlie says (113). The last part of the story shows the absolutely wrenching process of Charlie losing his intelligence and noticing the decline at the same time, helpless to change it.

Even so, I was relieved to see a future without those little orange Nardils. Unlike during that visit to my parents' house, this time I more wisely got off the drug much more gradually, over the course of many weeks. I was relieved to easily drop ten pounds immediately and hoped that the pattern would continue. I was also fired up to be drug-free, with some new philosophies having an influence. I had just gone on a research trip to California and visited with an old friend. She gave me a book by a researcher named Norman Cousins (1979), who had written about the power of the mind to influence the body and taking charge of your health on your own, without drugs. He had purportedly cured his fatal disease through the power of laughter by watching movie comedies.

I didn't find that my headaches got better with such activities, but I did have a new take-charge attitude. I decided to switch doctors at the Chicago Headache Clinic, to finally rid myself of the knucklehead assigned to my case. I was reassigned to a pleasant young woman doctor with stylish black shoes. She said that the good news was that there was a new class of antidepressants, the SSRIs, which had many fewer side effects and were being proven effective with headaches. She gave me a new one, Paxil. Even though my ideal was to be drug-free, the pain was so great that I had to be more open-minded. I took it and soon sank into the worst depression of my life. I called my mother for advice.

"Mom, I have been crying for the past few days," I said, plainly. "Do you think it may be this drug?"

I couldn't call my doctor, as it wasn't her day to receive questions, so my mom phoned a pharmacist, who read off a long list of possible side effects. The pharmacist was skeptical that Paxil was the culprit, as it was supposed to *improve* your mood, not bring you down. But she read down the list and said depression appeared there as a rare side effect.

On my own, I stopped taking the drug over the course of a week, which turned my work schedule upside down with insomnia and increased pain. Then I finally returned to a more normal mood and my previous level of headache.

At a subsequent visit, I asked the doctor what to do next, what her master plan might be. Well, she said, she hadn't one. I had to keep taking drugs and see which ones worked, if at all. But I should keep in mind that I did have "a very serious problem" and that treatment would not be easy.

Her honesty was both disturbing and refreshing. A very serious problem? Treatment not easy? Like Charlie of *Flowers for Algernon*, I finally lost my naïveté, or at least some of it. I realized how truly limited modern medical knowledge still could be. These doctors did know a certain amount, but once you complained about something that went beyond that boundary, you were on your own. And those borders were different for every problem and often seemed arbitrary in their placement. If you were infertile, there were endless things they could do, and you could go on for a while until reaching that edge, the end of options. If you were blind, you were more obviously hemmed in.

With some disorders—especially the unpublicized ones like chronic headaches—we patients typically don't know where the boundary is until we have reached it. We see this as a simple problem and are optimistic, especially after reading all the self-help books by doctors and seeing all those TV news features on "how far we've come" with migraines. But in reality, that edge comes up earlier when a headache is daily, and especially when it is constant. And butting up against such obstacles can be a rude awakening in this culture, where we expect technology and doctors to provide instant cures, and where we perceive pain as something optional, not as a given part of life on this planet as a human.

But this interminable pain, which blocked my thinking and sapped my energy, was hard to accept, as it was so intrusive in my daily life. Now I no longer had the energy to repress my mental and emotional reaction to it and just go on. For the first time, I realized that there might never be a cure for this problem, that it might never go away. I was being left alone with it, with no one knowing what I was going through. Compounding my sense of isolation was the thought that I was the only person alive who didn't respond to these drugs, whom the Chicago Headache Clinic didn't cure. I was personally responsible for not living up to the ideal of the Ortho Tri-Cyclen girl and her Siren associates in achieving glowing results.

Even though this was not a *real* illness, just a stupid headache, the possible consequences were crystal clear. My career, my personal life, and my financial life—the full range of life choices that had seemed so boundless just a short time ago—were all in jeopardy.

4

Those Summer Days

○ ○ ○ ○ ○ ○ ○ ○ ○

ALTHOUGH THE BEDROOM WAS DARK—its one small window was in the shadow of a brick wall inches away and was sealed off with a thick weatherproof vinyl shade—I sensed that it was probably about noon. I couldn't see the face of my watch on the dresser and had no desire to get up and turn on the light. That action would only disrupt my efforts to get back to sleep.

The question of the current time couldn't be confirmed by my alarm clock, either, the one with the lit-up green electronic digits. I had unplugged it, for health reasons.

You see, the acupuncturist I had recently seen had judged that the source of all my problems was an "electrical imbalance." He had advised me to stay away, at least eight feet, from anything plugged into an electrical outlet. I thought that was probably impossible in this day and age, unless I moved to Amish country and took up a job as a quaint country cobbler or canner of fine jams for tourists. After I had questioned this request as impractical, the doctor told me, well, at least unplug everything in your bedroom.

I did the math in my head to see if I qualified to get out of bed. Let's see, I had gone to bed at one in the morning, probably had fallen into a light sleep about three-ish, but I wasn't sure since I hadn't let myself look at the clock beyond a certain hour. Doing so only made me tense. As often happened, the sleep I did get was light and fitful, not of a great quality, so I probably had to factor in more total hours to make up for it. If it was noon now, that meant I'd been in bed for eleven hours. If I'd slept, well, 60 percent of that time, I'd have gotten the equivalent of roughly six hours of sleep. Six hours? Not great, but nonetheless, I calculated that I'd had enough of an investment in sleep to justify getting up.

As I recently had come to realize, if I got fewer than eight hours of sleep total, the Headache (which by now had earned its capital-H significance) would be especially grinding and I probably wouldn't be able to work the entire day or would have a much more difficult time doing so. Also, even if I had gotten plenty of sleep the night before, sometimes staying in bed an extra hour or two would make a great difference for the rest of the day, reducing the overall pain a notch. I wasn't sure what my brain secreted as I slept, but I wouldn't have been surprised if it were opium.

Once I was up, it was time to berate myself for going to bed so late. But, I thought in my own defense, I had been taking advantage of an opportunity. Because of the pain, I had not been able to do much the day before until about 9 P.M., when it gradually subsided to a more manageable level. As I had reluctantly become nocturnal, reverting to my most primal tendencies, this had become my pattern. I'd feel slightly better as the day went on and would therefore start to work as day unfolded into evening. I wasn't really fooling myself; I knew I wasn't getting much accomplished. But even filing articles I had collected—the easiest part of my book project—gave me the illusion of making some progress.

I thought of my old self from three or four years back, the woman who without complaint woke up at 5 A.M. to go to a reporting job and then often covered meetings at night. I wondered if I had imagined that person, if she had just been a dream.

All this summarizes a typical morning of unprofound thoughts, drug-addled ramblings, random anxieties, and self-recrimination in the still largely unrecognized world of chronic daily headache. In a typical journey, I was coping with both the limits of alternative medicine, which I was just beginning to try, and, most of all, the continuing and seemingly boundless pharmacopoeia of Western medicine. Much of my suffering stemmed not from the pain itself but from the constant roller coaster of frustration, shame, and havoc that it created in so many areas. Everything now was a challenge, from completing the most routine chore to making plans with friends and keeping them. I was always in conflict about pushing through the pain, or if I should just "give in" to it.

There comes a point when all sufferers of chronic illness fully enter that subculture, when the adrenaline to function in the outside world runs out. For me, this started to take place during the summer of 1994. That was when additional problems commonly related to pain fully kicked in, including insomnia and fatigue, only increasing the feeling that my life was spinning out of control. Now my old self was gone, torn asunder, and I had not yet figured out how to piece together a new one to replace it.

On an average day, my most difficult challenge was usually just leaving the bed, as this was the time of most severe and heavy pain. I would wake up lying on my back with my head pressed into the pillow, feeling as if a huge nail had been pounded into my left eye and stuck through the bottom of the bed, pinning me firmly in place.

If I was especially sluggish and late in gaining consciousness, I assumed it was raining or snowing outside—and I was usually right. On days like this, it felt like the force of gravity had gone up tenfold and was vacuum-sucking me down to the bed. At first, this effect seemed so bizarre to me that I didn't quite believe it. As with other "triggers," I was slow to recognize the weather as one; it happened to become clear to me as the months passed.

I was far from alone in experiencing this effect. You don't need a neurologist to tell you which way the wind blows. In fact, as I read later, the ancient Greeks observed the effect of "hot and cold winds" on pain and illness. During the U.S. Civil War, physicians noted that amputees experienced pain in their phantom limbs as the weather changed. One of the most famous and oldest medical case studies of a constant headache, from Dr. Thomas Willis, in the 1685 text *London Practice of Physick*, cites the weather as a part of an arsenal of aggravating triggers in his chronic daily headache patient, which included "the changes of the Year, and of the Air, the great Aspects of the Sun and Moon, violent passions, and errors in diet" (384). Other patients I have met through the years who suffered a variety of different problems—from multiple sclerosis to asthma to arthritis—also have described to me these aggravating effects of the weather.

Doctors have been slow to recognize this phenomenon of the weather as a trigger and have long discounted it because of conflicting evidence in studies. Many have also written it off as gloomy weather inciting gloomy moods. But in the past several years, despite varying study results, the evidence has stacked up.[1] Researchers now are able to explain that *changes* in weather are the culprit, not the actual bad weather itself. Changing precipitation, winds, and temperatures are all sources of this pain-aggravating barometric pressure—mainly as it falls, and sometimes as it rises. One theory about why headache sufferers feel this pressure shift so strongly, along with other common external triggers, is that our brains are slower to adapt to changes, and also that the weather pressure adds additional stress to already inflamed, overly sensitized, and swollen areas.

Although I had no insight at the time into the science behind these effects, I later recognized that heat was also likely to keep me down. The chugging box fan in my window did little to improve the situation. So, to lower the pain a notch, I often sought refuge visiting others or spending time in movie theaters with central air conditioning. In particular, I greatly feared the *humidity* of the summer. Was I so sensitive that even the weight of the most seemingly inconsequential and ephemeral elements—air and water vapor—was a threat? As I was also finally able to articulate at that time, humidity would often trigger an odd additional broken-glass feeling in my eye, which was more severe and debilitating than the regular headache and would last nonstop for about three days. (At least I wasn't like other migraineurs whose pain was aggravated in dry, cold air—a state which characterized my dream days, relieving like an all-body icepack. And I wasn't like a cluster headache patient, whose worst seasons are often spring and fall.)

As a result of this common weather influence, pain patients often find themselves obsessively following weather forecasts, with the same anxious interest as a farmer worrying about drought or floods or swarms of locusts jeopardizing crops. But of course, we can't control the weather. In the Midwest, where the weather fluctuations are intense and highly irregular—manic and depressive—even in the same day, I often felt my life stop and start again according to the whims and mood swings of the latest barometric shift.

On second thought, my experience with the weather is controllable, to some extent. I could always move to a tropical region near the equator, where weather shifts are less dramatic. But needless to say, moving into a hut in Ecuador is about as practical for me as the idea of moving to an Amish village to escape electrical current. Besides, some researchers say that the body eventually adapts to changes in a milder climate and then reacts just as severely to those new shifts in weather.[2]

However, sufferers can moderate other common headache triggers, unlike the weather. We sometimes can avoid people who cause stress; caller ID is one of the greatest pain-relieving medical inventions of our era. And we can try to steer clear of certain types of aggravating foods, which contain unpleasant chemicals like tyramine (in wine) and phenylethylamine (in chocolate). We can even avoid specific environments, for example, those with harsh sounds or harsh lighting, to which we can be overly sensitized. Individuals' triggers differ. My personal list of such pain-inflaming places is pretty idiosyncratic: the University of Illinois at Chicago library, with its grating combination of fluorescent lights on concrete in its appropriately named "brutalist" architecture; Filene's Basement on Michigan Avenue, with its low fluorescent ceiling; and the Au Bon Pain on Washington Street in the Chicago Loop, with its tiny checkerboard black-and-white tile.

That morning, as I often did, I wondered if it was unnatural to consider summer one's least favorite season. And more specifically, the really gorgeous clear, mild, and sunny days. In Chicago, where those days are in the minority, and especially in the youth-oriented North Side Lake View neighborhood, where I had recently moved with a few friends, it seemed like everyone felt compelled to get out and have fun, fun, fun. When I found myself stuck inside and not frolicking with the others, the contrast seemed the most extreme. I thought how winter, despite its own share of barometric shifts, was so much more pleasant, with much less social pressure on single people living in densely populated urban areas. Then, outside my door were mercifully few bikers and roller-bladers, the most supremely confident and daring of them all.

On this morning, after finally getting out of bed, I went to the bathroom and weighed myself. Then I took a shower, which often gave temporary relief to the viselike pressure on my neck and shoulders. But showering, in and of itself, was yet another hazard. I had to be extremely cautious not to get any soap or shampoo in my eyes, as that could result in a lasting sensation of broken glass lodged in the left eye. On the way to the shower, I would very likely stumble over piles of *New York Times*es, still wrapped in their little plastic blue bags. (From time to time, I would get a burst of energy, usually at night, and tear through a pile of these logs, at last focusing on them clearly enough to read them. I often found out about news events six weeks after they had happened, but it was better than nothing.)

I might then go downstairs to retrieve the mail and would always be confounded to find there what seemed like a daily issue of *Cosmo* or *Glamour*, both of which I was using in my book research on young women. Perhaps the July issue would arrive, but I could have sworn that I'd just got the February issue yesterday, or was it the one from last November? The days were blending together. Worst of all, a July issue meant that I had missed another deadline. I had told myself and my editor that I would definitely be cured by July, that by June I would have at least a first draft done, that by July my health issues would all be figured out. For me, thick, perfumed slabs of women's magazines featuring cover photos of beaming starlets in low-cut slip dresses and yet more Ortho Tri-Cyclen ads represented the fleeting sands of time, ticked off one month at a time.

At some point, I would turn the ringer of the phone back on. I had learned that when it woke me up too early, I could be assured of a worse headache that day and reduced productivity. Little did that telemarketer know what havoc he or she caused in my life.

On what was left of these afternoons, I would go back to the bedroom, find clothes, and put them on, usually losing momentum when it came to the pulling-on-of-socks part. Sitting on the edge of the bed to get leverage, I might feel the temptation to rest and would let myself fall backward, often staying that way for a very long while, still clutching a ball of socks in one hand.

If alert enough, I sometimes went swimming at the public pool on Broadway. This was a highlight of my weekdays, great for energizing me and toning the still untamed flesh. It was an especially luxurious experience because most of the people there during the day were gay men, actively socializing with each other on the edge of the pool. Not only did I have a lane to myself, but I lorded it over my own private women's locker room. The only hazard was letting chlorine get into my eyes, especially on humid days, which would, again, unleash the broken glass.

And then, at some point during the day, I would try to start writing, to meet the newest extended book deadline. But I was unable to even begin forming a coherent thought. Writing, unfortunately, is something you just can't fake. Headache pain, like all pain, inhibits work. But pain like this, felt at the core of one's being, in the brain, carries an added challenge in interfering with how you think.

Others have made similar observations. "There is something devilish about pain arising in the face and head," writes Dr. Frank Vertosick, a chronic migraine sufferer, in his book *Why We Hurt* (2000). "They strike us at the geometric center of our beings. Our consciousness resides, after all, within the confines of our skulls. A leg pain arrives in our consciousness telegraphed from some friendly but vaguely distant land, while the severe headache or face pain barges into the mind's home like an unsavory intruder. When our head or face burns, *we* hurt, and in a very profound way" (64, 65).

Other common health problems also created their share of ups and downs, adding to my frustration and anxiety about how delicate my entire body had become. Every minor glitch caused a worse headache. What had been just life's minor bodily annoyances in the past, such as PMS or a cold or a sore neck from sleeping the wrong way, were now completely derailing. It wasn't that they were disabling in and of themselves, but that they made the pain worse, by far the worst part.

And very often the pain would get worse for no apparent reason at all, even if I "did everything right," if the weather was clear and crisp, if the planets were aligned, if I hadn't been "too busy" the day before. In those cases, giving in to the added handicap of drug sedation, I would just lie down all afternoon, watching TV: *All My Children* at noon, *One Life to Live* at 1 P.M., *thirtysomething* on Lifetime at 2 P.M.. I felt guilty, but I knew that these days were in the minority.

Another typical added stress from these dog days was sheer paranoia. When I would get any other minor health ailment, I worried that, like the Headache, it was an omen of an intractable, highly suspect, and mysterious problem to come. That pain from the twisted neck or that cold that lingered a little longer than it should have had the potential to irrevocably imprint itself on my central nervous system, as the Headache had done. If the Headache hadn't gone away, why would these other things?

I even sometimes felt paranoid when the ailment was not physical, for example, when my computer broke down. I pictured going to an endless string of skeptical repair people, who would just shrug and tell me, "I have done all the tests, which all show that there is nothing wrong. Maybe it's time you went to a therapist." I was always amazed when they fixed it.

In sum, I simply had no more energy to deal with other unpredictable forces in my life. The Headache was all I could handle. In the chronic pain world, this type of worrying behavior is called *catastrophizing*. It's a natural response to give a larger symbolic meaning to the pain, to worry about its greater significance in the future. Indeed, my greatest fear was over what had *not* yet happened. A quote from Soren Kierkegaard, which I read in a book of daily thoughts for pain sufferers, sums it up well: "We frequently see those who in life conquered every battle; when it was a future enemy they had to deal with, they became powerless, their arms paralyzed."[3]

Unfortunately, even the very rare better pain days carried their own types of anxieties. Feeling thrilled to seem more like my old self, I would naturally overwork, to try to make a dent in my workload, and then would feel worse pain and fatigue the next day. Sometimes, when I found myself acting "normally" and having a good time out with friends, I would stop abruptly and worry about how much I was going to pay for it with future pain. For the rest of the evening, a cloud of dread would envelop me. As I was finding out, there was a price for everything.

As another pain sufferer related to me at the time, in an elevator leaving a doctor's appointment, it was like having a very limited amount of marbles as currency. And I had to be extremely careful and stingy about how I rationed them out. For every plan I made, I had to map out a complicated equation of variables and what exactly *X* and *Y* should equal. I figured out that before the days of pain, I had probably ten marbles to work with on any given day. But now I had a strict limit of three to five, depending mainly on weather and sleep levels. So, a plan to go to a party, requiring about four marbles, would mean a major commitment of bodily resources. If I did make it to that event, I knew that other activities, such as calling back Person A (one marble) or grocery shopping (two to three marbles) or working (four marbles), were out of the question for that day. After all, you are only given a certain number per day, period, and you cannot will more to come to you. The supply, ultimately, is finite. True, sometimes you can shift them around a bit, get extra marbles on credit or layaway, but you must always pay in future installments, at a very high interest rate. So if you exert yourself to turn a four-marble day into a seven-marble one, you will have virtually no marbles to work with the next day or even for much of the next week.

Adding to my overarching feeling of helplessness was the fact that I simply could not be productive without being in pain. Ironically, if I wanted to work, I had to *avoid* taking painkillers, because they made me very tired (and often with minimal accompanying pain relief). Besides, I had to limit their use or risk greater "rebound" headaches in the future. Many of the effective analgesics like Norgesic Forte (with a muscle relaxant) and Fiorinal (with a barbiturate) contained caffeine, and they would keep me up much of the night, also causing worse pain in the long run. Even those strong painkillers that didn't contain caffeine, such as Percodan, Darvocet, and Vicodin (all narcotics), made me too tired and "dumb" to work. And then I was subject to the additional wasted time and frustration of a fuzzy hangover the morning after. Of course, the hangover was never preceded by any kind of buzz; the pain seemed to suck up any high I might have gotten from it.

In any case, my ultimate euphoria was during those very rare moments when I didn't feel clouded by drugs and serious pain, and I simply felt like my true old unencumbered wide-eyed self. As I had my whole life, I equated happiness with lucidity and awareness, not numbness.

But then, the "preventive" drugs I took raised an even greater barrier, wasting even more of my time. Like Klonopin, the one I was on that summer, they typically caused fatigue and light-headedness and then brought on compounded troubles during the withdrawal process. I found this was especially true while I was trying to get off an ineffective drug. I could handle typical withdrawal symptoms, such as dizziness, insomnia, fatigue, and depression. But what was more difficult was the added vicious and raw level of pain that this drug-weaning process caused, as the brain adapted to its new chemistry.

One of my greatest challenges was with side effects from Klonopin (clonazepam), which is a member of the benzodiazepine tranquilizer family, which I had started taking that spring. It also has antiseizure properties, used to calm the hyperactive nerve activity in the brain, which has been implicated in chronic headache pain. Like many patients, I had no idea that it was addictive nor how high my doses had become. But I was alarmed when I told a group of friends about it and one grad student gasped and told me that they use it in the mental hospital where she works to pacify problem patients.

The long-drawn-out pattern for trying out this drug was typical of what I had experienced in the past with many others. After weeks on the initial dosage, I really didn't feel any effect, besides sedation, and so I called the prescribing neurologist at Northwestern University. She told me to double my dose and then call back a month later. This process of raising the dosage would gradually ultimately go on for a total of five months, until fall of that year, when I finally spent months getting off the Klonopin. Meanwhile, time was passing at warp speed, and deadline after deadline that others had set and, even worse, that I had made for myself, rushed by.

During the past year, I had tried a bevy of other typical preventive drugs from a variety of doctors. They mainly gave me antidepressants, which, as discussed earlier, are also widely taken off-label for chronic headaches. As is typical, most antidepressants, even at reduced doses, made it nearly impossible for me to sleep, causing me to feel even greater pain the next day. I would try to keep taking the drug, as I was again told that it would take awhile to kick in and that side effects would eventually subside. But then I finally, invariably, gave up after a week of hardly sleeping and suffering the ensuing aggravated pain, meanwhile never failing to notice how much potential work time was passing me by.

But sometimes, my sheer force of will did triumph. Even in some of the most trying circumstances with drugs and pain, I could occasionally push myself through some other less mentally intense work, such as doing interviews and transcribing them afterward. Early that year, in 1994, while on a trip to San Francisco, I had for the first time tried Sansert, a longtime migraine abortive drug (and relative of LSD) given off-label for headache prevention. In possibly the least fun drug trip imaginable, even the half dose floored me, making me feel lethargic, dizzy, and dumb. Lying face up on the kitchen floor of the friend's apartment where I was staying, I found the name of my new neurologist in my little phone book and called him.

As is typical of many headache specialists, who are bombarded with calls, and as a matter of policy, he wouldn't speak to me in person. So I waited awhile, still posed there on the cracked linoleum, for the receptionist to call me back. This was a common way I passed my days, in that pre-cell-phone era, just waiting. If I missed the call, I would have to possibly cancel my plans for the next day and wait by the phone. The most frustrating part was that I was never able to talk to a headache specialist directly. Because they get so many calls from headache patients, who have many questions about the inadequate drugs they are taking, these specialists often impose strict measures to guard their time and have nurses and secretaries field questions.

And I mean strict. In contrast, in my reporting career, with some polite persistence and various degrees of skulduggery, I have always been able, by deadline time, to get through to CEOs, mayors, best-selling authors, rock stars, and those accused of major crimes. But I have come up empty-handed every time as a headache patient wanting to ask about how best to taper a benzodiazepine. This is despite trying every trick in the book to reach the doctor personally, such as faxing over short lists of questions or offering to stay on hold for as long as it takes. But in the end, conceding to forces greater and smarter than I (the gatekeeper receptionist), I have had to resign myself to just greatly boiling down the question, passing it on to a third party, and then receiving a simple answer with little opportunity for follow-up questions. And then I must wait three months for personalized follow-up care at my next appointment.

On that day in San Francisco, the nurse finally called back and gave me one short message, to stop taking the Sansert. Although she had been pleasant during our earlier conversation, now she had a new level of irritation in her voice. She delivered the doctor's message so accurately that she had even taken on his tone.

Then, following what had become another regular routine in my life, I weighed my options in canceling what I had to do that day. I still wanted to go through with my interviews for that night, which my friend Steve had taken pains to help me schedule. So he accompanied me in the cab and stayed to help with follow-up questions, those I hadn't written out in advance on my sheet. Here, again, the drugs were more of an impediment to my functioning than the pain.

As a result of this constant uncertainty about how I would feel from day to day and the inevitable "paying for" everything afterward with more pain, I grew more anxious and protective. I was always on guard against something that would derail my present work, along with my entire range of choices and obligations for the day. However, in some ways, I was actually luckier than most chronic pain sufferers. I worked from home, was in charge of my own schedule, and had the option to collapse into a heap when I wanted and work when I felt up to it, even if that was the middle of the night.

Not that money wasn't an issue. I had gone through whatever I had gotten up-front for the book and was earning only a little through small grants and temp work and freelance writing of very small assignments. But I was also more fortunate than most of my age group to have the best type of financial, and emotional, security: largely nondysfunctional middle-class parents. This made all the difference, because, of course, it's one thing to be poor with no safety net, and it's another thing knowing that you will never go hungry or homeless, at least in the short term.

As a saving grace, I always had the option of seeking lodging with my parents, rent-free, no matter how dreadful the prospect of being in the suburbs and losing all independence seemed. But I still had the incentive to work to avoid that change of residence. I most feared it because I knew it would be tough to escape, without the constant struggle to pay rent and utilities. I also knew that I had to stay independent in the city for my sanity, to maintain ties to my "normal" life of friends and urban culture, and not to surrender every last thing to the Headache.

My parents weren't rich—my dad was a professor and my mother had stayed home to take care of us—but they were willing and able to help. I drove my dad's old car. And then, at some point around then, my dad helped me greatly by taking over paying my health insurance, which kept going up, as I was put into increasingly higher-risk pools. (If I ever get assassinated, the number one suspect will be my insurance company, which has paid for one too many two-thousand-dollar MRIs, which, unfortunately for them, were all negative. But then again, I doubt they would be organized enough to carry that off.)

Still, I found even this dependence difficult to bear. Besides the guilt of depleting my family's scrupulously managed and hard-earned resources, it made me feel even more out of control than before, intensifying the stultifying effect of the pain and IQ-reducing drugs. Part of this dread of dependence is cultural, as we expect everyone over eighteen to be completely self-sufficient, no matter how disabled the person really is. And chronic pain and fatigue, particularly, don't seem "legitimate" enough in society's eyes to warrant much pandering.

Unfortunately, regardless of pressures to conserve money, not only are people with chronic pain often dependent on others for the basics, but they also may have greater needs for money than before. And not just for health care.

At that point, my insurance covered most services involving bona fide doctors (even osteopaths) and drugs. But I had a strong desire to shell out constantly for convenience, which would save me marbles at the end of the day. Money does not equal happiness, but in my case it did equal pain reduction. When I traveled, I felt guilty paying for hotels instead of staying with people, but I had to be able to control my all-sacred sleep schedule. I longed to hire cleaning help, and to move to an apartment with central air conditioning, which, in Chicago, even in our era, is generally available in only a minority of new (and more expensive) buildings.

Even the smaller expenses add up. The average life span of an umbrella, a pair of gloves, a hat, a tote bag, or sunglasses was about a month. I habitually left them in buses and trains, sacrificed forever to the gods of the Chicago Transit Authority. On days when I was almost doubled over in pain, I would constantly make choices that saved me the most minor effort, such as when I went to the laundromat and forgot the bottle of detergent in my car in the parking lot outside. Rather than go back and retrieve the detergent, I would instead pay a few bucks for little boxes of powdered soap from the vending machines. On a visit to Whole Foods, I accidentally poured myself an entire bag of pine nuts from the bulk-foods bin, which came out in an unexpected avalanche, instead of the handful I had planned for a single recipe. I didn't want to go through the aggravation of tracking down a store worker, who was nowhere to be seen, so I just went to the checkout line and bought the entire bag, costing twenty-five dollars, making that my most expensive purchase of that week and one of the most valuable items in my apartment. I considered buying a safe just for storing it.

In my brain fog, I did what I could to earn money. But these efforts usually did not end lucratively. The articles for newspapers, quirky small magazines, and progressive publications, at which I was most skilled, paid little. The corporate writing, such as for brochures or press releases, came in at a trickle.

I tried doing articles for glossy high-paying women's magazines, but that always ended in disaster. Once an editor at *Cosmo* invited me to stop by the office when I was in New York to look through the magazine's famous three-ring binder of story ideas. I could pick one and give it a try. I was intrigued, expecting the office to be a plush 1960s-style sex den, perhaps resembling the inside of the *I Dream of Jeannie* bottle, with pink fur walls and fringed throw pillows scattered casually about. But, alas, it was a regular, sterile corporate office, like any other.

As I later learned, this visit to the three-ring binder was a rite of passage for young women freelancers. The magazine's legendary editor at that time, Helen

Gurley Brown, had a formula for what worked in this highly profitable magazine she had helmed since the 1960s, and she naturally didn't want to stray
from it. So the only article ideas green-lighted were ones that she had conceived of herself, typed up in breathy summaries, and rubber-cemented into
the pages of the binder. Most of them blended together in content and had absolutely no time hook to and recognition of the outer world whatsoever. I finally found one that sort of related to the topic of my book, something about
popular knowledge of the biology of the female body, so I could accomplish
multiple tasks with the same set of marbles. I wrote it up and inadvertently
turned in an article that read like a satire of Helen Gurley Brown's girlish
voice, with plenty of phrases highlighted in italics, like "This *outrageous* move
will drive your man *absolutely wild*. I know that it earned me *at least* one mink
coat and *several* pairs of *diamond earrings*." They ended up rejecting the article
and paying me a "kill fee" of a few hundred dollars for several weeks of work.

The temp jobs—when I could do them—also did not pay. The fact that I
could no longer handle even the most basic assignment alerted me to how
low my mental faculties had sunk. On perhaps one of the most humbling
days of that year, I was actually demoted as a temp job receptionist at a
bank for not being able to keep up with the phone calls, and then I was
sent home early. But most depressing was the "payback" for this day of
minor effort. I was so fatigued from just taking the train downtown and
back and waking up early and working for four hours on that stormy day at
the bank that I couldn't do anything the day after. I realized that in this
state, there was no way I would ever be able to work a nine-to-five job
again. And a newspaper job, with its unpredictable deadlines, was definitely out of the question.

I could find absolutely no silver lining. I couldn't even make a token
amount of money by being a research subject in pain studies because I was
"too chronic." I saw an ad in the alternative weekly, the *Reader*, wanting
headache sufferers as subjects in medical experiments. But those were limited to people experiencing headaches a maximum of three times a week. At
that time, a market researcher called me; he was looking for subjects for a
study, which happened to be on over-the-counter pain relievers. Hot dog, I
thought. He rattled off the questions and stopped when I told him how often
I had pain.

Worrying about my financial survival and wanting to decrease my dependence on my parents, I had to swallow my pride and apply for disability payments from the government sector in charge of doling them out, the Social
Security Administration, a division of the Department of Health and Human

Services. I knew the money would be no more than $550 a month, but it would help.

As it is for many people, applying for disability was a profoundly disturbing idea. I hated to label myself with the stigma of "welfare recipient" and, worst of all, admit that I had a lasting problem. But I thought I should at least try it. Since I had only earned about six thousand dollars in the past year, I thought I was a shoo-in candidate. I was almost smug as I filled out the form, detailing how poor I was, how pathetic my situation was.

Drawing from the worst stereotype possible, I had anticipated a long and drawn-out process of having to wait in line for hours in a dimly lit, cramped government office teeming with hordes of the indigent, each lined up with their twelve different kids from twelve different fathers. I imagined I would have to fill out countless forms in triplicate—one in canary yellow, one in blue, one in pink—getting dizzy from inhaling carbon paper vapors. Then they would copy everything on a stinky mimeograph machine, the type they had in my grade school in the 1970s.

Instead, I filled out the form and mailed it in, and I got a quick phone call soon after. They had assigned me a "Miss Crabtree,"[4] whose throwback prefeminist title and prim WASPy name evoked images of JFK's and Lyndon Johnson's call to duty—and the well-meaning college graduates they inspired to visit newly minted housing projects in droves, dressed in their pillbox hats and white gloves.

But my romance with Miss Crabtree soon ended with her first question: "So, how long have you had your drug problem?" She had confused me with someone else.

Soon after, I got a form letter informing me that Social Security had turned me down, explaining that I wasn't "disabled under our rules."

I called Miss Crabtree and asked why. It turns out an income of six thousand dollars made me a high roller in the disabled world. To qualify as disabled, you have to have made no more than eight hundred dollars—*in the past year*—from the time of becoming disabled. Miss Crabtree pointed out a particularly offending and red-flagging job, a report I had written subcontracting through a friend, a freelancer for Arthur Andersen's corporate communications department. Over the course of one weekend, he had paid me forty dollars an hour, a total of eight hundred dollars, to rewrite some employee materials on "continuous improvement." Summoning all my strength, I had fought bitterly to complete it through a haze of Klonopin withdrawal and distorted vision. On the Social Security form, I had been proud to list that work, seeing it as proof to the feds of how hard I had indeed been trying, showing that I wasn't a layabout.

I had missed the boat. Miss Crabtree explained that to qualify for disability, you have to be *totally* disabled and not be able to do *any* job of any kind *at all*. This is despite the fact that most people with chronic pain, and indeed chronic illness, are not *completely* disabled. In fact, the American Chronic Pain Association lists ten distinct levels of disability, the first being totally incapacitated, and the last being, in lay terms, ready to party. Most of us fit somewhere in the middle. So chronic pain patients are often in the impossible position of passing themselves off as more disabled than they are to get disability and health care benefits and totally retreating from society—or pushing themselves through the rigors of a nine-to-five job, embroiled in a constant and bitter minute-by-minute struggle (at least in cases where they are able to find an employer who will tolerate them).

And so, my dream of being a welfare queen was quashed.

In addition, I felt terribly humbled. I was no better than Goldie Hawn at the beginning of *Private Benjamin*; she arrives in the army with a warped fantasy of how the "other half" lives. I wondered what would have happened to me without my parents, how I would have had to force myself to work a full-time job being that sedated and in that much pain. And even if I had made no more than the required maximum of eight hundred dollars gross for one year, how would I have even survived during that time? Where would I have lived? Where would I have gone? How would I have paid for my health insurance, not to mention my pine nuts?

Is It Just a White Middle-Class Female Thing?

I now recognize that I was in an especially strong financial and educational position compared to the general population of chronic-daily-headache sufferers. Although the stereotype of such patients is that they are affluent whiners with nothing better to do than to think about themselves, studies have shown the opposite: This population is generally less educated (and of lower income) than the general population. In fact, education and gender are the two main variables determining who has chronic headaches. In a recent study, the odds ratio of CDH was almost three times as high in patients with less than a high school education than in those who have graduated from college.[5]

(continues)

(continues)

Part of the explanation might be that these problems are a self-perpetuating cycle, with those in pain (and also with depression) lacking the wherewithal to get education and better jobs. And the stresses of being poor in the first place—including money woes, lack of preventive health care, and straining physical labor—can certainly exacerbate chronic pain. And with better access to health care, people from more prosperous backgrounds are more likely to get an actual medical diagnosis of migraine or chronic daily headache.[6]

But while working on this book, I saw that chronic pain's not being limited to the whining elite—and actually disabling poor people in greater numbers—is far from common knowledge. (This, of course, is also true of the misunderstanding of other largely women's ailments like fibromyalgia and chronic fatigue syndrome.) The most common question about chronic pain from those I have just met has been the suspicious "Hmm. Does this happen just to a 'certain type' of patient?"

Even more troubling, I have also wondered about this point privately, of my greater privilege to complain. I have thought back to my immigrant grandparents, who would never have had the nerve to dwell on such things, which they would have seen as "just life." I assume they did not have migraine or other headaches, but I really do not know, because more basic issues of survival were more on their minds. My dad's father didn't even complain when he had "real" problems, such as when he got shot and stabbed and was seriously injured in robberies at his small West Side butcher shop in the 1930s. My mother's father, who also had escaped penniless from Russia in the 1920s, suffered an even worse fate in one of America's inner cities. In 1973, he was shot and killed in a robbery in Milwaukee, while working as a late-night grocery clerk.

Reflecting on this extreme generational contrast in affluence levels, a (former) friend enjoyed pointing out my relative self-indulgence in complaining about headaches. He would say something like, "Do you ever think about your ancestors, who survived countless horrors, of famine and slavery, of rape and pillaging, of ghetto walls, of restrictions throughout the centuries to full participation in the societies in which they lived? And do you ever think how you are one of the first generations to be free from all that, to reach the Promised Land of America, to be able to work and study and worship as you please—and now you are waylaid with a headache?"

This hurt because it reflected my own self-doubt. Yes, I have certainly asked about myself: Why now? Is this complaining of mine a result of our self-absorbed culture? Are we less able to tolerate the natural problems that arise in life, such as chronic pain, depression, and fatigue—even when they happen in extremes?

After pondering these questions for years, I can finally confidently answer: Yes, it's true. We do tolerate less. Compared to past generations, we are pussies.

Our society's currently high rate of divorce is another example of that sense of entitlement to a better life. Today, women, who are the ones who mostly initiate divorce, do have less tolerance of mistreatment, and even unsatisfying relationships, for better and for worse. But that doesn't mean that we have a moral defect for not "biting the bullet" and are not addressing real problems. The same could be said of surgery patients in the mid-nineteenth century after anesthesia was invented, who literally were not biting the bullet anymore. They could have been called "weak" for having anesthesia, which their elders could never have imagined as an option.

I do credit myself for one major accomplishment during that year, which I didn't fully appreciate at the time. Over the course of three months, I got myself off the Klonopin, tapering it off very slowly, much more slowly than directed by the doctor. By that time, I knew that the most agonizing part about the Headache was the trauma of getting off drugs. And I was learning that doctors paid minimum attention to the nuances of that process. In contrast, getting patients on drugs was a high priority.

Soon after, I learned more about the high addictiveness of Klonopin in particular while watching a VH1 *Behind the Music* special about Stevie Nicks of Fleetwood Mac. In the absence of getting such information from doctors, that show had become a Physicians' Desk Reference of sorts. Nicks had said that, in her case, getting off Klonopin required her being institutionalized, as well as going through a longer time of suffering and withdrawal in seclusion for several years on her Arizona ranch. In fact, she said that getting off Klonopin was much more traumatic than detoxing from years of intensive cocaine abuse. "Those prescription drugs are worse than anything," agreed one of her band mates in an interview for the show. The camera ominously pictured a vial of Klonopin, bathed in eerie dark shadows.

As I went to sleep that night, I knew I had done the right thing, although I suspected that my days to follow would be no different.

5

Bridal Bingo

○ ○ ○ ○ ○ ○ ○ ○ ○

AND THEN, AS IF ALL THIS WASN'T BAD ENOUGH, there were the bridal showers.

I was suddenly attending so many in the mid-1990s that they became almost a part-time job on the weekends. They were disproportionately and oddly troubling because they were strongly symbolic—as most disproportionately and oddly troubling things are. I didn't really envy the getting married part, although I was impressed by my friends' fiancés and impossibly ideal partnerships. (That was before I knew that at least half would be divorced within seven years.)

No, what bothered me was that these tuna-salad-soaked events represented others moving forward with their lives of affluence and fulfillment as I watched from the outside, frozen in limbo. These friends, whom I had known from grade school and college, and who came from middle-class or more modest backgrounds, were now entering the upper middle class with careers and ambitious professional husbands. And I was aspiring to get on the dole.

On second thought, I do admit that I did feel some intense small-minded envy at those events. For the flatware. This forbidden desire often cropped up as I made countless trips downtown to Crate and Barrel to study the seemingly endless pages of my friends' registries. I considered the gorgeous "Stelvia Vetreria Tulip Individual Bowl 6". Price: $6.95. Wnt 12. Rcv 4." I scanned the list and considered what I could really use but couldn't afford, the "Krups Blender Power X Plus 14-Spd Wht. Price: $49.95. Wnt 1. Rcv 0." But ultimately, I got whatever was on sale and most compact, which was easiest to lug home on the el.

Making me feel more out of rhythm with the others was that most of these showers were morning affairs, which meant less sleep and more pain. Creating more strain, they were usually way out somewhere in the dreaded suburbs. My "disability" was most glaring and troubling at those times, at social events on the weekends. In contrast, when I was in the privacy of my own home, I naturally had fewer struggles with the pain to keep pace with others. While alone, I could lie down when I felt the worst; in these social cases, I had to put my own needs second and instead engage in polite conversation about house remodeling.

Actually, I was no stranger to this amplification of a disability in social situations. I knew about it intimately, as a lifelong sometimes-stutterer. Of course, to an even greater extent than with chronic pain, the most unsettling aspects of stuttering are experienced with other people—not bothering me much when I'm alone. Through my life, this has been mostly a minor problem, happening a vast minority of the time when I speak. But it grew to become more of an issue at that time, exacerbated by my growing anxiety and sense of self-doubt. Because of the pain, I was losing all confidence and any idea of who I was. As the weeks passed and I felt more isolated, I felt as if I was forgetting how to talk coherently to others.

So, at the showers, when we went around the table to introduce ourselves, I would say something that sounded to me like "Mmmmubba dubba dooby Kamen." (In retrospect, I realize that I probably sounded fine, just a little worse than a "normal" person, but I had taken every last disfluency to heart.) As a result, as I sat there feeling some of my most severe pain and frustration of that week, I had the darkest thoughts of all. They surprised me, as my mind had not worked that way in the past. While the gifts were being opened, I thought of how I could most painlessly and quickly kill myself—a stabbing with "Pizza Wheel OXO, Chicago Cutlery. Price: $7.50. Wnt 1. Rcv 1," or instant strangulation with the cord of the "Processor Classic 7-Cup Cuisinart. Price: $179.95. Wnt 1. Rcv 1," perhaps? Was that "GE Tster Oven. Price $59.95. Wnt 1. Rcv 1" big enough to accommodate my head? These thoughts especially raged after I had heard endless chatter about having to fit into a size 2 wedding dress handed down from one's great grandmother, who had come of age at a time when Americans were about half their present weight. I tried to be supportive and suppress my urges for self-destruction when three friends of the bride trotted out at once to model their similar-sized bridesmaid dresses and complained about how expensive Vera Wang was these days.

I gave myself away at some of the other showers by not fully cooperating in playing the long rounds of bridal bingo, the ultimate communion of weddings and consumerism. That game involves filling in a blank bingo card with names of gifts you think the bride will receive, like a blender, towels, vase, and so on, and then checking off the corresponding square when she opens that particular gift. The person who gets "bingo" gets a prize. Over and over again, an overzealous cousin or aunt of the bride who was choreographing the game would lean over, see my blank card, and chastise me for not playing along. As another hint that I was living on a different mental planet, I was invited to a "recipe" shower, requiring buying the guest of honor all the kitchen tools she wanted to complete a particular recipe. I was the only one who didn't get the hint and just literally brought one recipe on an index card, and nothing else.

These showers, where I struggled to fake it and fit in, represented a struggle I was having with friends, even though they didn't necessarily know it. On one hand, I really wanted to continue my previous life and maintain connections. Also, as with other events, not going would have meant "giving in" to the Headache.

But I also had a strong desire to be alone, to save my marbles. When it came to socializing, I sometimes feared the Headache as a controlling, clingy, needy antisocial boyfriend, the kind who hates your friends and just wants to stay in on Saturday nights and rent videos. And sometimes it's just easier to give in to that seductive impulse. Instead of bothering to go out, it beckons, why not just stay here all comfy on the couch, make microwave popcorn, and order out from that Thai place you like so much, while comforted by cold packs stacked against the neck and shoulders.

If I went out, I was drained. If I canceled plans, I felt detached and guilty. When you're in pain, hell is other people, and hell is also the absence of other people.

The stark reality is that you basically have to suffer your pain alone and in silence. In the beginning, you can talk about chronic pain to friends, but then it gets old, fast. You feel like a character in one of those sitcoms that has stayed on the air way too long, having exhausted the same old story line to the limit and becoming a caricature of oneself. (Like during the last few lame seasons of *Happy Days* when Richie had split and they made Jenny Piccolo and Chachi major characters.)

In contrast, other people's problems had definite beginnings, middles, and ends. They would suffer crises—breakups, parents getting divorced, parents getting sick, parents coming out of the closet—all of which ran their course. My problem was hopelessly postmodern, without a linear narrative structure and devoid of the least hint of a conclusion. So as not to drive people away, I stopped talking about the Headache with all but my closest friends, although it raged on worse than ever. At most, I just touched on the topic, such as with "Yes, I still get migraines sometimes. And how are you?"

In an effort to be upbeat and nondepressing, I even often tried to be cheery about how things were improving, being overly optimistic when I would get a short-lived bounce from a drug. But because chronic pain is invisible, and I often looked happy and was not outwardly miserable all of the time, friends and family continually assumed my pain was in the past. To my great annoyance, they regularly brought up the problem in the past tense, as something I had already overcome. With all the best intentions, they interpreted some of my "odd" behavior, like my penchant for sleeping late, as a bohemian eccentricity.

However, as is common with such invisible illnesses, people I didn't know as well interpreted my pain-induced behavior more negatively. This was especially true of people I met professionally, with whom "coming out" immediately can be more awkward. In a late-morning playwriting course, a teacher singled me out for not participating enough in the group discussion, as if I were being rude. In reality, I was using all my energy just to be able to follow the conversation, much less comment on it. What was more worrisome, my book editor was beginning to think that I was careless about deadlines, and she was clearly losing patience with me. After all, as her attitude suggested, plenty of people have "migraines," but they still manage to do their work. And I kept making matters worse by promising to finish the book "in the near future," especially during those rare optimistic periods when the pain got (temporarily) better.

At about that time, I got a rare honest view of what some of my peers thought of chronic headaches when I wrote a short story addressing the topic for my fiction-writing group, which had been meeting irregularly at cafés for years. Just to get it down on paper, in one sitting, I wrote a stream-of-consciousness autobiographical story about the typical day of a twenty-seven-year-old woman on the North Side of Chicago who had a constant headache (which I cribbed for this book as the intro to the previous chapter).

The group immediately launched into a discussion about the symbolic meanings of the headache:

"Well, it's obvious that this headache is a metaphor for the character's mental problems."

"Clearly. But which ones exactly?"

"Perhaps some type of immaturity, dependency, sexual repression of some sort."

I countered, "Why does it have to be a metaphor for something? Can't it just be a physical problem that this character has?"

The group considered this suggestion a second and then went back to their debate, homing in further on the character's mental imbalances.

Of course, I don't blame them. In literature, a character's physical ailment is often a major metaphor. For example, in Jim Harrison's 1990 novella, *The Woman Lit By Fireflies*, at the onset of a migraine, a woman uses the insights from her "pain-ridden consciousness" to realize she must leave her husband. In these cases, a headache isn't allowed to be just a headache but serves instead as a vehicle for expressing some other, and more compelling, underlying theme.

Much of this lack of understanding is rooted in a great absence of public understanding and knowledge of the neurology of chronic pain, not to mention chronic daily headache. And some of it is just a question of human nature. People's empathy for others' misfortunes, especially those that seem totally random and inexplicable (and therefore may possibly happen to them), is always in short supply. This is one of the main lessons of the Book of Job in the Old Testament, one of the most famous meditations on pain and its meaning or, rather, its common lack thereof. Almost every pain book seems obligated to offer an interpretation of this biblical classic.

(A refresher: In that story, God makes a bet with Satan that Job, a prosperous farmer, will not turn against him if he makes Job's life absolutely miserable. God kills Job's entire family and his farm animals and, to add insult to injury, covers him in "loathsome sores from the sole of his foot to the crown of his head." At the end, in what seems like a tacked-on Hollywood ending, Job keeps his faith in God—and God gives him a brand-new family, twice his original number of sheep, and heals his painful sores.)

In addition to being a parable about pain and faith, Job's story highlights the unfortunate but common lack of sympathy from onlookers. Job's neighbors ramble on and on, for pages and pages, about how pain has to have meaning, how God rewards the just and punishes the wicked, so Job must be wicked. "Miserable comforters are you all," replies the frustrated Job. "Shall windy words have an end?" (15:16). In reality, his pain has no meaning as a rebuke to him personally, as the book repeatedly calls Job "blameless and upright."

In her classic 1930 essay *On Being Ill*, migraine sufferer Virginia Woolf recognized this universal lack of empathy for the chronically ill, like herself—

but wasn't bothered by it. She reasoned that just as people aren't naturally happy for you when good things happen, they also don't get too worked up about your losses. She reasoned that if we all felt every shred of the pain and discomfort of others, civilization itself would fail to go on. She cheered on the unsympathetic but productive "army of the upright' in the world of commerce and consigned the burdensome task of sympathy to the "laggards and the failures, women for the most part (in whom the obsolete exists so strangely side by side with anarchy and newness), who, having dropped out of the race, have time to spend upon fantastic and unprofitable excursions" (10).

I add that it's probably good that people have so little empathy for those in pain. If people had really understood my struggle at that time, no one would have asked me to do anything, and I would have been more isolated.

But an irony is that those who are invisibly ill often crave sympathy. It is sweet and rare nectar, a balm, a tonic, more healing than the purest spa waters at Lourdes. Whereas those with visible disabilities have long campaigned to "fit in," others who are regularly mistaken for "normal" may long for at least a shred of recognition of what they are going through. This would provide a modicum of validation, which we are often lacking in a skeptical "bootstrap"-mentality society. This doesn't have to be done with Mother Theresa–level prostration, but with just a casual comment, as when a friend told me, "Gee, last month I had a migraine that lasted, you wouldn't believe it, three days! I thought, boy, how does she do it?" Ah, what ambrosia, this thing of empathy.

Yet, in addition to validation, sometimes we need more concrete help from friends and family. And there's the rub. Though I had many friends, partly the result of staying largely in the same metropolitan area for my entire life, I found it impossible to ask anyone to assist with daily chores, for fear of being a burden to them. Perhaps I would have felt different in a temporary crisis, such as recovering from knee surgery. It's one thing to ask if a friend can go shopping for you once, but it's another to ask, "Uh, well, do you mind going shopping for me . . . like, for the rest of my life?" I also was very careful about calling in favors and was saving them for only the direst circumstances. In asking for help, I also would have crossed a line and changed the power dynamic of a friendship, one perceived as based on mutual support—and not on my dependence and neediness, far less noble traits.

Over time, tension grew with friends over my relative unreliability when it came to making and keeping social commitments. Not able to relate to the fatiguing factor of chronic pain, people often failed to consider it a valid excuse not to do something. So, ironically, they let me off more easily with a temporary and visible complaint with which they could identify, such as a cold. "Ah, the common cold is so elegant, so simple," I marveled to myself, heeding their gentle ministrations in those cases to "just rest and take it easy and enjoy life without all the expectations that you normally have." Yet the discomfort of a cold was, as a rule, much less intense than that of a headache, even on the best of days.

In deciding whether I would cancel a date, I also had to figure out my friends' individual tolerance levels for such an action, the availability of a lot of other friends to fall back on, their hassle level in rescheduling (finding a baby-sitter, for instance), or their controlling nature. But now, looking back, I am amazed by all the times I did *not* cancel and went out until late at night. Sometimes doing so was like torture, as I fought through the pain for hours and put on a happy front. But other times, especially when the pain was on a lower level, I was distracted enough by the events around me, such as a party or a concert or a play, to get through. And sometimes that would provide a needed antidote to depression, to not dwelling just on myself.

Indeed, my "trooper" quality sometimes backfired. One of my new roommates would observe me going out at night and then wonder out loud, "How much pain could you really be in?" If you're not visibly miserable all the time, people are suspicious.

The Gate Theory Revisited: Pain in the Head, After All

At the time, I really couldn't explain to skeptical friends why distraction by something pleasant, like a movie, did sometimes provide relief. But now I better understand how thoughts and emotions can affect how the brain modulates pain—at least in the short term.

One of the best explanations I have ever read of this phenomenon is in Atul Gawande's chapter "The Pain Perplex," in his book *Complications* (2002). He discussed the case of a prominent Boston architect who was crippled by back pain. But his wife expressed doubts and thought he was "faking it" when his emotions influenced his pain, such as when a depressing thought made him feel worse, and he canceled plans). But "among chronic pain sufferers," Gawande explained, "his case is altogether typical" (118).

He described the pain-relieving or exacerbating effect of emotions by evoking the same 1965 gate-control theory I had studied so long ago, for my sixth-grade science project. That theory had been revolutionary in demonstrating how other biological input, such as temperature or a touch, could block pain signals from reaching the brain. This theory related specifically to blocking signals at the spinal cord. Examples of this effect are

(continues)

(continued)

someone's hitting a hand with a hammer and then instinctively sucking on the hand to divert pain signals, or someone's soaking sore muscles in a hot bath, its temperature temporarily relieving discomfort.

Gawande further pointed out how one of the gate theory's two originators, Ronald Melzack, expanded the theory in the late 1980s to focus more on the brain's ultimate role in modulating pain. Just as there are "gates" that block and filter pain at the spinal cord, the brain has its own set of controls. To be sure, the brain is not merely a passive transmitter of physical pain signals, but an active interpreter and filterer of a wide "symphony" of input, from sources physical, mental, and emotional. As a result, that architect's negative emotions, such as disappointment about a loss, could actually make his physical pain worse by interfering with how pain signals were processed in the brain. The fluctuations were real; he was not "putting on an act."

Indeed, biologically speaking, wrote Gawande, "all pain is 'in the head.'" The bottom line is that no matter where the pain is felt in the body, pain is ultimately processed in the brain. In other words, if "a mad scientist reduced you to nothing but a brain in a jar," Gawande wrote, you could still feel pain in other areas, such as the limbs or back. As further "proof" that the brain is the command center of pain, most people with amputated limbs continue to feel "phantom" pain in those areas because the neurological signals related to that area of the body are still active in the brain.

Despite these stresses, I somehow was still able to have some good times during that period, even on days that started out as afternoons. I was surprised that instead of falling apart, my quality and quantity of friends were not only undiminished but increasing, plenty still being single and without a really good set of flatware. I always had a social life, although a slower one. This is probably one of the biggest ways I contrast to the typical pain patient, who often can't spare the energy for a social life, as the sheer survival of oneself and one's family is the foremost priority. It takes all their energy just to make it through a nine-to-five job, and then all they want to do is crash. That is how they spend their marbles.

But this contact with friends, coupled with a decent sense of humor and absurdity, is what kept me going. Despite the ever-present pain, I had many moments of genuinely enjoying their company and their jokes and their outrageous stories, and it showed. I soon realized that friends that couldn't handle what had happened to me really hadn't been that prominent in my life to begin with. And I strengthened many friendships with a new level of honesty in communication; and in return, they opened up about things I had never expected, such as a period of past depression.

I never got too isolated, as my roommates were intensely social, always knowing about a party or comedy show that they were involved in. It was a very good time to be in your twenties in Chicago, a time when the music, poetry-slam, and theater scenes were exploding, and the living was relatively cheap.

My roommates even found humor in my situation, as when I walked around wearing a blue "ice hat," an ice pack in the shape of a bathing cap. One time, as we were watching television, one asked me why I was vibrating, and I pulled up my shirtsleeve to reveal a TENS (transcutaneous electric nerve stimulation) unit, a black box about the size of a cell phone. A wire led from it to a "pressure point" between the thumb and forefinger of my right hand—the same one used as an acupuncture point to thwart headaches—where it was affixed with a gel-soaked pad. Theoretically, it was supposed to be the "gate theory" in action, blocking pain signals by sending alternate vibrations to the brain.

In other settings, my sister had to laugh when my dad kept asking me if I had ever "considered getting a vibrator," meaning something (cheap) with which I could massage my head and get relief. "Maybe that would help your headache." He usually brought up this question when we were sitting in a public place, such as a packed doctor's waiting room.

Some friends just made accommodations for me, not making a big deal about it, taking my different pace into consideration. When together, as for a weekend, we could plan around my worst time of pain, the mornings. The best example is when I would go with a friend to visit another in Madison, Wisconsin, several hours away. They would both wake up at a "normal" hour, such as 9 A.M., and go out for breakfast without me, leaving me alone in my own room in the morning. Then they would plan to meet me for lunch, and our day together would begin. I would get up when I wanted to, without embarrassment or self-doubt. That was a sign of my beginning level of acceptance and "coming out" to others with pain. But these were options that I had barely begun to explore.

6

Sex and the Single Migraineur

○ ○ ○ ○ ○ ○ ○ ○ ○

PERHAPS THE GREATEST PUBLIC SERVICE I can do for chronic headache patients is to clear up one major myth—about the Excuse.

After all, the "Not tonight, dear, I have a headache" response is a cultural cliché, employed as an easy punch line everywhere from a Beetle Bailey–level cartoon strip to garden-variety sitcom. In the beginning of the movie *Annie Hall*, Woody Allen flashes back to an attempt at intimacy with his ex-wife, which is frustrated by her migraine. In fact, Allen uses the fact that she is a headache sufferer as dramatic shorthand to characterize her as neurotic and the marriage as a frustrating failure.

But as easy as it is to imagine that migraine sufferers are antisex, established academic research shows that sex can actually *relieve* women's migraines, not worsen them.

One major study, summarized in a 1990 issue of the journal *Headache*, surveyed 82 women with episodic migraines. Backing up previous research by the same team, the survey found that about half of the women reported some improvement in their headaches after sex, with about 12 percent (or 10 subjects) reporting "complete relief" or "remission of headache." In contrast, only about 5 percent (or 3 subjects) reported that the SI (sexual intercourse) made their headaches worse. "The mechanism or mechanisms involved in relief of headache are unclear but may include the activation of endogenous [brain-centered] pain control systems," explained authors James Couch and Candice Bearss.

This same research was presented by Couch and Randolph W. Evans in the May 2001 issue of *Headache*. "Dr. Couch's data suggests that some

women who decline, 'Not tonight, I have a headache,' may be avoiding an effective treatment," reads an uncharacteristically wry introductory editor's
note. The authors added that this effect has not been as well studied in men
but is thought to be evidenced in "occasional anecdotal information." One of
these doctors noted that he had recently found that "orgasm would relieve [a
male patient's] cluster headaches."

In fact, other surveys do show a worsening of headache with sex, but that's
mainly for *men*. The typical sufferer of what has been called *coital cephalalgia*
or, as more recently classified in 2004, *primary headache associated with sexual activity*, is male, middle-aged, mildly to moderately hypertensive (with
high blood pressure), and often in poor physical shape and overweight. And
he usually has a preexisting migraine disorder. The male-to-female ratio for
sexual headaches is four to one.

Researchers have actually spent a lot of time classifying various types of
sex-related headaches, which can happen whether with SI or masturbation.[1] One of the most common, now called *orgasmic headache*, was titled
explosive headache. It comes on suddenly near or at the time of orgasm and
may last from less than one minute to three hours. In the past, it has been
classified as a subtype of "exertional" headache, which can also be brought
on by exercise or even coughing. Up to one-third of these patients also suffer similar headaches as a result of physical exertion. This headache is a
type of sudden-onset or "thunderclap" headache. (A nonbenign form with
the same patient description can be triggered by a more ominous cause, a
brain hemorrhage.)

The second type of primary sexual headache, *pre-orgasmic headache*, is
characterized by a dull ache in the head and neck that intensifies as sexual
excitement increases, and that can last up to several days. Not surprisingly,
sexual headache and the exertional types are thought to be related to "hemo-
dynamic changes," or changes in blood circulation and muscle contractions.

But as one advantage, one thing these men do *not* have to worry about is
being told "it's all in your head." They have to deal only with the explosive
pain, not with social recrimination. As far as I know, psychologists have not
attributed any specific meaning or symbolism to sexual headaches. And you
don't have to be a radical feminist to assume that is because this type of
headache is primarily male. If it were primarily female, Freud and his followers would have written about it at length a hundred years ago in famous trea-
tises about how this pain symbolizes some type of female sexual immaturity
or indicates past sexual abuse or a childhood hang-up with masturbation. In
contrast, with this male coital cephalalgia, a cigar is just a cigar.

Of course, whatever endorphin rush sex may bring, the obvious truth for women is that headaches can diminish sexual desire. It is just common sense that even relatively minor pain can have a real negative influence on both the desire and the experience, its quality and frequency. Needless to say, this is especially true when the pain is severe and when the patient suffers other common "sickly" symptoms of chronic headaches, such as an aura, vomiting, and nausea—all undeniable buzz kills. And yes, a headache can cause libido-deflating depression and anxiety, as well as fatigue and preoccupations with other more pressing matters in our hierarchies of needs, such as increasingly overdue bills. Of course, other types of chronic pain—in the back, for instance—may actually preclude the physical act itself.

For the single woman with chronic daily headache—the kind that stays relatively constant with a moderate level of pain—there is a different story, one you won't find in the medical journals or textbooks. Unless the headache is severe, the single female headache sufferer can usually muster up the energy for SI, borrowing whatever "marbles" are needed from the days or even the weeks to come. In fact, as I've learned anecdotally, few cases of pain can stop her if the moment is opportune, especially after a long and dismal dry spell; then she will mortgage whatever marbles she needs—from her next life, if necessary. One motivation is that, at least when done right, sex can be an endorphin-rich activity that may actually relieve pain, not to mention provide a valuable distraction. In an article reprinted in the *Utne Reader*, migraine sufferer Holly Harden (2003) listed masturbation as a part of her arsenal of pain-relieving techniques, to get rid of the swarm of "silverfish" she describes as characterizing her own migraine aura. "Masturbate until your arm tingles and you think you feel a shark born of your head going after those blessed little fish," she says (46).

Indeed, the main question is not being up for sex but having the energy for all the stuff that leads up to it: the dating part.

And dating takes energy. Single women typically endure at least two to eighteen hours of one-on-one dating time, commonly involving two to three separate meetings, before they get to the point of going to bed with someone. Even the most "liberated" woman usually wants to spend at least that amount of time with the potential sex partner, not necessarily to fall in love, but just to make sure he is someone she likes, a much more realistic standard to maintain. Of course, that's also the time to look for red flags warning about one's physical and emotional safety, such as explosive anger toward the ex-wife or effusive Jovan Musk.

Although possibly very interesting, the hours of conversation can be tiring for chronic pain patients, who may swing many times in the course of the evening from a wry Bridget Jones to a tortured Frida Kahlo. As her trigeminal nerve seems to thrash about like a burning live wire behind her eye, the urban neurologically challenged single gal maintains a relaxed expression and casually pursues answers to her preferred dating questions. In cases such as mine, these may include elaborate discussions of each party's career trajectory, the assets and drawbacks of living in Chicago and not New York or LA, the assets and drawbacks of each person's current urban neighborhood, the assets and drawbacks of Trader Joe's versus Whole Foods, and opinions about the Middle East crisis—Do you have any ideas?

And these pleasantries often are not enough. As I've more recently observed, men now expect something much more adventurous and compromising than mere discourse leading to intercourse. In high-achieving and youth-worshiping urban settings, there is a new ethic that incorporates taxing athletic activities into a date. One party will suggest that they bike to a museum, instead of driving there, even though the destination is many miles away and the ground is covered with ice. He lobbies that they train for a marathon together, with a series of six sessions on consecutive Sunday mornings starting at 6 A.M.. "Let's go get some fudge," he suggests, to her delight, adding, "We'll just kayak to Mackinac Island to buy it!"

I certainly don't object to working out, as it can be a major pain-relieving strategy, but not in extremes as a required dating activity. This makes one pine for the old days when all we had to worry about in dating was stalking, rejection, sexually transmitted diseases, frustrated religious-conversion attempts, and unintended pregnancy.

A friend of mine with chronic fatigue syndrome, Rivka, who recently reentered the dating world, made this same observation on her own. She lamented that she just wants someone to have a chat with and share some physical intimacy with, not reenact a *Survivor* episode or do Outward Bound. She said that in the online profiles, men in their thirties describe sport after sport that they want to take part in with a woman. "They want to ski, and mountain-climb, and camp for days, and live off the land. And all that hiking," she said.

"Yes, all that fucking hiking," I replied.

Even if the single invisibly ill woman in the city is able to get over the high-intensity athletics hurdle, another basic challenge is just being able to keep a date. As in other areas of life, a perennial problem in times of a physical flare-up is whether you should cancel. A consideration, of course, is:

What if another flare-up happens at the time of the rescheduled date? And that time, the pain could be worse. Then the guy will think you're a total flake. But if you show up, you won't be at your best. Sometimes the best excuse is to just play the "I have a cold or flu" card, which is always an acceptable excuse. Certainly, it's simpler than the truth, which would go something like this: "Sorry I can't go out, because not only do I feel as if a railroad spike is piercing my retina, but I am suffering withdrawal from an addictive anticonvulsant/tranquilizer/mood stabilizer and would probably distract you with my delirium tremens and profuse sweating. Ironically, for me, it will be a double date because I may see two of you."

And it's common for someone with chronic pain not to want to even mention the topic at all, especially as an excuse for canceling a date, in the very beginning. For one thing, as in other areas of life, even if one came out of the closet with chronic daily headache, most people would not be able to sympathize. And besides, no one wants to start a relationship with a negative spin and mention pain, even as something episodic, for fear of becoming the dreaded "headache girl." You don't want to join the pantheon of undesirable freaky "types of women," such as those characterized on *Seinfeld*, from the "low talker" to the one who always wears the same outfit.

After all, the women with headaches in pop culture and literature do not provide any positive role models. I keep thinking about the self-absorbed, vindictive, distant mother character in the best-selling novel *Atonement* by Ian McEwan. She spends most of her time nursing her headache alone in dark rooms, while also plotting against the other characters. More ubiquitous is the specter of Omorosa of *The Apprentice*, who in 2004 was one of the most well-known contestants (and villains) of reality television. Omorosa was widely ridiculed after she complained of headaches triggered by plaster falling on her head at a construction site. "I have plaster fall on my head all the time, and it's fine," commented the highly unsympathetic Donald Trump, before giving her the axe. Even country singer Toby Keith complains about this irritating sort in his 2001 hit "I Wanna Talk About Me," which begins with the lyrics "We talk about your work, how your boss is a jerk. We talk about your church and your head when it hurts." In the video for this song, the woman is yakking cluelessly away, boring not only Keith but also a hapless criminal stuck in the back of his police car.

Other obstacles to getting to the sex part don't have anything to do with pain or physical disability. Drugs often have libido- and orgasm-dampening side effects. Of 327 chronic pain patients who took part in a study published in an issue of the *Clinical Journal of Pain*, about a third were taking drugs with the potential to impair interest in sex and to reduce satisfaction. And about 20 percent were taking drugs that could impair performance.[2]

Often, doctors overlook these sexual side effects as a concern, especially for women, for whom these side effects can signify a real loss. We are not informed of the risks to sexual desire or function, such as the possibility of having to work full time for at least twelve hours to have an orgasm. We are lucky if doctors consider this matter, even as an afterthought. A typical medical journal will devote pages to clinical observations relating to men and perhaps tack on a cursory paragraph about how, well, the same conclusions could apply to women, but the topic hasn't been studied that much.[3] Just as in the broad field of disability and medical research itself, pain researchers have been slow to include gender as a variable or an object of study, this emphasis only recently taking off in the pain field in the early to mid-1990s.[4]

Even if this issue isn't being studied, men and women themselves more widely report sexual side effects with commonly used antidepressants. These include the tricyclics, most commonly used for headaches, and especially the newer SSRIs, like Prozac. Studies reveal sexual impairment side effects happening in women patients from a minority to up to 80 percent.

And of course, the challenges for the headache-afflicted single gal go well beyond sex and dating. Indeed, because of effects on one's appearance and functioning, chronic pain can become a major issue in forming life partnerships for young women, who are in the age group most affected by headaches.[5] That is probably why God created casual sex, but of course, for many, that is not a satisfactory option.

The female pain sufferer, of any type, may need even more energy and patience to deal with another type of typically male figure in her life: the neurologist. As writer (and diagnosed "female hysteric") Alice James confided to her diary in 1890, "I suppose one has a greater sense of intellectual degradation after an interview with a doctor than from any human experience."[6] Unfortunately, as I found out in one particularly jarring instance, the old-time Victorian prejudices about women and illness, bolstered by pseudoprogressive postmodern cultural theories, are still alive and well today in the examining room. They compound the guilt and shame that chronic pain sufferers may already feel about our "deviances," pushing us deeper into the closet.

Part Two:

THE BURDEN OF PROOF

7

The "Pleasant" Patient

o o o o o o o o o

Reading Between the Lines

ONE OF THE MOST IRRITATING PARTS of getting a constant headache is not the pain, nor is it the resulting isolation and impoverishment. It's the frustration of it all, of always feeling as if you're near a cure, but not quite there. As the months passed, I grew more and more incredulous that doctors did not know how to cure such a banal problem, that there was not one simple thing right under my nose that would do the trick.

After all, I kept asking myself, wasn't this like what happened to Underdog, in the cartoon we watched as kids? I remembered him wondering aloud, "When I bend over, I'm as right as rain. But when I stand up, there is a stabbing pain." And then, at the end, he realized some villain had planted a sword in the back of his shirt, pointing downward. Problem solved.

Was the solution for me just as obvious? If I just saw *one more* doctor, I asked myself, wouldn't he or she be bound to find it, just through sheer common sense? If not a doctor, was the solution elsewhere? Wasn't there someone out there in a lab somewhere slicing up a stem cell for my benefit?

Wasn't there some service journalist publishing an article with an uplifting case study exactly similar to mine, with a 1-2-3 bulleted plan?

In other words, I wondered whether I had been the victim of a huge bureaucratic misunderstanding, involving some kind of simple clerical error. With more explanation and patience, and perhaps a conversation with someone's department manager, it would all be cleared up—in the same way that I straightened out the matter of an overcharge on my phone bill. It should be just a matter of communicating clearly and directly.

But the harder I tried, the more Kafkaesque the journey became. Despite fears that I was getting paranoid, I increasingly suspected that doctors were my adversaries, that my negative experience with my first doctor at the Chicago Headache Clinic was not a fluke. They listened but never seemed to hear or understand what I was saying. Most annoyingly, when doctors heard the particulars of my story, such as the description of chlorine in a pool triggering a headache, they just shrugged and said that they had "never before heard of anything like that." End of conversation.

Worsening the situation was my growing despair. I wasn't sure if my listlessness was a result of the pain or the drugs, or if it was just me. I was also always aware that my book, which had become a symbol of how much "in control" I was of my life, was now more than a year overdue, past the original deadline. I knew it was impossible to work substantially on it in this state. At that point, I couldn't even swim anymore because the chlorine in the pool now triggered that broken-glass sensation *every time* I went swimming, instead of just occasionally, as before. Even the simplest pleasures had been stripped away from me. And taking their place was a new stream of dark thoughts, about programming Jack Kevorkian's number on speed dial on my phone. I knew in my heart that I would never take such action, but I was still alarmed to find my mind wandering in that direction.

I can't say that I was depressed; it was more like being broken. As someone who had not lived before with major depression, I didn't know how to go on coexisting with it. Very simply, we had battled and it had won.

But despite much self-blame about my state, I also became curious about whether the depression *wasn't all me*. I wondered if I was going through stages common to people with chronic pain, just as mourners typically experience a discrete set of stages. I thought that if I could get insight into my distress, I could get a more objective perspective on what was happening to me, to distinguish between what was a "normal" reaction and what wasn't. Then I would know what attitudes I had to work on personally to change. At last, I concluded, it was time to stop being defensive and see a therapist.

The only therapist I could afford was at Jewish Family Services downtown on Wells Street, right off the el. They charged me five dollars each time, as a token payment, to acknowledge that I appreciated their time. The therapist, who was about my age, fumbled her way through our sessions and didn't say much of value. I finally decided to protest when I told her about my discovery, the Internet, *and she had never heard of it.* (This was late 1994, but still.)

"So," she said, with a deliberately neutral and nonjudgmental tone, after I had mentioned my discovery of the online world. "You turn on your computer and talk to people? What do these voices say to you?"

"They're not voices," I answered. "We type to each other."

"OK, you say you type things to each other," she said, making a note in my chart. "What do you type to each other?"

"Answers to each others' questions. They also have special chat rooms where you can go and talk to a lot of people at once."

"Your computer has rooms in it?"

"No, not real rooms. It's all electronic. No one is in the computer. They are all communicating from their own homes, all over the world."

"You say these are real people?"

"Yes."

"From all over the world."

"Yes."

"But you're not leaving your apartment?"

I tried to explain more about how this all worked through the phone lines but could tell she was still confused.

Soon after, I found out that she was an intern. At my request, I was reassigned to an older and more experienced social worker. I told her about my waking up late and my pretty much not being able to write. But she apparently didn't know about the complexities of pain and blamed my growing "labile" depressive state for *causing* the pain and my current work impasse.

As I've come to find out, this is a very common problem faced by pain sufferers seeking help. Therapists and doctors, who haven't had the pleasure of knowing you in your past life, prepain, are likely to judge your current unstable state as defining your nature, as the Real You. They are likely to see this depression as the natural root of your problem—and not as the *result*. I had to explain to this lady that I had never been clinically depressed before all this happened. I was a lot of fun, a regular riot, the life of the party, a barrel of laughs, you should have seen me then.

I also pointed out that I was not depressed, and was even elated, on those rare days or in those rare hours when the pain was diminished and manageable.

I still had the full will and desire to go on with life, even if I didn't have the energy for it. If I had been a depressive, wouldn't I have been the first to know about it?

The traditional therapist I visited at Jewish Family Services also tried to point to family origins of the pain. Although my family is by no means perfect, I had never been more grateful for having a relatively trauma-free childhood.

In fact, I wanted to call my dad and thank him—for never molesting me. Not because of the ordeal of being molested, but because of all the money and time in therapy it would have cost me to analyze it as a source of the headaches. Since therapists tend to single out sexual abuse above all other types of trauma as causing every physical problem imaginable, that would have been a tough red herring to bag. In addition, a history of abuse in my life would have halted all other investigation into possible causes of the Headache, along with reducing the urgency to treat it medically.

I was further dismayed that even the brand-new wonder drug of that time for migraines, Imitrex, which seemed then to be working for everyone else, had failed me. As the result of a mammoth marketing campaign in 1993 and 1994, which included articles about Imitrex sent to me by relatives and friends across the country, I had been curious to try it. What was the harm in it? However, the neurologist I was seeing at the time did not want to give it to me, thinking my pain was too chronic for it to work (and he was right).

So, my well-meaning mother suggested that I go with her to an internist whom she had seen in the south suburbs and had liked, on a day when I was visiting there and was in an especially severe amount of pain. At that time, Imitrex was just available as an injection, unlike the myriad of more accessible forms that triptans come in today, from nasal spray to tablets that dissolve under the tongue. But after the injection, I merely ended up with an uncomfortably warm and fuzzy feeling in my head.

Even worse, the internist got into an altercation with my mother about our "real" motives: After he had left the room, she asked me about how I would deal with the pain that day, and I said I had no idea. She asked if I needed a refill on the Norgesic Fortes or Esgic Plus, which sometimes helped provide temporary relief. "Sure," I said, humoring her, not even sure what I had in stock. She then called the doctor into the room to request a prescription for one of these painkillers. He recoiled in horror.

"Mrs. Kamen! That's a narcotic! I can't do that!" he gasped. "So this is what all this is about." He called in the nurse and ordered her to immediately discharge us. Then he left, shaking his head in disbelief. As usual, a request for a drug that works is regarded as suspicious, but a request for a drug that merely makes you uncomfortable (Imitrex) is completely understandable.

My mother looked at me, confused. The idea that my mother—in her sequined Jewish-suburban-mom sweatshirt—was a drug seeker, was absurd (even though I know such people come from all backgrounds). If I hadn't been so embarrassed, I would have found it funny. Instead, expressionless, I led my mother to the receptionist's desk. Besides Imitrex not working with the pain, its failure also meant that my journey to "legitimize" my problem would continue.

Still, I had no choice but to trudge on, following all paths possible. The next step was to visit a neuro-ophthalmologist at another prestigious medical center, a base I had yet to cover. I had decided to see him to measure pressure behind the eyes and rule out a type of constant headache that typically hits women in their twenties and thirties, a result of "benign intercranial hypertension," that describes increased spinal fluid volume or pressure. It was a long shot, since most people with that disorder get a worse headache when they exercise, and I was the opposite. But it was a common question that doctors asked again and again, just as they asked about TMJ (temporomandibular joint) disorder, for which I had tested negative. And it was a way to avoid the other major diagnostic procedure for my problem, the evocatively named spinal tap (or as it is properly termed, the lumbar puncture).

Luckily (or unluckily, as this problem is treatable), the test was negative. But the doctor had an idea. He suggested that I see another headache specialist he knew at the medical center.

My mother and I returned for that appointment in the first weeks of 1995. I admit that I had looked better in my life and wasn't in the ideal frame of mind. I had been up for about three nights straight with insomnia, the side effect of another drug, an antidepressant that I was trying. I would have gotten off it sooner, but I had thought it was my last hope for pain relief and tried to stick it out as long as possible, until I absolutely couldn't stand it anymore and was a danger to myself and to others. The stormy weather outside also made matters worse, riling up the nerve storm inside my head and giving me one of the worst headaches of my life. In other words, to quote W. C. Fields, "Even the two-headed boy at the circus never had such a headache." In most cases in public, I had put on a good front, with no one being able to tell that I was in pain, but this time, I could only clutch my head and stifle tears.

When we got to the medical center, the nurse told us there had been a misunderstanding, that the headache specialist was out of town, and I was to see another doctor, a general neurologist. Since we were already there, we agreed. This doctor seemed skeptical from the beginning, asking a lot of questions about my work life and how I was getting help from my parents. Meanwhile, he sketched down notes and, in the interim, twirled his Princeton class ring.

I continued to earnestly answer his questions, often needing my mother to confirm the dates and places and drug names of my past. By this time, they were all a blur in my mind. He ended the visit saying he would prescribe Depakote, an antiepilepsy drug commonly used for chronic headaches, an obvious one that I had never tried. (I found out later that patients who take it call it "the instant middle-age drug," since common side effects are weight gain and hair loss.)

When I got home, I took a full dose and was, again, vegetized, feeling as if I had entered a stupor. Once again, I wouldn't be as lucky as Underdog. I went to sleep, unable to do much else. The next day, I called and left a message with the nurse about what had happened, and she said she would tell the doctor and have him call me back. He never did. Feeling an odd vibe about the whole experience, and with little strength left to deal with the matter, I decided to let it go.

Eight years later, I understood finally what had happened between that doctor and me and realized that, yet again, I had been on trial. In 2003, I stumbled upon a letter this doctor had written about me to the neuro-ophthalmologist who had referred me to him. I had requested most of my medical records to use as background for this book.

What drew my attention to the letter was length and great detail; it more resembled a legal brief than a medical document. The Princetonian gave an almost word-by-word account of our visit, starting with naming the numerous drugs and doctors I had tried, and then quoting my descriptions of adverse reactions: how one drug "worked at first" and another made me "physically sick." He made a note about my "not working" since May 1993 because of the headache problem, when the Nardil allegedly pooped out. Then he led up to commenting about my mental state: "Physical examination reveals an awake, alert, apparently uncomfortable young woman who is moaning intermittently during the interview and examination. . . . The mental status was normal, although the patient's speech did appear pressured and rapid at times."

I skimmed, wondering why he was commenting about my speech, and then read on: "The patient's mother frequently answered questions directed to the patient. In addition, the patient often looked to her mother for answers to some questioned [sic]. . . . Ms. Kamen's neurologic examination and MRI scan are within normal limits and I see no evidence of a structural neurological problem to explain her persistent headache."

And finally, here's where all this was leading: "I believe it is possible that there may be severe psychiatric issues present which could be contributing to the patient's overall problem. It is difficult for me to assess the significance of these factors during one office visit. I discussed this with the patient and she was quite resistant to the notion that psychiatric issues could be contributing to her headache problem. . . . After much discussion, the patient agreed to a trial of Depakote, but when I subsequently spoke to her on the phone, she decided not to begin the medication. . . . Thank you for referring me to this pleasant young lady."

After reading that letter, almost a decade after it was written, I felt violated (despite being thrown a few crumbs and being called "pleasant," meaning that I was compliant). I had gone to a doctor in good faith to seek understanding about a medical problem and instead had been secretly psychoanalyzed and my "real" motives for the pain questioned. Used as "evidence" was everything I did and said during that one visit. Even disfluencies in speech were suspect. (Later I found out that "pressured speech" is one way to diagnose bipolar disorder.) Also incriminating were the facts that past drugs hadn't worked (which is, actually, common in chronic daily headache patients), and that the MRIs had been negative (as they are in 99 percent of cases of headache sufferers). It turned out that he thought I was behaving erratically and mistakenly believed that I had not even tried the drug he had prescribed. He also interpreted my financial dependence as some kind of motivation for the so-called pain. And he saw the presence of my mother— oh, the poor mother, always an object of blame in psychoanalytic theory—as signaling some kind of warped and stifling relationship, instead of one human helping out another in need.

But in the end, I was grateful to have seen this letter, as both a patient and a researcher. Besides explaining what had happened with that strange doctor, it also explained the dismissive behavior (although not as blatant) of some other doctors from the past.

The letter also served as a jumping-off point for exploring a bigger and timelier story beyond just me, about doctors' traditionally adversarial relationships with women pain patients. I interviewed more than a dozen other chronic headache patients (whom I quote in the final chapters) and doctors, and then read some basic history of pain medicine. I learned that I was not alone, and that many greater social forces were at work to create such seemingly bizarre episodes with doctors. I also discovered that as a mainly female illness, "headache" has been a lightning rod of prejudice. Even in modern times, it carries much of the stigma that the word *hysteria* did during the Victorian era.

Today, these prejudices specifically remain strongest with chronic daily headache in particular, which is not as treatable nor as common as episodic migraine. But changes have at least been made in how the verdict is delivered to these "problem" patients. Most doctors are politically correct enough nowadays not to directly state that it's "all in our heads." Instead, such discussion goes on between doctors behind closed doors, often couched in "code words" about the patient's real underlying motive and mental state, such as *dependent, difficult, histrionic* (hysterical), *conversion disorder, somatization, psychogenic, emotional overlay,* and *secondary gains.* And resisting these opinions is often futile, or even more damaging to one's case. The more effort a patient makes to get adequate medical treatment, with her original doctor or others, the more likely she is to be classified as a "thick folder patient," or one who is making it all up.

Some of this prejudice may be a special shock to younger women, who may not even be aware of these subtexts occurring in their medical examinations. As someone who grew up taking the women's movement for granted, I personally was surprised to read, in medical sources, about these blatant opinions, even when they were portrayed as existing in the past. In a report from a June 2000 meeting at the National Institutes of Health, I read a common introductory remark: "Migraine, we used to believe, was a disorder of anxious, neurotic women whose blood vessels overreacted," said Dr. Stephen Silberstein, neurologist and cochairman of the U.S. Headache Consortium.

He went on to explain: "Migraine is not that. Migraine is a neurological disorder of the brain." He went on to voice current scientific theories about headache that have yet to fully catch on among doctors, as well as the public at large.

The stigma has been so significant and influential on treatment that even the most current medical textbooks feel obligated to acknowledge it. "Headache is the Rodney Dangerfield of medical maladies—it gets no respect," Dr. Silberstein and his coauthors observed in *Headache in Clinical Practice* (5). In another 2003 textbook, *Reducing the Burden of Headache*, the three editors, all renowned neurologists, wrote positively in their preface of new advancements in understanding the origins of headache but added, "The bad news brought by this book is that physicians are slow to accept headache disorders as biological and to see a need for and apply modern treatment."

The Yentl Syndrome: "Doctor, Can You Hear Me?"

No wonder studies have shown that women pain patients are more likely than men to be inadequately treated by health care providers. Although emotional and mental factors can certainly contribute to pain, doctors too readily use that as an excuse to undertreat the patient, often without realizing their biases. Authors of a major review of recent pain literature on women, published in the *Journal of Law, Medicine and Ethics* in 2001, summarized the conflict. Diane E. Hoffman and Anita J. Tarzian (2001) wrote:

> First, women are more likely than men to have their pain attributed to psychogenesis whether or not that is in fact a cause of their pain.
> Secondly, for those women whose pain *is* exacerbated by emotional disorders, the health care provider's bias against psychological contributors to pain may lead them [*sic*] to undertreat the pain. (20, 21)

And the more women verbally express the pain (i.e., with moaning), the more they are likely to elicit such an opinion. These authors added that women "are more likely to be diagnosed with histrionic disorder (excessive emotionality and attention-seeking behavior) compared to male chronic pain patients" (20).

As a result, gender is the number-one variable in the undertreatment of pain (which studies also ascribe to other "vulnerable" classes of patients, according to race, social status, disability level, and age—if they are children or elderly). As a multitude of studies have shown, women are not given painkillers as often as men. Instead, they are more likely to be prescribed sedatives and referred to psychotherapy. In fact, as I have noted, the pain examination for a woman is more like a trial, where she must put forth extra effort to "prove" that she is as sick as a man in a similar situation. Hoffmann and Tarzian referred to this extra work to be adequately treated as the "Yentl syndrome" in women's pain care, named after Isaac Bashevis Singer's story (and the Barbra Streisand movie), where the main character has to masquerade as a man in order to be taken seriously as a scholar.

Unfortunately, the role of cultural critics, mainly of influence on the intellectual set and then trickling down to the masses, has also been negative. They have argued that pain is largely a subconscious emotional response. Part of this all-encompassing explanation is an extreme reaction against the "organic theory of pain" established in the seventeenth century by René Descartes, and embraced in Victorian times. In an effort to bring "reason" into the process of understanding pain, Descartes declared that pain has nothing at all to do with emotion, that it is a mechanical process of tissue damage firing signals to the brain, period. The nerves then produce pain, "just as, pulling on one end of a cord, one simultaneously rings a bell which hangs at the opposite end," he explained in *Treatise of Man* in 1662 (270). In response, present-day historian David Morris (not a doctor), author of *The Culture of Pain* (1991), even suggested that we should return to the era of centuries past when pain was seen as a "mystery" beyond our understanding, not as a puzzle to figure out.

But another cultural critic in particular has been instrumental in doing the opposite of rejecting the "meaning" of illness. In her classic and invaluable 1978 essay on the topic, *Illness as Metaphor*, Susan Sontag exposed the dangers of ascribing too much meaning to disease—and gave lessons that can be well applied to chronic pain and other "invisible illnesses." In general, Sontag explained how a medical problem becomes most vulnerable to metaphor when its origins and treatment are "unknown." Unable to cure the patient? Then blame the patient. The less doctors know about a problem, the more psychological, spiritual, and moral meaning it takes on.

"Theories that diseases are caused by mental states and can be cured by will power are always an index of how much is not understood about the physical terrain of a disease," Sontag wrote. "That ineluctably material reality, disease, can be given a psychological explanation. Death itself can be considered, ultimately, a psychological phenomenon" (55, 56).

As a cancer patient herself, Sontag critically examined at length the "cancer personality," which was widely thought to be at the root of cancer "in one that suppresses violent feelings." A result was added shame in coming out with cancer, as well as the risk of not treating it aggressively enough with Western medicine (which she ended up following). She detailed the highly illustrative similar phenomenon of portraying tuberculosis in both medicine and literature as an affliction of the poetic, overly emotional, and sensitive personality. That was until 1882, when "Robert Koch published his paper announcing the discovery of the tubercle bacillus demonstrating that it was the primary cause of the disease," she wrote (54). Then scientists developed a vaccine that could kill the disease, taking the metaphor along with it into the dustbin of history.

Turning patients' headaches into metaphors has serious medical consequences for the chronic-pain sufferer, beyond just imposing guilt, shame, and confusion. One result has been a systemic failure to devote resources to research and to treating patients adequately. According to a 1995 *Consumer Reports* survey, chronic headache was the ailment most likely to indicate a patient's status as "dissatisfied" with medical care in the past year.[1]

Another consequence is the failure, until very recently, to formulate adequate clinical terminology and classifications. "Over the past decade, there has been some progress in diagnosis and management of migraine, but important challenges remain," stated a 2001 report in the journal *Clinician*, presented by the National Institute of Neurological Disorders and Stroke of the National Institutes of Health. "Several barriers may continue to undermine the prospects for optimal patient care, in many medical circles; for example, migraine is still not accepted as a legitimate medical disorder, because it cannot be evaluated using objective tests, is not life threatening, and is episodic rather than chronic. The reluctance to view migraine as a legitimate disorder may also be influenced by gender bias, as migraine is more prevalent in women than in men" (3).

As a result, besides receiving inadequate treatment, women pain patients typically develop and harbor a great deal of hostility toward doctors. According to recent studies, they commonly have to go through the hassle of seeing a dozen doctors before getting adequate medical treatment.[2] Another result of the metaphor-making is plain dishonesty on the part of the patient, who does not want to be categorized as a complainer or, worse, hysterical. At about this time, for comfort, a friend lent me her copy of Siri Hustvedt's novel *The Blindfold* (1992), which speaks to this irony, of a woman in a headache clinic acting "antihysterical," to the point of denial: "With Dr. Fish, I was always cheerful. I joked about my nerves. I smiled even when the headache raged and I had to hide my trembling hands by clasping them tightly together. Concealing illness from a physician is absurd, but I couldn't bear to be seen for what I was—a person going to pieces" (94).

In a way, I cannot blame anyone for using metaphors with me and doubting the physical basis for my extremely cockamamie headaches. After all, since the day they started, I have had almost all of these thoughts on my own. No one has ever had a judgmental thought about the nature of my headache that I had not had first.

As a journalist writing about social issues, I'm a critic, of sorts, and what critics do best is read subtext. So this "narrative" of the Headache was no exception, and I subjected it, too, to analysis. After all, critics make their living from saying what something *really* represents beyond the surface: A theater reviewer talks about how the playwright was *really* discussing his repressed homosexuality in the story about the man who loved fancy hats, and a music critic talks about how the rock singer was *really* criticizing the record industry for ripping him off, not firing missives at a jilted lover, as it seemed. I agree that this cultural analysis can be valuable in many cases, and that the subconscious and the emotions can certainly contribute to pain, but academics writing on the topic often overstate that influence.

My isolation and lack of education on the topic also exacerbated my self-blame. It was as if I had invented this deviance on my own. I compare this state of isolation to that of a gay person in a small town in the 1950s. Like that person, I hesitated to "come out" to others with what they would see as a sign of mental illness. And I also internalized a lot of the prejudices against us: as neurotic, too driven, too lazy, too dramatic, and so on. Indeed, some of my greatest conflicts with headaches were not with more concrete things like work or money or friendships, but with my own personal prejudices against headache sufferers.

But despite these mental detours, I fundamentally continued to believe the Headache was "real" in nature and biologically based, even if stress was an exacerbating factor. For one thing, it hurt like hell. Besides, I experienced many external triggers—an obvious case of cause and effect. I shared too many patterns with other headache patients, which we all couldn't have just made up by ourselves in one big conspiracy. We never met, shared a secret handshake, and vowed that our headaches would all come on at about the same time in life, in our teens or twenties, peak in the thirties and forties, and then taper off in menopause, as often happens, God willing. I thought it couldn't be hysteria, because hysteria, at least by the definition of boomer feminist and cultural critic Elaine Showalter, in her influential 1997 book *Hystories,* usually means that you have been influenced by external cultural forces, such as media hype making you think you have a certain malady. And I had never even heard of someone with constant headaches before I had them. At that time no article on chronic daily headache even existed.

When medical "proof" of the legitimacy of one's illness is missing, often it is just a matter of waiting for technology to catch up. Ten years later, after this experience with the Princetonian, I now have the aid of more advanced objective research from medical journals to validate my experiences.

Thankfully, because of very recent medical science, doctors no longer have to just take patients' word for it in order to know that chronic head pain is biologically based. Now we have some concrete proof: pictures. They come from advanced types of brain scans, such as high field magnetic resonance imaging (MRI), functional MRI (fMRI), and positron emission tomography (PET). These scans have the ability to penetrate many layers of skull to identify structures, pathways, and functions in the brain involved in the pain process. Much of this work is in tracing blood flow, which is linked to nerve cell function, revealing which parts of the brain are activated when the patient reports feeling pain.

Such scans have proven invaluable in the research lab to reveal the plethora of neurological activity surrounding a typical migraine (which, unlike chronic daily headache, has a beginning, middle, and end). In 1995, Dr. C. Weiller and his colleagues in Germany made a breakthrough, imaging a migraine attack in progress with a PET scan (used in clinical settings to detect cancer). This scan traced the origin of migraine to a dysfunction deep in the central nervous system, in the brain stem, where doctors actually triggered a migraine by stimulating that area. The scan showed that basically, during a migraine, areas of the brain stem are active and remain so even after treatment, which suggests that the brain stem may not be functioning properly. Perhaps, the "migraine brain" fails to adapt to changes, either external (weather, stress) or internal (hormones) in origin. Instead, overreacting to the trigger, the brain "freaks out," sending a sometimes violent cascade of neurological signals through the brain, resulting in pain, visual aura, nausea, neck pain, sinus congestion, a sensitive scalp, vertigo, and/or other related events. With chronic daily headaches, it appears that this process gets stuck in a loop, like an old vinyl record that keeps stopping at the point where it has been scratched.

"Migraine is—I see it as a physiological maladaptation of the brain to change," explained Dr. Nabih Ramadan, whom I recently interviewed at the brand-new campus of Rosalind Franklin University of Medicine and Science in suburban North Chicago, Illinois. A distinguished brain researcher, he has published his own notable work about headache, including the role of magnesium in migraine, the relationship between migraine and stroke, and the value of preventive drugs in migraine treatment. He has also suffered from various forms of migraine, which runs in his family. During his childhood in Lebanon, he watched his mother pressing a whole lemon against her eye socket, as a way to relieve the pressure of a migraine.

He said, "And some of us who have the genetic disposition, the appropriate triggers, particularly [a number of them], will mount up to develop this recurring condition. And we are rather maladaptive in the sense that we don't know how to turn off our brain reaction to a stimulus as well as somebody who is not predisposed to migraine."

Dr. Ramadan explained how research into headache and pain has illustrated other basic concepts behind chronic headaches in recent years. Referring to the groundbreaking insights of Dr. Rami Burstein and his colleagues at Harvard Medical School, doctors call this cycle of the brain being overly sensitized to pain *peripheral and central sensitization*. This can happen during a single migraine episode, revealed externally by the pulsation of blood vessels felt to be painful (peripheral sensitization) and areas over the face and body becoming painful to the touch, when normally they are not (*cutaneous allodynia*). This happens to some degree in up to 80 percent of episodic migraine sufferers. Others have built on this concept to explain the less visible mechanisms behind chronic daily headache, where this process of central sensitization becomes progressive. As the pain goes on, the central nervous system may become more and more sensitized to it, changing its wiring to interpret the pain as a "normal" event. "Frequent stimulation results in stronger brain memory so that the brain will respond more rapidly and effectively when experiencing the same stimulation in the future," wrote Dr. Dawn A. Marcus in the fall 2002 newsletter of the American Council for Headache Education. She compared this process, of the brain becoming more sensitive to pain, to "learning a new skill," such as mastering a new language or playing the piano: "Repeated practice changes the brain, so that messages within the brain are sent more efficiently and seem to become more 'automatic.'"

After learning about these theories and doctors' general work with brain scans, which have mainly centered on migraine, I naturally wondered about the use of these tools to detect (read: provide some real "proof" of) chronic daily headache. Dr. Ramadan pointed out two major studies on chronic daily headache, elucidated by work with fMRIs, that point to progressive changes in the brain in such patients. The first study was published in 2001 in the journal *Headache* by Dr. K. Michael Welch (who, coincidentally, had just moved to the Chicago area to become the president of Rosalind Franklin University). It showed that patients with chronic daily headache have increased amounts of iron—a potential sign of neuronal damage, which could interfere in pain processing. This iron irregularity is present in a certain area of the brain stem, the periaqueductal gray, which is thought to be where headaches are generated or modulated. As quoted in the *New York Times Magazine* on January 12, 2003, about that study, Dr. Silberstein referred to this effect as "brain rust."[3] Another study, published in 2002 in the journal *Headache*, reveals "decreased platelet serotonin" reception, or suppression of brain-based chemical pain control systems, in the brains of chronic daily headache sufferers. This process, over time, can facilitate "central sensitization," again, basically the brain becoming unreasonably oversensitive to stimulation.[4]

Other encouraging news is that imaging-related studies on headache and chronic pain in general keep multiplying, giving more concrete clues about these mysteries (with too many from the past several years to mention here). The January 28, 2004, issue of the *Journal of the American Medical Association* printed a report by Kruit et al. on a study from the Netherlands, conducted with a highly sensitive type of MRI that found increased brain lesions in migraine sufferers, particularly in women and those with visual auras. "The findings of this study will change the common perception that migraine only is a 'trivial problem' with only transient symptoms, into [seeing] that migraine may be a chronic-progressive disorder that may cause permanent changes in the brain," Kruit told WebMD. Specifically, they found more "infarcts," or areas of dead brain cells.

In response to this article, leading headache specialist[5] Richard B. Lipton and Julie Pan wrote in the same issue of the *Journal of the American Medical Association* about the urgency of caring for headaches aggressively when they start. This evidence of brain lesions characterizes headache as a progressive disease, with the potential to be slowed down or possibly nipped in the bud. Indeed, writing the patient off as "just neurotic" can have serious consequences in delaying important medical treatment.

But such studies have limits. Unfortunately, researchers are just at the beginning stages of tracing the origins of chronic pain with brain scans. Yes, they have homed in on the areas of the brain that generate it, but they still do not know what gets the process going in the first place.

Also, more important, these results have had little practical application to chronic daily headache treatment so far. Even if one finds evidence of "central sensitization" in one's head, it may not be possible to do much about it. This is especially the case among those with constant pain, in whom the cycle is harder to break. Also, this concept of central sensitization and its related serotonin deficiencies in the brain is still a "theory du jour." And in truth, every current test for pain has to be interpreted. Even if doctors find physical irregularities, such as brain lesions or "brain rust," they can't prove that this is the source of headaches, just as X-rays of most people's spines reveal some irregular bulges, which may or may not contribute to back pain.

"Is there any evidence that people who have abnormalities on their functional MRI or PET are more or less likely to be disabled than the ones who don't? We don't know the answers to that," said Dr. Ramadan, who is also the vice president for Clinical and External Affairs at the university.

After I interviewed Dr. Ramadan, I walked around a bit trying to process all these data. I was in that type of haze that you feel after talking to someone who is obviously a hundred times more intelligent than you are.

First, as I headed down the gleaming new hallways of the university, I mused about the coincidence that this is where my uncle had gone to medical school (when it was based in Chicago and called the Chicago Medical School). This was truly a democratic and enlightened place, from the start, standing out even in the early 1950s for its lack of religious quotas.

I then wandered down to the Scholl College of Podiatric Medicine, which has long been part of the school. And then I spotted an actual footwear museum there! Open was an interesting permanent exhibit, "Feet First: The Scholl Story," about Dr. William M. Scholl, who had his start in Chicago and had founded the school in 1912. On the way to the exhibit, I walked through the museum by rows of antique shoes, such as a curled Turkish boot and a flat Eskimo snowshoe. And then I wished that I were studying the foot instead. You have the heels, the toes, the soles, and that's about all you need to know. Very straightforward. By the look of the diagrams on the wall, feet looked so much simpler than the brain, the seat of consciousness, where so much research remains to be done.

But insight that exposes false metaphors about women and chronic pain is not something we can gain just in a laboratory. Another method of investigation, which I am more personally equipped to do, is to question the concept of headache as metaphor as a journalist, as Susan Sontag did in her book. This investigation involves looking at a little history and asking some extremely basic questions.

8

"Hysteria" and the Founding Fathers

○ ○ ○ ○ ○ ○ ○ ○ ○

JUST WHY, DESPITE VAST SCIENTIFIC EVIDENCE to the contrary, do so many doctors (and the general public) still view chronic headaches as "all in one's head"?

As in many cases, a good place to start for answers here is at the top.

Widespread views of chronic head pain in women as mainly psychosomatic in nature, and hence "hysterical," can be traced to no less than the founding fathers of modern medicine and psychology. They include, most notably, Sigmund Freud and others influenced by him in many fields, including psychiatry, pain management, and neurology. Indeed, although these leading figures of the past hundred years have also made many notable contributions to their areas of studies, they have also all played key roles in creating and reinforcing myths about pain.

It isn't that these men did not consider migraine "real," or at least partly based in genetics. The majority of these thinkers that I am about to describe—including Freud, Harold G. Wolff, and Oliver Sacks—all have suffered from migraines themselves. But they seemed to be more judgmental in the case of women patients. Their most fundamental theories on the female sex deeply influenced how they have perceived—and belittled—the female chronic pain patient. Although they were correct to point out that emotion and stress can certainly contribute to pain, they (and even more stringently, their disciples) erroneously assumed that women's pain is largely psychological in nature, and that when there is a psychological component, medical treatment is not necessary.

Women of our time may be surprised to learn just how commonly the dismissive label of *hysteria* was used as a medical diagnosis and, as feminist historians have pointed out, as a justification to keep women in a second-class position in society. But if one has any doubt about how powerful and widespread the concept of hysteria was in Victorian times, the best way to get the real story is to visit a medical library. We need to examine the old textbooks in order to write the new ones.

That is just what I did for this chapter. I spent much time in the basement of the Galter Health Sciences Library of the Feinberg School of Medicine at Northwestern University in downtown Chicago, from where I often returned home with my hands caked in black dust. This floor houses the "retrospective collection" of textbooks, dating from before 1985. It includes several volumes published before the turn of the twentieth century, which evidently had not been opened in years. Sample books in the neurology and pain section are *Sexual Neurasthenia* (1887), *La Fatigue Intellectuelle* (1898), and *Insanity and Women* (1871). Apart from the potential of these titles to be lent to avant-garde films, this collection reflects the prevailing beliefs of their time that women's chronic pains were no more than a major component of hysteria (or neurasthenia, the higher-class version).

The word *hysteria* is taken from the Greek root *hyster*, which means "womb." In ancient times, doctors believed that the cause of *hysteria* was the womb's wandering loose through the body. Then, in the Victorian era, doctors regarded hysteria as the result of an imbalance between the woman's sexual organs (including the ovaries and uterus) and her brain, each of which could drain the other. Besides headaches, the body could react with other types of pain, fainting, hallucinations, emotional disturbance, breathing problems, fatigue, and more. Problems that we today regard as associated with hormonal fluctuations, such as PMS irritability and postpartum depression, were also prominent in the diagnosis of hysteria.

But headaches stand out as especially stigmatized among other "hysterical" women's complaints. One reason is that they are literally in the head, the center of imagination. Another is that hormones, long considered a source of hysteria, are often involved in causing headache pain or making it worse.[1] In a typical medical commentary of the Victorian era, a prominent British doctor, H. G. Wright, made this connection between hysteria and women's headaches: "The ordinary Nervous Headache most frequently occurs in persons . . . whose spirits are variable, easily elevated, and easily depressed; whose tempers are fickle, and their sensibility very great. The Nervous Headache is of frequent occurrence in girls and women of hysterical tendencies."[2]

Silas Weir Mitchell (1829–1914)

Indeed, the history of pain treatment in women is intertwined with some of the most deeply entrenched sexism of the Victorian era. To illustrate this, one has to look no further than Silas Weir Mitchell, known as the father of modern neurology. He is the author of a large row of once-best-selling books in the Galter Library basement. Many in the pain field justifiably paid homage to him for his valuable and pioneering work with nerve injuries suffered during the U.S. Civil War. However, in the 1970s, feminist medical historians began to offer much harsher words about him, portraying him as Public Enemy Number One. They lambasted him as the single most prominent "expert" of that era to justify women's intellectually restricted roles, including his invention of the notorious "rest cure." In their critiques, these feminists went back to analyze Victorian texts on hysteria, in which the woman (usually the patient) assumed the "child" role and the man (the doctor) that of the parent. In fact, in the influential 1978 critique *For Her Own Good: 150 Years of Experts' Advice to Women,* Barbara Ehrenreich and Deirdre English credited Weir Mitchell personally with "the development of the twentieth century doctor-patient relationship" of female subservience and male domination (132).

One of Weir Mitchell's most famous books, *Doctor and Patient* (1887), discusses women's proper gender roles, even beyond the examination room. He was reflecting a desire for clarity and order in this era of confusing social turmoil, when men and women were testing out new roles in the industrialized era. "Experts" like him were advising that the home was woman's "natural" sphere, and that the man belonged out in commerce and industry, in the outside world.

Doctors were at the center of such power struggles, trying to assert their new authority and ensure control of their growing medical institutions. Part of that task, for example, involved pushing out female midwives from medicine. At the same time, select groups of "New Women" were making waves in taking advantage of new opportunities to attend the emerging women's colleges, such as Smith, Wellesley, and Mount Holyoke, in addition to others that had originally been established for men. Ehrenreich and English argued that to make sense of all this upheaval and assert control, male doctors assumed the role of "expert" and consigned women to the role of the subservient patient, a relationship the wider culture was ready to embrace.

After reading *Doctor and Patient*, a thin volume of essays brittle with age, I see their point. Weir Mitchell praised the "good patient" as one who is seen and not heard: "Wise women choose their doctors and trust them. The wisest ask the fewest questions. The terrible patients are nervous women with long memories, who question much where answers are difficult, and who to-gether one's answers from time to time and torment themselves with the ap-parent inconsistencies they detect" (48).

He continued, justifying the long-standing complaint of paternalism from the female pain patient, of their doctors' not being direct with them, to the point where many would perceive them as downright deceitful. He expressed his pride in secretly giving a woman a placebo instead of an opiate for pain, when he feared she was addicted. "Another form of trouble arises with the woman whose standards are of unearthly altitude," he added. "This is the woman who thinks herself deceived if she does not know what you are giving her, or who, if without telling her you substitute an innocent drug for a hurt-ful one which she may have learned to take too largely, thinks that you are untruthful in the use of such a method. And you would indeed be wrong if you were of opinion to tell her the whole truth, and invite her to break the habit by her own act" (48, 49).

For whatever women's ailments he treated, his concept of a "rest cure" was central to treatment. In this book and another one, the 1877 *Fat and Blood: An Essay on the Treatment of Certain Forms of Neurasthenia and Hysteria*, Weir Mitchell promoted the rest cure as combating the dangerous drain of the female intellect. In fact, at that time, he imposed this "cure" on some of the most prominent female intellectuals of the era, including activist Jane Addams, poet Winifred Howells (daughter of novelist William Dean How-ells), and writer Edith Wharton, all of whom made pilgrimages to his Philadelphia offices. One patient, Charlotte Perkins Gilman, a very well-known writer and activist for women's rights, modeled her classic and still much-studied 1892 story "The Yellow Wallpaper" on her own true-life experi-ences with him. (She even mentioned Weir Mitchell by name in the text of the story and wrote in her memoirs that she had sent him a copy of the story. She received no reply.[3])

Feminist writers like Gilman perceived the rest cure as a type of ritual, or social theater, in which women were controlled through isolation—at this time when the New Woman seemed to threaten the status quo. Weir Mitchell's solution to pain was for women to act as traditionally "female" and passive as possible, and to be confined to bed and restricted in all mental and physical activity. He stressed that this treatment involved a firm and authori-tative doctor who would seclude the patient from others, even removing her from her home, safely away from the enfeebling influence of a sister or mother, whom he described as having "the grip of an octopus."[4]

Sigmund Freud (1856–1939)

No discussion of blaming the mother would be complete without mention of another influential neurologist, Sigmund Freud.

Instead of the "rest cure," Freud prescribed a different remedy for what he saw as pain rooted in the mind: the talking cure. This shift in the late 1800s to an emphasis on the psyche as the cause of chronic pain was gradual. Ironically, this change can be attributed to movements to treat pain more "scientifically." It was the era of early microscopes, which could detect germs, and doctors were starting to insist on more concrete visual proof for pain, just as with everything else. The increasingly accepted theory became that if you cannot see the source of the pain—if not with the naked eye, then at least with the ultimate technology of a microscope—it must not exist physically. A pain with concrete causes, such as a gunshot wound or a tumor, was biologically "real"; other types were pushed aside into the psychosomatic category. So the types of pain ordained invisible, and thus "inorganic," were left to the alienists (asylum keepers) and psychiatrists. That was very bad news for those with many forms of chronic pain, such as chronic headaches, whose roots lie deep in the not-so-visible neurology of the central nervous system (spinal cord and brain).[5] This mode of thinking became so well accepted that this standard for pain, of a visible nerve "lesion" or "organic disease," was not revised in the official diagnostic criteria of pain until 1973.

In fact, the concept of hysteria in particular, with pain as a major component, became prominent in the formulation of the most basic psychoanalytic theories of the day. Freud's explanations of hysteria actually provided the framework for his very influential theories of the subconscious mind—how our motives, even if they are not consciously known to us, can indeed influence our behavior and cause us pain. He emphasized early childhood experiences, including sexual abuse, as the source of pain in his most famous and most studied patients. He presented some of his resulting basic psychoanalytic theories in the very influential 1895 book *Studies in Hysteria*, coauthored with his colleague Josef Breuer.

The first patient described in a case study, Anna O., had "left-sided occipital [face] pain," among many other disturbances. Freud analyzed these disturbances as being caused partly by a "monotonous family existence" that restricted her from expressing herself intellectually (which may explain why many feminists, in fact, embraced much of Freud, for acknowledging the harm to women of repression, both sexual and intellectual). Freud and Breuer explained the leg pains of Emmy von N. as subconscious resentment of a long series of care-giving sessions to a sick brother.

In an influential 1901 essay "Fragment of an Analysis of a Case of Hysteria," Freud analyzed Dora, who suffered from migraines, among other problems. He attributed her continuing physical problems to sexual confusion in her family. In detail, Freud described how Herr K., a friend of her father, had made repeated passes at her, confusing her all the more, because Herr K's wife, Frau K., was Dora's father's mistress. In short, this whole drama, forming the base of modern psychiatry and chronic pain treatment, reads like a Viennese *Young and the Restless*. Although it may seem obscure, this history still profoundly shapes the experience of the patient seeking relief. (See the sidebar.)

A major problem is in the *interpretation* of these theories, more than in Freud's original ones. In calling pain psychosomatic, Freud was still acknowledging it as "real," even when he saw the mind as being its generator. He also discussed pain as originating in a real "biological" problem (but then being perpetuated by the psyche). In this case, his phrase to describe that "motivation" for the patient was "secondary gain." In any case, whenever he recognized a mental component to the pain, he did not "blame the victim" or see it as a moral failure. But even today, his followers have taken his theories to the extreme, seeing *all* chronic pain as purely psychological in nature, and then dismissing it as not "legitimate." They also fail to recognize that Freud was constantly reevaluating and revising his ideas, seeing them as works in progress.

Harold G. Wolff (1898–1962)

Indeed, Freud's theories provided the framework for many experts who later emerged in the pain field. In the area of headache, researchers built on his ideas of underlying psychological motivations as root causes of chronic pain, including in crafting specific ideas about the "migraine personality." This was a major thrust of chronic headache research of the past century. These experts reasoned that migraines were more likely to emerge as society became more sophisticated and people evolved so that they did not directly express

The Legacy of Freud: Gentle Tips to the Headache Patient

A June 22, 2002, cover story in the *New York Times* "Women's Health" section on women and pain contains many alarming points about women's frustration with doctors. But probably the most revealing interview was with a pain specialist at Northwestern University, who went to the extremes of *coaching* her female patients before referring them to other doctors. This way, they would act less "emotionally" with doctors and would therefore have their pain treated more seriously. And so, considering my own experiences, and those of other patients cited in such research, I give the following simple advice to the woman about to start her trial of the medical system:

- Don't be shy.
- Don't be outgoing.
- Don't be understated about the pain, or else they won't believe you.
- Don't be expressive about it, or else they won't believe you. (That is known as a *pain behavior.*)
- Don't joke about anything, just as you would not joke nowadays about carrying a bomb while going through airport security.
- For God's sake, if you're a woman, wear a skirt. Listen to your mom and put on some lipstick. Speak in comforting soft tones. Wear a wedding ring, even if you're not married. (In other words, give them more Laura Bush—and less Hillary Clinton.)
- If you're gay or bi or transgendered or butch or just not having sexual intercourse on a regular basis, *hide it at all costs* (if you don't want just to be dismissed as a wacko and then spend the next twenty years of your life in shock therapy and zoned out on lithium, à la Janet Frame in *An Angel at My Table*).
- And no matter how weak you feel, if you don't have a husband to go with you to the appointment, go alone. You are allowed to be dependent on him, but not on anyone else, especially your mother, who probably caused all your problems to begin with as a result of her emotional detachment, overbearingness, or neglect in breast-feeding or toilet-training you.

primitive emotions. Instead of moaning or growling, they could just get a headache to express their distress. This was a theory popularized in the 1930s and 1940s by Dr. Harold G. Wolff of the Cornell Medical School, known and respected as the father of headache research. In a very influential argument, he contended that the migraines were an expression of repressed anger and hostility. Without the help of today's modern brain scans, he was unable to find the neurological source of the well-known fluctuations of blood flow experienced during migraine attacks. So, like others in the past (and in our own era) who trust their best diagnostic tools as definitive, he suggested a mainly mental source of the problem. Nine-tenths of his own migraine patients, he said, were perfectionistic, obsessive, driven go-getters.

Some of this description was indeed complimentary, but then he shifted gears to be more condemning when applying it to women. Suddenly, sexual dysfunction became a major issue in his analysis of women patients, although he did not significantly report that problem in the male migraine sufferer. University of Michigan sociologist Joanna Kempner summed up his view in a recent essay in the book *Migraine in Women* (2003): "He described 80 percent of his female sample as sexually dissatisfied, particularly because of dissatisfaction with sexual experiences. 'Orgasm was seldom attained and the sex act was accepted, as at least a reasonable marital duty.' Furthermore, the migrainous woman was sometimes 'reluctant to accept . . . the consequences of maternity.'"

Later scientific studies contradicted Wolff's influential conclusion about the prevalent "migraine personality." In the 1960s, Dr. James Lance of the University of New South Wales in Australia notably found in research that 25 percent of migraineurs were obsessive, just like 25 percent of the population. "The U.S. National Health Survey uncovered no link between chronic headache sufferers and either intelligence or career success," mused journalist Edwin Kiester, Jr., in *Smithsonian Magazine* in 1987. "Researchers reached the obvious conclusion. The movers and shakers didn't have more migraines. They were just better able to afford treatments."

Today, although much progress has yet to be made, doctors of influence in the field of psychiatry and pain management tend to exercise more caution than their predecessors. They are more likely to subscribe to the more commonsense theory that mental disturbances can help trigger headaches—or coexist with them as a result of the same root chemical imbalance—but do not cause them. An example occurs in the 2000 volume *Personality Characteristics of People with Pain*, published by the American Psychological Association. In that book, a longtime supporter of Freud and expert on the topic of "hysteria," the very influential Dr. Harold Merskey, whose own teacher had been taught by Freud himself, admitted that previous psychoanalytic theory had been overstated: "Resentment and aggressive behavior are thought to be common among patients with chronic pain, and these findings bear them

Shifting Metaphors

As patients of all backgrounds should be aware, the culture at large ascribes different meanings to the same type of physical pain at different times. Much of this shifting analysis relates to concepts of class, which determines one's "vulnerability" to certain maladies. In the Victorian era, male "experts" had actually cultivated a reverse prejudice about and even glorification of migraine sufferers, referring to them as suffering from the high-class "neurasthenia."

"The sufferers possess what is called the nervous temperament; their brains are very excitable, their sense acute, and their imaginations free," wrote Cambridge doctor P. W. Latham in the late 1800s about headache patients. "Attacks are induced by prolonged mental work, protracted mental excitement, or any intense strain on the feelings."[6] Other writers today wonder if migraineurs were praised as imaginative high achievers because so many headache doctors and researchers tended to suffer from the problem themselves.

This elevation of sorts contrasted to the widely negative views of epileptics, also suffering from what the distinguished British physician Edward Liveing called "nerve storms" in the head. (He was more than a hundred years ahead of his time, having made a connection of shared neurochemistry between epileptics and chronic headache sufferers that is widely accepted today.) Doctors judged epileptics to be of a lower stock, with their unsettling and rather inelegant "fits" and losses of consciousness.

out. Part of the resentment can be attributed to experiences of unsatisfactory treatment. . . . It is not surprising that people with chronic pain become irritable and perhaps resentful and difficult. A new, deeper explanation may not be necessary" (32).

And the List Continues . . .

However, intensifying at the height of Freud's popularity in the 1950s and continuing today, one particular type of headache sufferer has been singled out more negatively, as suffering from mental problems and secret motives. That is the person who suffers what is termed today *chronic daily headache.*

I did not realize the full extent of this distinction until I read Oliver Sacks's classic text *Migraine,* first published in 1970. Of all the books I knew I would read for research in the past year, I had been looking forward to this one the most for elucidation and validation. I recognized Sacks as the beloved, intro-spective, and conscientious hero of the movie *Awakenings*, played by a cute and cuddly and bearded Robin Williams. I took the book off my shelf and curled up with it and a nice cup of tea on the sofa, under a comforter. If I had had a kitty, he or she would have been sitting in my lap, purring.

All was well until Chapter 9, "Situational Migraine." It starts with a lofty quote by G. Groddeck about the challenge of looking into our inner psyches for answers to our problems: "The *causa interna* . . . we have forgotten. Why? Because it is not pleasant to look within ourselves." Then Sacks launches into a discussion of the type of headache patient not suffering periodic migraines, but "a large group—who suffer from repeated and unremitting attacks for no reason which is immediately apparent."

He then reasons that if a person's head pain is severe enough to interfere with her or his life, then it is logical that she or he must have an internal mo-tive for perpetuating it. Sacks does concede that episodic migraine sufferers have biological problems, as proven by the effectiveness of the popular drug of that time, Sansert. But he offers no such reasoning for more chronic cases for which Sansert would not work. In those cases, he speaks in the language of a trial: "These possibilities will be considered and given a fair *hearing* [ital-ics mine] by the physician, but by degrees it will be borne in upon him that the vast majority of patients with incessant unremitting migraines are not the victims of such physiological stimuli or sensitivities, but are caught in a ma-lignant emotional 'bind' of one sort or another, and *this*, he will come to sus-pect, is the driving force behind their migraines" (165). Specifically, Sacks reasons that patients with headaches that are severe enough to interfere with their lives are looking for a way out of their present routines: They "may be *at-tached* to their symptoms, in *need* of them; the extent to which such patients may *prefer* the migraine way of life, with all its torments, to any alternative which is felt to be open to them" (236).

Sacks goes on to reject Wolff's migraine personality theory. Instead, he reasons, the motives of each person in perpetuating her or his headaches vary widely. Migraines, he argues, are not just the province of the hard-driv-ing Type A personality alone. He then offers about a dozen case studies, all involving some kind of hidden agenda on the part of the patient. Most dis-turbingly, especially in the case of women, the patients' sex lives are of prime interest in his analysis. This angle reveals the enduring influence of Freud, whose popularity reached its height in the middle of the twentieth century.

To wit: Case 62, a fifty-five-year-old woman who is indicted for helping to take care of her parents and for having more than one physical ailment.

Unmarried, and the only daughter of parents who had always been compelled to work at two jobs, for a total of 14 hours daily, to support the household. She had no friends, no social life, and had never had any sexual experience. She felt it her "duty" to support her parents and to be with them whenever she was not working.

At one time, indeed, she had made pathetic efforts to establish an independent existence, but these had been foiled first by parental intervention, and subsequently by her own discomfort and guilt if she went out alone. In the past 10 years, she had lost all choice in the matter, for she had suffered severely from migraine, ulcerative colitis, and psoriasis, not concurrently, but in a never-ending cycle.

Comment: This pitiful case-history illustrates the sacrifice of a life, and the trapping of this patient at three concentric levels: an intolerable domestic reality, an intolerable neurotic conflict, and an intolerable circle of psychosomatic symptoms. (171)

Of course, Sacks originally wrote this case history awhile back, more than thirty years ago, I thought, when people did not know any better. He was just expressing the ideas of his times. So, I expected that Sacks would recant in his updated 1992 edition of *Migraine.* He does start out, in a revised chapter, discussing the scientific advances of the past twenty years, furthered by brain scans, which helped scientists trace the neurological origins of migraine. As a result, he concedes that migraines are "a real and morally neutral event" (267). But in the end, he stays true to his original theory about singling out those with more severe headaches as seeking an "illness lifestyle": "For migraine, when frequent, is not just a disease, but a whole way of being, which forces the organism into special adaptations and identities" (268).

Unfortunately, placing blame on sufferers of chronic daily headache is not a relic of the past. Recently, as I was paging through a September 2003 journal, *Headache and Pain,* looking for another article, I saw a case study that stopped me in my tracks: "Woman with Nearly Continuous Headaches for Whom 'Nothing Has Worked.'" A red flag was that the patient was being quoted, as I remembered from my case in that letter about me from the Princetonian neurologist. That quoting of the patient is usually given as "proof" of her mental imbalance. And the word *woman* also tends to give away that the psyche will be emphasized over neurology.

The doctor writing the article, Russell C. Packard, is a scholar in the psychiatric aspects of headache management. He described his patient's "host of prescription medications," all of which were typical for chronic daily headache. Later he discussed the results of a psychiatric evaluation, in which the patient "blurted out" that she experienced some "good" headaches that sometimes offered her "only time out" to relax and not work. Needless to say, the doctor ended the case study with a psychosomatic slant, blaming the patient's alleged headache on her subconscious avoidance of stress. And like the "experts" of the past, he cited the patient's "unresponsiveness" to drugs as evidence of a psychological condition. "We have a wonderful menu of medications available to combat headaches," reasoned Packard, before delivering his conclusion: "One thing I have learned: when patients describe their headache as 'good,' there is usually something in their life that is worse" (113).

I do not disagree that personal motives can play a part in pain as triggers, and they should be examined—openly with the patient. Freud made many valuable contributions, introducing the concept of the subconscious to a mass audience. Certainly, stress can be a major exacerbating influence for many people, and reducing it can often relieve pain. But in reality, Packard indicted, if not convicted, his patient on thin and circumstantial evidence.

Instead, here is my take. Recent studies have revealed the inadequacy of the current drugs available to prevent chronic headaches. If they don't work, it's more often the fault of the drug than the patient. And with enough psychoanalysis, *every* illness can be portrayed as helping the patient "get out of something" he or she doesn't like to do. I could even go through the obituaries and pick out for any of those deceased "real" motivations for dying, what they are craftily avoiding, from doing their taxes to shoveling the driveway. Besides, this diagnosis of stress avoidance can be applied to the majority of today's working mothers, who are juggling many areas of life and for whom sickness indeed would provide a rare excuse to stop. Does that mean that in every case of a woman with a stressful life, stress gets blamed completely and the woman's pain doesn't qualify to be treated medically?

Although terminology may differ, this specter of hysteria is still alive in other forms, creating more suspicion of chronic headache sufferers. The patient with multiple forms of pain is the most suspect; the "logic" is that after a certain level of symptoms, the patient is just a complainer. The terminology for this form of hysteria has changed through the years. From about the 1950s to the 1980s, the term *Briquet's syndrome* was used to describe a patient with many types of pain. Now this kind of case is officially listed as *somatization disorder* in the fourth edition of the *Diagnostic and Statistical*

Manual of Mental Disorders (DSM IV). To qualify, the patient must fit at least twenty-five of a list of medical symptoms named. In other words, we are now most likely to consider pain hysterical when many types of complaints accompany it. In addition, the patient's being "dramatic" about the pain is another major way to diagnose somatization disorder. (By this standard, I could be diagnosed with this syndrome just by the act of writing a book on my pain.)

With this concept of somatization, patients with chronic daily headache are at greater risk of misdiagnosis than other types of headache patients, once again. The reality is that these patients are more likely to have other physical problems—such as fibromyalgia (a disorder characterized by pain throughout the body), fatigue, sleep disorders, depression, and anxiety—which may be the products of the same types of chemical imbalances. Doctors even have an increasingly used term to describe this phenomenon: *comorbidities*, or illnesses that are likely to coexist with others. Unfortunately, multiple "complaints," as in Sacks's "pitiful" case study above, often stand as "evidence" that the complaints are all fake.

But there is hope. Despite lingering superstition from the past, chronic daily headache is now at that stage of being understood where other neurological disorders, once perceived as having "no physical source," were decades ago. These include multiple sclerosis, autism, and Tourette's syndrome, which also carried great stigmas as revealing deviant personality traits and early childhood trauma. A chilling documentary on PBS, "Refrigerator Mothers," by Hanley, Simpson, and Quinn, reveals that influential Freudians in the 1960s blamed autism on mothers, for being too cold and emotionally withholding. The theory was that a mother's lack of warmth created the child's inability to connect with others. In earlier times, suspicion of psychiatric disorders was used to explain other problems with unknown origins, such as tuberculosis, asthma, and ulcers. A neurologist I just met told me about a patient of hers who had received a psychiatric discharge from the U.S. Navy in the 1950s for "turning away from life" with his dystonia. Now dystonia is solidly classified as a neurological movement disorder.

These examples illustrate that doctors in each era, including our own, tend to consider their diagnostic tools definitive, and they are likely to include drug responsiveness as an important measure of validation. They assume pain is invisible and thus purely subjective, at least until a more sensitive type of brain scan is invented to refute that assumption. They insist that the current drugs are effective, at least until a new drug manufacturer—or their sales reps—come along to campaign against that opinion. What is a "subjective" illness with "no physical source" in one generation becomes a visible one the next. In the meantime, if any doubt arises, in any possible situation, doctors can always easily get off the hook by finding or inventing a "hidden motive" on the part of the patient.

For too long, the field of neurology has questioned patients' motivations— instead of those of the doctor. This approach has had dire consequences. After all, doctors are the ones who fundamentally validate pain as "real" in our society. This is what they expect of themselves, and what we expect of them, as all-knowing heroes always able to control the body. In our society, a pain is not considered real until doctors say it is; the word of the patient is immaterial. In her book *The Rejected Body* (1996), Susan Wendell gives the example of a small percentage of advanced multiple sclerosis patients through the years who had been told the pain in their bones and/or skin was "impossible." Later, they were told that this was indeed "real" when more recent medical studies confirmed it (125).

On a one-to-one level, we also need to set a new standard for doctors' directness with pain patients, discouraging doctors from secretly turning a neurology appointment into a mental-health evaluation. We also have to give them the permission to actually tell a patient, "I don't know," and admit to gaps in their knowledge. If not, the impulse is to turn around and blame the patients, telling them that it is "all in their heads."

We have to join some of the more enlightened researchers on gender and pain, who go a step beyond in sophistication, to recognize the effects of *both* biology and one's environment in shaping the pain experience. Although pain can be genetically based, it would be simplistic of me to swing to the opposite direction from the Freudians and say it *never* has a psychological component. Indeed, as researchers are now saying, stress from one's environment can exacerbate pain and, in some cases, even influence the wiring in one's brain.

Taking a more balanced view, many in the pain field are now adopting the noncondemning "biopsychosocial" model of explaining pain. This looks at how *all* these factors—biological, social, psychological—contribute to the pain experience, with all taken seriously as creating "real" pain. As researcher Roger Fillingim explains in his 2000 book *Sex, Gender and Pain*, he and his colleagues are finding it harder to make distinctions between these parts of the self: the biological, the social, and the psychological. An example is depression and anxiety, which can be seen as chemical in nature, just like physical pain, which can fluctuate according to external pressures. And even when psychological problems are seen as contributing to the physical pain, does that indicate a moral failure? We cannot assume that the mind can always "control" the body. Even if an aggravating source of stress has been discovered, it doesn't mean that chronic pain is automatically reversible, that the patient can just be cured through "mind over matter." No matter what the "cause," the chronic pain still has a biological presence, and real medical treatment is in order.

But one difficulty in putting this model into practice is that it is complex. It does not reduce the pain patient to one easily identifiable mental patient stereotype. In other words, the "biopsychosocial" model takes time for a doctor to implement, to actually communicate with and get to know the patient, without judgment. The old tactic, simply reducing the patient to a "hysteric" or "migraine personality," is so much easier.

Although this time-consuming multidimensional approach is often not practical for many pain doctors, an increasing number of their patients are recognizing it as a necessity. At this time, in early 1995, I noticed large numbers of patients taking action, to seek more holistic forms of treatment. Fed up with fighting the condemning and tired ghosts of the founding fathers, I became all too eager to ascend from the depths of legend and myth to join them. There had to be another way.

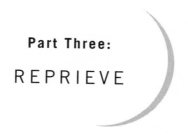

Part Three:

REPRIEVE

9

Recreational Medicine

○ ○ ○ ○ ○ ○ ○ ○ ○

IT WAS MOVING DAY, IN SPRING 1995, and a friend was helping me by sweeping up the now-empty apartment. With an amused grin on her face, she approached me with the dustpan, wanting me to take a look. There among the dust balls were dozens of pills—of every shape and size, from biscuitlike three-layer pastel white, blue, and yellow Norgesic Fortes to those little orange Nardil pellets. Over the past two years, just the occasional pills dropped behind the couch had become plentiful enough to form colonies.

She had argued with me in the past that I should lay off the drugs, and now she had a visual aid for her argument, how extreme it all had become. I explained that I hadn't known of any alternative.

Yet, as I packed up, I did feel definite change in the air, about the move and beyond. I was now about to live on my own for the first time, seeking more peace and quiet in a much less densely packed neighborhood. With our rent going up because of the growing local economic boom, my two roommates had spurred the move, deciding not to renew our lease.

I agreed that this was a good idea. After all, I was gaining some new priorities. I newly craved stillness and space to focus on a more "natural" and conscious form of healing, away from drugs. And I was not alone. At about that time, in the mid-1990s, my options suddenly seemed to expand with the growing phenomenon of alternative medicine, a new type of nonopiate for the masses. I joined millions of other Americans, most of them women, heading hopefully down this path. Illustrating the inadequacy of Western medicine to treat chronic pain, a whopping 89 percent of sufferers turn to alternative treatments. Such usage is most common for those like me with ever-present pain and exacerbated times of flare-up.[1] The most common use of alternative medicine, in fact, is to treat chronic conditions like headaches, depression, back problems, and anxiety.

With the same intensity that Freud's theories had permeated popular culture in the 1950s, alternative medicine was suddenly in the air. From all directions, I felt beckoned to try it, with best-sellers on the topic topping the charts, articles being spawned in virtually every women's magazine, and Bill Moyers's extended blockbuster documentary series on the mind-body connection, *Healing and the Mind,* playing on PBS.

But my greatest attraction to alternative medicine was not the hype. It was that it was indeed an *alternative* to regular medicine. It appealed precisely because it was *not* Western medicine, which I had grown to revile and fear. In contrast, as far as I knew, these "new" (but actually very old) treatments did not involve invasive procedures, covert psychiatric exams, stultifying side effects, endurance tests to stay on unpleasant drugs, hours spent on the phone on hold begging to talk to a doctor, and the need for very large pastel clothing.

Also, in its accessibility, alternative medicine had another appeal: It was punk rock. Just as punk rock had come on the scene in the late 1970s to counter the dinosaur and bloated music establishment, alternative medicine was emerging in pop culture to fill gaps in Western medicine. Where popular music had grown bloated and out of touch and formulaic, punk rock was infused with rebellious and exciting energy. Whereas popular music increasingly became a profession practiced by only rich and well-connected professional performers, punk rock was supposed to be truly democratic, for everyone, thriving with a DIY aesthetic.

At the start of 1994, I had taken some beginning steps in that antiestablishment direction. I saw a few chiropractors and acupuncturists. But despite some initial short relief, their work seemed to lose effectiveness after a few visits.

Yet, by the next year, other forces cultivated my optimism about such treatments. I went to a massage therapist, whose treatment actually was the opposite of my experiences with neurologists: It was *enjoyable*. This was the beginning of what I called a foray into "recreational medicine."

Now, I could really understand why massage was becoming so popular, as one of the most commonly practiced types of alternative medicine. (In fact, by 2002, it accounted for almost a third of the business of alternative medicine, involving about 18 percent of the population, spending a total of about $4–$6 billion in 2002.) And like anyone else, I would want to get massages even I weren't in pain, at a spa in my leisure time, then wearing a very thick robe. And as a bonus, like other alternative healers, the masseuse even had free herbal tea in the waiting room!

From the start, noting the extreme amount of tension I carried in my neck, back, and shoulders, the massage therapist, a former nurse, was optimistic, saying that if I came twice a week, the pain would be relieved in a few months. The cost was high, about sixty dollars per session, adding up through the month to my share of rent at that time—but if that got rid of the headaches, of course, it would be well worth it. Actually, if it got rid of the Headache, I'd promise her my first-born child.

Ironically, this massage therapist working out of her basement in a modest neighborhood was much more costly for me than the prominent neurologists I had seen on the Gold Coast. And this type of cost differential is not unusual. One reason is the typically large amount of time the massage therapist must invest, with hour-long sessions as the norm. Another is the lack of reimbursement from insurance. Like most other Americans using alternative medicine, I covered the expenses out of pocket.[2] In contrast, my private insurance—actually a throwback to another era, not a restrictive HMO—would cover about anything with an M.D.'s imprimatur. In that case, someone could rotate my kidneys or pound a nail into my forehead and call it a lobotomy—and it would all be covered (or at least the portion of it that was considered "reasonable and customary").

Indeed, about the only threat that alternative medicine posed to me concerned my financial well-being. I wasn't yet sure if I believed in the mind-body connection, but I was certainly convinced of the mind-wallet connection. In this true marketplace of ideas in the world of alternative medicine, some ideas cost more than others.

As with my brief forays into acupuncture and chiropractic manipulations, the pain was relieved temporarily, usually for a few hours immediately following the visit. The massage therapist told me to have patience, that it would take time, that it was a matter of retraining the body slowly. Even with this temporary relief, I was encouraged to see some undeniable connection between muscle tension and my head pain. I saw the two were clearly related. When the masseuse dug her thumb and first finger in deep to pinch on and release a tight, rubbery muscle in the left side of my throat, the pain behind my left eye intensified. And when she did the same thing on the right side of the neck, I temporarily had a similar pain behind my right eye. Then, after continued pressure applied to that "trigger point," it hurt less in both places. (A trigger point is a site of contraction or a knot that "refers" or channels pain to other areas in the body.) This baffling and intangible pain problem—which Western doctors have viewed as being rooted in neurology, neurotransmitters, neuropeptides, and the overall "neuromatrix" (pain pathway networks) of the brain—now seemed treatable and concrete, as something that could actually be touched, manipulated, and kneaded, like a Friday-night challah.

But despite all these enchanting new theories I was learning, the pain-relieving effects seemed to wear off. After three months, my checking account had emptied to a new low, and I reassessed the situation. I was now having the same "honeymoon effect" with this work as I had had with every other past therapy, including drugs. In the beginning, it seemed promising, but now I could not tell if it was helping. Would the periods of relief have come on anyway?

In the past, when I had realized I was hitting a dead end with a neurologist, I had just drifted away, silently, without any explanation, like with two people after a so-so coffee date who immediately forget about one another's existence. But I felt a personal connection to this massage therapist; she had shown me genuine compassion on such an intimate level. So I "broke up" with her to her face, sitting with her on her couch in her waiting room, honestly explaining the situation.

"I guess it's time to give up," I said, finally defeated. "Now I have tried everything."

"No," she replied, quite presciently, turning from looking at me to facing the horizon out the window ahead. "There are *plenty* of things left."

I got more encouragement in that direction while on a trip to New York soon after. I met a writer friend for lunch and mentioned the pain as a reason why I was running late, even though I did not know her very well. I was deeply discouraged about how intensely I'd struggled just to meet someone by

Massage and Acupuncture in the Lab

Many forms of alternative medicine have recently started to prove themselves in scientific trials—as activating the body's natural pain-relieving mechanisms. This is true despite the ongoing challenge that every practitioner does them differently and they are not standardized in treatment, unlike drugs. Years after my first experiences with massage, while attending a 2003 presentation by Dr. Serge Marchand of the Faculty of Medicine at the University of Sherbrooke in Quebec, I learned more detail about the actual physical mechanisms that may be involved.[3] He explained that massage works on many different levels. First, the vigorous work of pressing on and then smoothing out the trigger points "can recruit inhibitory pathways from the brain stem"—or activate the body's natural analgesic endorphins to spread throughout the body.[4] Second, the soothing and more gentle movements help to activate the pain "gate," which, as discussed earlier, sends sensory signals to the spinal cord that temporarily block pain signals from getting through.[5] (After a little while, though, the brain gets "bored" by these new signals and goes back to interpreting the old painful ones.) And third, the massage oils used may actually provide relief by soothing the limbic system, the primitive part of the brain associated with pain and emotion. Interestingly, Dr. Marchand found this effect of odors most true in women.[6] Also, the undeniable psychological effects of human touch are a factor.

In the past several years, more progress has also been made in scientifically testing acupuncture's effectiveness and mechanisms of action. In 2004, Dr. Bruce Rosen, a radiologist at Harvard Medical School, found that acupuncture reduces blood flow and increases pain-relieving dopamine to the limbic part of the brain, according to a functional MRI.[7] Another study, published in the *British Medical Journal* that year, revealed relief with acupuncture for chronic headache sufferers, mainly migraine sufferers.[8]

And thankfully, with increased U.S. government support in recent years, the research will continue to investigate the effectiveness of a wide variety of nondrug methods to relieve pain. Hopefully, it will further develop to track pain relief in the long term, which matters most to chronic pain patients, especially those whose pain is the most severe. As Dr. Marchand stressed, this research must also fundamentally study the body's natural pain-relieving mechanisms, to determine how to better apply these methods.

noon, Eastern Standard Time, across town, and I was unable to put on a brave front.

In response, she instantly shifted from a light chitchat tone to one of dead seriousness. She related a story about her severe back pain, which had gotten so bad that at times she had to lie down on the subway to find a tolerable position. For relief, she had visited an eccentric elderly psychologist with a home-PC-sized biofeedback machine, actually one of the leading nondrug methods for treating pain, since it had first been developed in the early 1970s. He hooked her up to measure tension levels, and she realized that when she thought about her mother, the beeping of the monitor went off the charts. He taught her how to relax certain muscles, to self-regulate tensions that she previously had not consciously noticed, and to hold her body differently. And better yet, he gave her therapy about how to deal with her mother. "I know this sounds crazy and way too simple to believe, and I wouldn't have believed it myself if someone had told me this, but it worked," she said.

The moral of the story: "You have to take responsibility for your health," she said. "According to what you have told me—with the doctors, the chiropractors, the massage—you have just gone to someone wanting that person to *do* something to you to make you better. Such people can help you heal, but it's ultimately up to you to take an *active* role in the process."

(The moral can also be that therapy can indeed be useful in some cases of pain relief when a particular stressor—like her mother—is the main trigger of this biological process. Alas, I didn't have as much of a problematic relationship with my own mother, and I had to look to other avenues for relief.)

One way to start was yoga, which also involves becoming more conscious of tension in the body. She told me about the Wild Onion yoga center on Sheffield Avenue, where she used to attend classes when she lived in Chicago. If I looked on the top shelf in the dressing-room area, I would find the pair of green yoga pants she had accidentally left behind. I could keep them, as a gift.

I took her words of advice seriously and, as the months passed, learned more about what she was talking about. The turning point in understanding these concepts was when I met Dr. Chung (not his real name), a highly recommended acupuncturist downtown, whom I had to wait months to see.

Immediately, when my mom and I entered the room for the first visit, I knew that I was dealing with someone entirely different. Mainly, I noticed what he was missing: an ego. His manner was meditative and understated, not the commanding and abrupt authority of the neurologists I had met. But ironically, this man's reserved manner commanded even more respect.

Although he was a trained internist, he had been greatly influenced in spirit and philosophy by his practice of Chinese medicine, which his elderly parents also practiced in the same office as he. In a profile of him in the alternative weekly *The Chicago Reader,* which was posted on the wall of his office, he said that his parents had been pathologists, getting their medical training in China. Then, when his father's shoulder pain did not respond to Western medicine, they tried acupuncture and were stunned by the positive results. Afterward, they devoted themselves to the practice of acupuncture. In the 1980s, Dr. Chung made several of his own journeys to study in China.

On a personal level, I also related to him better than even to the few other acupuncturists I had seen, who were foreign-born. The other two were older and spoke little English. They had just stuck me with a few needles after I gave a minimal explanation, and I left feeling unimpressed. But Dr. Chung was not much older than I, in his mid to late thirties, sporting a ponytail. As a first-generation American, he spoke to me in the same easy tone and manner as my friends did.

He started our appointment by asking me about my health, and I spat out quick answers. I had expected him to be like the others, spending a few minutes with me before whipping out the prescription pad with one hand and pushing me out the door with the other. But I soon realized that he wasn't going anywhere and slowed down in answering his questions. In total, he spent about a half hour in conversation, an amount I saw as impossibly long. Some questions were standard, including when the pain started, what it felt like, and so on. But he also had some strange ones, speaking matter-of-factly about other bodily functions, such as stool color schemes and menstrual flow consistencies. And then he asked me in great detail about my life and any pressures I was facing.

After the conversation, Dr. Chung gave his opinion of what I had and how to proceed, which totally changed my perception of the Headache— and disease itself. I had told him I wanted to "get rid of the headache," and he responded that it was a symptom of a larger problem, a greater weakening of the body. I had suffered a physical breakdown but didn't know it. According to Chinese medicine, we're all animated by an essential life force, *chi.* When balance in the body is disrupted, the *chi* gets stuck at a preexisting weak point in the body (like around the eyes in me), and pain and dysfunction result. The acupuncture actually unblocks *chi* (or sends out endorphins, if you follow a Western model). This was the first in-depth discussion I had ever had about the philosophies behind alternative medicine, and his words rang true.

Dr. Chung's description matched what my headache felt like: a blocking of energy. Besides the pain, another component, which I hadn't ever really articulated, was a sense of heaviness that I was always pushing through, to think and to exercise, such as when I struggled to run a short distance at the indoor gym track. On days when that "blocking energy" was more severe, I ran much slower and for shorter distances, as I watched the people passing me by many times over on the inner lanes. The gradual dispersion of energy in a typical day helped to explain why that heavy feeling was strongest when I woke up, and also why I felt most clearheaded at night.

Instead of describing the Headache as something to fight and my body as the site of a "battle," he taught me about how the body could actually have the wisdom to repair itself and correct present imbalances. This philosophy went against other models of health care, which dictate that you see a doctor only when you are in extreme crisis, and then you treat just the problem that caused the crisis. His view, in the Eastern tradition, was that health is a "practice," a constant object of attention, the work that maintains a healthy lifestyle that prevents getting to the point of crisis. His philosophy of a doctor's personalized treatment also especially made sense in connection with efforts to control chronic pain, which is different in every patient and demands tailor-made treatment.

Back then, this way of thinking seemed more controversial. At that time, in the mid-1990s, alternative doctors and Western doctors seemed to fall into two distinct camps, being more at odds with each other than today. Alternative medicine was later called complementary and allied medicine (CAM), as it was used more in conjunction with Western medicine. However, that term seemed a bit off to me. After all, the alternative practitioners that I had met in the mid-1990s were anything *but* "complimentary" in their words about "regular doctors."

Again, in the examination room, while dishing out more criticism of the Western medical system, Dr. Chung blamed the drugs that I had been taking for worsening my problem. He explained that these agents had been taxing the liver, the source of health problems having to do with pressure, such as headaches and menstrual irregularities. I felt validated; I felt that my problem with drugs was possibly *not* just me personally being "unresponsive," that these drugs had some real limits over time.

My mother was naturally skeptical, repeatedly telling him that my liver had been thoroughly tested in blood tests, and that nothing was wrong with it. Dr. Chung responded that what he was describing was subtler. But I decided to take a different approach. I totally suspended disbelief, as you do when you watch a play. You can somehow get yourself to believe that a bunch of twenty-two-year-old actors wearing gray wigs really are old people from eighteenth-century France.

Then Dr. Chung gave me a sheet outlining foods to avoid that were "phlegm-forming," that is, inhibiting the action of the liver. The list included red meat, milk, and, worst of all, coffee—even decaf. He also encouraged me to look at how I had been living my life, explaining that lifestyle changes are a basic part of Chinese medicine. I needed to exercise more and take a break from deadlines, to restore myself, he said. Indeed, I needed to put my current book project on hold for at least a year.

"I can't do that," I said.

"Why?"

"That is too big a risk. I would lose control of it."

"Why do you think you ever had control of it to begin with?" he asked. "You could turn it in and it could be rejected or your editor could get fired and no one would be there to look after it. Or it could get bad reviews and no one would read it."

He had a point.

"But what about all I have invested? I can't just give that up."

"I had a friend who went through medical school and dropped out in the last year when he realized that medicine wasn't for him. That's a part of life."

He offered to sign a letter of explanation to the publisher asking for an extension, if I would write it. I said I would consider making this request, although the idea set me on edge.

A few minutes later, I calmed down greatly with the help of Dr. Chung's acupuncture treatment itself. The process involved the insertion of needles in the face, hands, arms, and toes, all parts of the "liver meridian." He flicked them in deeply and decisively in a single quick motion, as in an unchallenging game of darts, where the target is just a half-inch away. Although I had read that this didn't hurt, it actually did, especially in the more nerve-dense areas of the toes and hand. A *desirable* goal was for me to feel a "shock," which felt as if some kind of electric channel or nerve was being hit.

But unlike with the head pain, I knew that effects from the needles would be temporary, and I soon felt a buzz of relaxation, like the effects of a good tranquilizer, but with clarifying, and not stultifying, mental effects. Not even distracting were the electrical wires clipped to the needles—which doctors sometimes use to create an added punch—that created a pulsing sensation in my extremities. After the initial abruptness of insertion, I hardly felt the needles, only a dull ache radiating from some of them. Oddly, even though I'm typically impatient, I lay there serenely on the table in the dark for about forty-five minutes, not bored for a minute.

Overall, not including the shocks in my feet, acupuncture was enjoyable, like the massage. In fact, when I later described the process to a friend, she was disappointed that she didn't have any health problems that warranted her seeing Dr. Chung.

When I left after the first visit, the pain behind my left eye was diminished, staying that way for about a day. I looked forward to the next appointment, filled with hope that the effects of acupuncture would be cumulative and that if I balanced my life enough, I could get better.[9]

More than the surprise I felt with such a small reprieve, I was honestly stunned to get such attention from a doctor for my problem. This was something I had seen happen only on TV, not in real life, in commercials for large university medical centers, such as for those at Rush University Medical Center or the University of Chicago. This was the only place where I ever witnessed doctors declaring openly that they "cared," that they would go beyond treating just the illness, to also treat the "human spirit." I had never before met any doctors like this in person—or at least any real ones. Ironically, underscoring this contradiction was an actor whom I met several years later on the back porch at a friend's party, where he had gone to smoke. He had played one of those caring doctors in a commercial for a major university hospital. After he told me that, he asked me about the Headache. And then, just as in a real doctor, his eyes glazed over with indifference. Even the actor *playing* a doctor on TV didn't bother to feign concern about me, I thought.

Although Dr. Chung expressed caring with his actions, one of the most useful lessons he imparted was detachment, an essential concept for those dealing with pain, which I hadn't yet even begun to grasp. Although he was clearly devoted to diminishing the pain, he did not get agitated if it didn't happen. After all, to one who is following Buddhist thought—dedicated to achieving inner peace—pain and suffering are a part of life. The major challenge was how one reacted to it, with acceptance and even transcendence, instead of panic and denial and self-reproach.

Dr. Chung's lack of ego was a calming force. Only because of his example did I realize that in contrast, an underlying and subtle conflict with some neurologists and other M.D.'s had been the pressure to get better. A doctor who couldn't cure me had an issue of *personal* "failure." And rationally or not, I had felt partly responsible for the burden of supporting and affirming the doctor's efforts.

After that first visit to Dr. Chung, I sat down to draft a letter to my publisher to request a delivery extension. I knew that I was making the right decision, just because of the difficulty of writing one single page through the pain and fatigue. After I sent it to Dr. Chung, instead of feeling panicked, as I had assumed I would, I felt relieved.

Suspending my writing was only part of the plan for the next year. To support myself and keep ideas circulating, I would solicit more speaking gigs at universities about my first book, invitations for which had started coming in on their own. Although speaking to audiences used many marbles, I was able to rest afterward and somehow get through—and often even enjoy it. On a less glamorous note, I also started a small tape transcription business, realizing that this was something that I could not only do when in pain but, even better, could also farm out to others and still make a little money. It was the opposite of writing, totally passive and even a bit meditative. I wasn't in good enough physical shape to work as a temp, but I was hearty enough to boss others around. I would become like the surly older madam interviewed in a documentary on Hollywood madam Heidi Fleiss. She was over-the-hill and unable to walk but still confidently commanded others from her large frilly pink bed.

My journal entries from this time went from despair to hope, expressing pride in myself and how "hard I was working to get better" and achieve balance. I was exercising daily, avoiding phlegm-forming foods, and not mentally taxing myself, giving the brain a rest. Overall, although far from cured, without the drugs, I felt a degree better, enough to function on a higher level. My thinking got clearer, as in the old days, and I had the happy realization that it was the drugs, and not the pain, that had been the greatest obstacle to being able to begin writing seriously again.

If acupuncture and Chinese medicine worked, besides thanking Dr. Chung and myself, I knew I could credit one other person: Richard Nixon. He had opened the door to acupuncture's current popularity in the West in the 1970s when he visited and opened relations with China. He hadn't been so bad a guy after all, I thought.

Despite my new hope, I was not totally uncritical of Chinese medicine. A few weeks later, I went into Dr. Chung's office and recognized the distinctive sweet smell of pot wafting through the air. "Ah ha! This is why he was so mellow!" I thought, temporarily disillusioned. All that stuff he had told me about the *chi* was just the result of a Dead Head phase. I got more upset at the treatment, when he uncharacteristically forgot which side my pain was on.

But a few weeks later, my cousin, who is a chiropractor, happened to mention his use of acupuncture with the warming herb moxa, which smells just like cannabis. In the process of *moxibustion*, the burning of the herb heats the needles.

I also had to get used to Dr. Chung's directness and lack of euphemisms, such as when referring to my weight. "Look at *all this fat!* You have to lose it!" he exclaimed, blaming my weight on keeping my body in a state of imbalance and more vulnerable to external triggers, such as weather changes. With the weight now implicated in the pain levels, I had a new motivation to withstand the discomfort of dieting and being hungry while also hobbled by chronic pain.

Another strong recommendation was to learn how to relax. I realized that this task was not necessarily easy and that I wasn't quite sure what it felt like. But then, slowly, I picked up on it, what it was all about. In my journal I wrote about my epiphany: "I figured that being stress-free means being interested in, or not bothered by, *boring* things, like yoga, meat-free food, long walks."

But my vegetarian life was short-lived, lasting only about twenty-six hours (which surpassed my attempt to eat an even more restrictive macrobiotic diet, which clocked out at eight hours). As a vegetarian, I may have been eating healthier, but I was also losing the will to live. I also didn't have the patience to cook any more meals from my new, fussy Dean Ornish cookbook, which involved hours of shopping and preparation, including multiple steps of double-rinsing, chopping, seeding, parboiling, and bean soaking.

In future visits to Dr. Chung, I also had moments of doubt when the acupuncture got more painful. He tried more and more sensitive points in my toes. When I felt the resulting shock and jumped and sometimes cried out, I apologized to Dr. Chung, saying that he should continue, that this was not a complaint, that I would "do anything" to get rid of the headaches. "I know you would," he said, quietly. But then afterward, I felt a catharsis, as if I had let out what had been long bottled up, all the suffering alone in silence with the pain. I had heard about people having such emotional responses to deep-tissue massage, as all kinds of energies are released, and I wondered if that was also a part of the process of acupuncture.

I also spent time pondering Dr. Chung's more cryptic comments about my personality, such as "You are like a tree and don't bend with the wind."

Again, he was using an entirely different type of language, a seemingly nonjudgmental set of metaphors, to describe what was happening to me. He recommended that I read the *Tao Te Ching*, a foundation of Taoist philosophy by Lao-tzu, a fourth-century contemporary of Confucius.

But I had one problem: I was too stupid to understand it.

Maybe it was my book's particular translation, which was too authentic. I had to keep stopping to read footnotes that explained the varied meanings of words like *wind, note, sound*, and *straw dogs*—how they could actually mean something else in Chinese. Besides, the metaphors were so abstruse—for example, "governing a large state is like boiling a small fish"—that I couldn't begin to penetrate how they related to my headache. I felt as if I was trying to seek therapy by sorting through a text as accessible as *Beowulf*.

In frustration, I went out and bought a book for the lay reader, *The Tao of Inner Peace* (1991), by Diane Dreher, which conveyed these concepts in more accessible and convenient lower-IQ terms. Although it didn't say anything profound, it made sense. It set out the basics, Spirituality 101. I feel trite even discussing it here. But clichés are clichés for a reason, and it was still an awakening—the type others describe after their first visit to Alcoholics Anonymous, or after finding out about the "connectedness of things" by climbing a mountain or joining a particularly scintillating cult. They see another way of thinking, a way of approaching things less fearfully and of viewing themselves as a part of a larger process.

This spirituality had been a missing component in other headache guides I had bought, which emphasized lifestyle changes but did not discuss the philosophies behind them or actual ways to transcend the pain. And I see now that it was a vital ingredient, a source of strength and courage. It offered hope of success—in tolerating the intolerable, in living with the pain instead of being engaged in a constant war with it. This new understanding was a matter more of instinct than of intellect, going to another level of depth. It offered seemingly contradictory concepts of letting go to gain some control, and of nonresistance while still taking responsibility for improving one's health, which eased tension and relieved at least some pain. I had a very long way to go to understand these concepts, but the seeds had at least been planted.

Dr. Chung also directed me to buy the classic book *Between Heaven and Earth: A Guide to Chinese Medicine* by Harriet Benfield and Efrem Korngold, which maps out both abstract philosophies and specific remedies, a combination of plain old horse sense and ancient Chinese mythology. The book particularly stood out as provocative with its imagery of the five elements and how they relate to health. This active involvement of mine as a patient reveals another advantage of Chinese medicine: encouraging self-knowledge, which helps in being able to manage one's health. Although I was a stereotypically self-absorbed writer, I found that oddly, I did not have much self-knowledge, an entirely different thing.

In summary, the book explains that we all run on one of five basic operating systems, all dominated and symbolized by different types of major organs. I imagined this as sort of like five kinds of human Windows operating systems.

It turned out that I was running on Liver 5.0. I was a "wood," correlating to the liver, whereas "fire" related to the heart, "earth" to the spleen, "metal" to the lungs, and "water" to the kidney.

No one element is better than the other, each having pluses and minuses, says the book. In extreme and absurd forms, Adolph Hitler, Warren Buffett, Rocky, and the good literary agents are woods. A wood is thought to be a hard-driving "pioneer" or entrepreneur type who does not follow external rules, strives to achieve, and is driven by independent internal pressures. A negative, among many, is that the wood person often does not know when to quit and depletes resources. He or she often can't have energy without feeling compelled to expend it.

The remedy is to take herbs geared to the liver, plus acupuncture on points along the special liver meridians that run through the body. Wood also corresponds to the spring season, so spring foods, such as greens, are recommended.

This philosophy also gives guidance in structuring the most mundane aspects of life, a guidance that contributes to an overall feeling of order. I took the lead of the "wood" case study in the book: "Sally is at her best when the pace of her life keeps her engaged but not exhausted, defined by a clear purpose but not confined to an inflexible program. Permitting herself to moderate extremism and accept structure and discipline helps her to harness her drive" (163). Following this guide influenced my work and sleep schedule, which before had been chaotic. I now accepted that since I operated by cranking up my internal pressure, I needed the morning to get going, should do the heaviest work in the afternoons, and then cut off all taxing mental activity after dinnertime, to give my body the chance to wind down. From that time on, and still to this day, I avoided reading after 8 P.M. Gradually, I seemed to fall asleep more quickly.

One reason I was surprised by this "liver" person analysis is that I thought everyone thought and got through life that way, with this same "operating system." But learning about the other elements gave me some appreciation of other types of people, all of whom have their place in the universe. I'm sure that part of this interest in the elements was like the effect of reading a horoscope, where the descriptions are often so general that people can find themselves in any forecast. And many of the points are flattering: Oh, I'm such a pioneer, I'm such an achiever, I'm such an independent thinker.

But the parts I related to were provocative and even poetic in their imagery. And since birthdays are not involved as determining factors in the elements, I saw the elements as less wacky than astrology. I recognized this elements scheme as not a mystical and reductive test, but as a Chinese Myers-Briggs, a useful set of descriptions of different types of personalities that have been refined and tested for thousands of years. I found it similar to studying other types of philosophers to understand life, from Plato to Nietzsche, but with more of a spiritual twist. I explained to friends that it was like taking Psych 101 and learning the textbook difference between an extrovert and an introvert, which is useful in articulating patterns you have always known about but wouldn't have been able to define. Plus, I recognized that these descriptions are not definitive, that people are much too complex to be reduced to them, and that everyone shares features of the others. Dr. Chung said I should study how the water (the more serene and still and critical "philosopher" element) nourishes, literally and figuratively, the wood. You can imagine the rain, for example, watering the brittle tree.

He recommended building reserves of energy with waterlike meditation or yoga—or Chinese *chi gong*, which combines elements of both, like a meditative form of tai chi. I needed more stillness in life, even with things as minor as not always having the TV or radio on when I was at home alone. Dr. Chung handed me a copy of an article from a health magazine about stress reduction, which even recommended stopping listening to the news for a day or two. (In the margins, someone had crossed out "for a day or two" and substituted "every day.")

Although I felt newly enlightened by Chinese medicine, friends showed some skepticism, while reflecting some of my own doubts. One said this all-defining scheme of the elements sounded suspiciously like the all-defining four bodily "humors," invented by the Greeks about two thousand years ago. They had thought that the concept of the four types of personalities (with four accompanying types of health problems)—sanguine, phlegmatic, melancholic, and choleric—had gone out of style sometime in the, say, 1600s?

I was reproached again when talking at a bar to a group of friends and their journalist colleagues. The subject of the elements somehow came up, and I told the group about it. One friend approached me afterward in private to tell me that most of the people there, who had not met me before, thought I was "completely nuts." But he said he understood that I was, naturally, grasping at the irrational as a part of my desperate quest for answers. He still assessed my advocacy of the elements as being on the same level of wackiness as the advice of a mutual college friend of ours, who had told me that in her Italian culture, headaches were thought to be a result of someone giving you the evil eye. As a remedy, she had recommended my seeing some kind of mystic to reverse that spell.

All this made me wonder if this was a slippery slope, the beginning of my losing my edge. In the past, I would have made fun of someone like me, but I could no longer satirize anyone, because I had committed these unspeakable superstitious follies myself. Worst of all, this would definitely threaten my dating life, even more than the pain. I had become one of those New Age wackos whom I had long avoided. Everyone knew that a belief in alternative medicine could immediately discredit one. I later even read it in *Cosmo*, the Bible of such matters. In March 1999, the magazine ran an article, penned by a male, about "Nine Things You Should Never Tell a Guy." Second on the list was "your belief in alternative medicine. . . . When you tell us about your experiences with aromatherapy, reflexology or crystals, all we hear is *unstable, unstable, unstable*" (58). Years later, I even saw this warning being made more subtly, in the context of current events: In early 2004, in another major source of dating advice, the *New York Times*, I read about such fears in a profile of Teresa Heinz Kerry, the wife of then–presidential hopeful John Kerry. In a front-page story, the reporter discusses her "reputation as being offbeat if not a little odd," partly because of her exploration of alternative healing methods that "can leave her audiences as mystified as they are impressed."

Now, where would *I* personally draw the line? Colonics? Crystals? Scientology? Jews for Jesus?—although I still strongly remembered my Hebrew school assembly in the 1970s warning us against their lure. My new "psychospiritual" therapist, Lisa, was urging me to "get my chart done," which meant going to an astrologer to analyze what my date, place, and time of birth meant for my life's purpose. I was considering it.

I feared that I was crossing more into the margins of society when visiting another type of doctor in addition to Dr. Chung, actually a chiropractor, Bill. This is an ordinary course of treatment for a headache sufferer, chiropractics being the most common type of alternative medicine that we try.[10]

But this was no ordinary chiropractor. I knew this visit would be a different experience just by the hipness of the building his office was in—an old urban loft with exposed brick. When I met him in the hallway waiting area, I told him that this was quite different from the sterile medical buildings I was used to, and he said, "Wait until you see my office." He opened the door and revealed a wonderland of nature and ritual artifacts from multiple religions. There were lit candles on a minialtar, a bubbling tank with a few huge tropical fish, angels, Indian feathers, and a painting of the Virgin Mary. "Whatever happens, we've got our bases covered," the collection seemed to say.

Without having me fill out any paperwork, he sat down with me and asked me to tell him my story. I talked, and he listened knowingly, without taking any notes. Occasionally, I would stop and there would just be silence, with which he seemed very comfortable. I told him I was thinking about getting an MRI of my neck, since I was becoming more aware of my ever-present neck pain, on the same side as the headache, and was wondering if they were related.

He said an MRI wouldn't find anything, as it just captures the structural parts of the brain, and he launched into a discussion of energy, auras, and pulses, the hidden animating forces around us. He suspected this was the area where my problem resided. He said that my energy was frenetic and had preceded me into the room. He talked about how I harbored a lot of fear and was going through life like "a hamster on a wheel." Echoing what Dr. Chung had said, he mentioned that when one is not grounded or centered, the energy rises fitfully and gets blocked in weak areas. As I interpreted it, this all meant I had a case of "bad vibes."

After turning the lights down, Bill then had me lie on a table to do "energy work." This involved his placing hands and stones and other artifacts on me. This was one of the oddest experiences of my life. I feared I might be one of the biggest suckers of all time. But when I got up, I did feel the energy shifting, as after you get off a roller coaster. I was operating at a higher and more alert frequency. I made another appointment.

Gradually, I stopped being surprised by some of the surprising things that Bill said. During one energy work session, he put a heavy burlap sack on my stomach that reportedly had been used to deliver a baby in Peru. He also had me see a visiting native shaman from New Zealand, who gave me some very simple advice: Take it easy more.

Whereas Dr. Chung had described me as a "wood," Bill said I should follow the eagle totem (an ancient animal symbol used by Native American tribes), which represents people destined to fly above, occasionally get scorched by their ambition, and see "the big picture" in life. (As a freaky twist, while walking at Montrose Beach in Chicago a week later, I stopped and picked up a round gold plastic playing piece of a children's game from the sand, which had a portrait of an eagle on one side.) In contrast to what I had heard from Western medicine, this New Age wisdom was indeed flattering. Instead of being a pathetic and annoying "malingerer" and "drug seeker," I was now a wise, noble eagle, soaring above.

At each appointment, Bill would talk to me for about a half hour on topics such as how I should have more faith to work in a more grounded way and no longer associate work with fear and anxiety. This was actually more helpful than anything I had experienced in therapy. In the meantime, he sometimes wandered off into monologues about shamanic healing traditions that related to me, like the philosophy that my headache was like a fire, and I was being consumed by it, standing *in* the fire. I had to learn instead to stand away from it, removing myself but remaining close enough to still tend it and not ignore it. He was right that I had a very erratic energy, where my entire mood depended on the state of the pain: If it was bad, I was in despair, and if it was more tolerable, I was happy. The change could happen in a matter of minutes. I was living on a roller coaster of emotion. I always was in fear of the next inevitable shift, which I could not control.

So I learned, then, to distinguish between the physical pain and two other types that resulted. These were emotional pain, the "affect" involved, such as sadness or depression, and cognitive pain, the meaning that I gave to the pain. This conflict was evident in the most mundane aspects of life, such as when I had gotten upset by my difficulty in meeting a friend for lunch. In that case, I had suffered most not from the physical pain involved, but from anger at myself for being so weak and fear of what the Headache might indicate for the future.

This philosophy is not new, but is reflected in the old saying, "Pain is mandatory, but suffering is optional." Becoming aware of these thoughts and the difference between physical and mental pain gave me at least some feeling of power over this pain. This tactic of detachment from the pain still stood out as something I could use *in the long term*. Although not a panacea, it was something that had no side effects or future "payback." Therefore, it contrasted with other common pain-coping methods, such as short-term denial of the pain or distraction, such as going to a party or giving a lecture, for which I would suffer later. Of course, emotional detachment tactic was more easily said than done, but it was something, more helpful to me on a practical level than the drugs had been.

Bill also promoted prayer, a type of higher vibration, as "talking to God." But even more than that, he encouraged the practice of meditation—as "God talking back." To learn this skill, I saw an expert on the topic, a well-reputed psychologist who was affiliated with the Northwestern University pain clinic. My physical therapist friend, Elizabeth, had told me that in the entire Chicago area, maybe a handful of people knew about pain, and he was one of them. Although many health care providers had told me to meditate, I had never really known what that process involved or how powerful it was to help relaxation. I realized that I needed to talk to a teacher of meditation one-on-one to really learn the theories and physical techniques behind this process. (I describe the slow process of learning meditation as being like a woman learning how to have an orgasm. This is a culturally hidden mechanism of channeling energy that takes time and practice to master. Plus it's different for everyone.)

The psychologist explained that meditation, which is basically a practice of stillness to relieve one of the demands of one's thoughts, actually helps restore the nervous system, the way physical exercise builds muscles. One gets "in tune" with the body and "centered" by focusing on one's breathing. As in exercise, the effects are cumulative and not obvious right away. As I learned later, brain-imaging scans have shown that meditation can calm the limbic system in the brain, which affects pain and emotions. Meditation is also supposed to build an inner core of strength and awareness that carries over to times when the person isn't meditating—and keeps him or her resilient to the extreme ups and downs inflicted suddenly and at random by the outside world. The psychologist helped me get over one of my greatest obstacles: a wandering mind, which took my focus away from the breath. He advised me, instead of trying to fight these thoughts, to gently let them pass and then focus again on the task at hand, expecting this process to be a part of meditation. I figured it was like just pulling off to the side to allow an annoying tailgating car to pass, instead of having an emotional confrontation with that driver and then being more annoyed overall.

Like other treatments, this meditation therapy had its greatest effects in the beginning. I followed the psychologist's directions and soon felt more strength, at times waking up hours earlier the next day and being more refreshed. And very significantly, this process also somewhat relieved my depression by further making me realize that "I am not my pain," that I could separate my consciousness from the rest of my body even in the worst of times. The underlying commonsense tenets of meditation, of managing stress by not constantly locking oneself into a battle with it, gave me some needed peace. (These tenets are outlined in Jon Kabat-Zinn's 1990 book *Full Catastrophe Living,* which the psychologist had me buy after my first visit. Basically, this fourteen-dollar paperback, along with a meditation tape advertised for order in the back of the book, describes everything I learned from him in ten hundred-dollar-an-hour sessions.)

Interestingly, the psychologist demonstrated that this meditation technique may be more effective than biofeedback, which was also gaining ground in the mainstream pain field. He hooked me up to his biofeedback machine and measured tension levels after I had worked on relaxing for a while. Then he had me try the meditation I had learned, and the machine's reading of tension levels actually decreased further. So I kept practicing meditation at home, although, despite my best attitude, I found it more and more tedious, with flashes of boredom now commingling with the flashes of enlightenment.

As hopeful as I sometimes felt in their care, these alternative healers did raise doubts, even in my now-suppressed critical consciousness. I would tell my new therapist Lisa that I didn't know why a person I'd just met had strongly got on my nerves for no apparent reason, and she would respond, "Well, you probably had a conflict with her in your past life." I read through books recommended by Bill, such as *Vibrational Medicine*, which describes his healing practice of energetic medicine, and put it down after a passage on the wisdom we can learn from the Lost Civilization of Atlantis. He also raised some red flags for me when he recommended the use of Bach flower essences, a homeopathic remedy in which the essence of a particular plant is diluted to the extreme in a mixture of spring water and brandy. The remedies, sold since the 1930s, each address very specific emotional imbalances that are thought to get in the way of the healing process. He recommended that I buy Mimulus, which addresses the "fear of known things," and Oak, "for the plodder who keeps going past the point of exhaustion." Each one cost $8.99, sold in a tiny yellow milliliter dropper bottle. A dose was several drops. I did feel a bit relaxed afterward, but I wasn't sure if it was because of the "vibrational powers" or the brandy.

Although her spiritual wisdom was helpful, I also had mixed feelings about Lisa's explanation of the Headache—that this was a message from the body to be more meditative and not "live in the head." (The body could be quite literal in its messages, she explained.)

"See the headaches as a gift. This is the only way your body could get you to stop working so hard and reflect," said Lisa. On one hand, this was comforting, because it gave some meaning to the illness—an explanation of why it happened—and seemed to create the possibility for change if I rearranged my thought patterns. On the other hand, I felt guilty that I had brought this all on myself, and when I had pain, I felt that I wasn't working hard enough to change my attitudes. My most vexing thought was that if I took the time to be a yoga expert, which sounded incomprehensibly difficult to me, like trying to learn to be a rocket scientist, I would be better. It was just laziness keeping me down. As the heart seemed to be more valued than the brain, I started to fear the intellectual part of me as negative, as pain-causing.

Actually, Lisa spoke in terms very similar to those of the Freudians, framing physical pain as an expression of emotional pain. However, as she and many alternative healers interpreted and phrased them, these philosophies did at least seem less blaming. Doctors had used this symbolism to describe headache patients as "neurotic" and "attention seeking," but the alternative medicine practitioners had framed it as "not listening to the body's wisdom." This healing through the mind was, overall, an overtly spiritual matter, which imbued the process with a less "intellectualized" or clinical tone.

At the time, even in a state of desperation, I recognized many of these irrationalities. But instead of rejecting alternative medicine and New Age philosophies for these reasons, I took the opposite route. I made a very conscious choice to devote myself entirely to it, more than I had ever done with my religious or political beliefs.

I decided to just "give myself" to it, heart and soul, to have faith that it would work, despite reason. I would think positively, *believe* that I was getting well, and then I would be well. And I wouldn't let negative or critical thoughts or intellectual reasoning get in the way. As they arose, I would simply let them drift through me, like clouds you watch crossing through the tops of mountain ranges in the distance.

After all, I had no choice. I was a person in intolerable pain. This route was my only possible way out. I had nothing left to lose. Believe it, and I would get better. Believe it, and be it.

In the end, I still couldn't help thinking, even if this all was a bunch of crap, I'd be happy just if I could get some kind of placebo effect going. After all, like a lot of chronic pain patients, I had no other alternative but to agree with the words of physician and revolutionary Che Guevara, who wrote in his book on guerilla warfare, "The most important thing about a strategy is not that it is conventional, ingenious, or legitimate, but simply that it works."[11]

Besides, healing with the mind seemed to work for so many others. I had seen testimonials everywhere, especially in books like Dr. Andrew Weil's *Spontaneous Healing* (1995). They all came from other seemingly hopeless patients who had gotten better through positive thought and hard work. I

What Is Your Headache Trying to Tell You?
Illness as a Metaphor

My guilt about my headaches was compounded when I read one of the most influential writers of the New Age movement, the fantastically successful best-selling author Caroline Myss, a self-described "medical intuitive." I would classify her as a classic New Age healer, representing a basic "positive thinking" spirituality embraced by some parts of alternative medicine, which is actually quite diverse. In her 1988 book, written with Dr. Norman Shealy, *The Creation of Health*, she quoted the views of British doctor Edward Bach, the inventor of flower essence potions, who located the roots of illness in emotional blocks: "'There is nothing in the nature of accident as regards disease. . . . Disease in general is due to some basic error in our constitution.' By errors in constitution," Myss explained, "Bach meant defects in attitude."

Like many other types of New Age healers, who characterize the basic philosophies behind much of alternative medicine, Myss additionally sees each part of the body as expressing a different frustration. Basically, the body is one large decoder ring. Getting well is a matter of being able to read the body's messages about its spiritual and emotional crises. For example, heart disease may reveal issues with intimacy, and shoulder pain shows a feeling of burden. And one doesn't have to think much to understand what a painful head is trying to say: Don't live in the head so much.

In her book, Myss specifically explained the roots of migraine as emotional and mental—in almost the same language used by the most orthodox Freudians fifty years ago: "Migraine headaches develop in response to an attempt to control one's emotional reactions of anger, frustration, rage or other emotions containing the same quality of energy. By control, I am referring to someone trying to prevent an emotional explosion from occurring externally, and, thus, it occurs internally. The need to control is the major characteristic of people prone to migraines" (265). She also defied basic science in her explanation of phantom limb pain, recognized by neurologists as being caused by the still-active but confused centers in the brain that ultimately program sensation in the limbs. Instead, she sees such pain as a case of the body teaching the patient an emotional lesson about the emotional pain of "letting go": "Phantom limb pain is created as a result of the person not coping with or accepting the reasons why the amputation occurred in the first place, and it is also a substitute for the more authentic issues that arise, which are vulnerability and inadequacy. This type of pain is fairly clear evidence that 'cutting away' the problem does not resolve the cause of the problem'" (267).

didn't want to be the only person in America left with pain, as everyone else had apparently been cured through this route.

I also valued alternative medicine for adding dimension to my life with a new sense of spirituality. I had not been at all spiritual before this, but now I had no choice; I needed spirituality just to get through each day. This knowledge is something that, quite honestly, my traditional religion—at least in the forms that I had known—had not offered me. I thought back to the Torah portion I had read for my bat mitzvah, talking in detail about procedures for conducting animal sacrifice with goats, the types of prayers to say, the slaughtering instruments, and so on. That may have been interesting how-to information at the time, say near 1000 B.C. and might convey a basic lesson about God's being the boss, but it was not very relevant to my life then in the suburbs.

Instead of just Jews as teachers, I wanted *New Age Jews*, like Lisa and that couple, Harriet Benfield and Efrem Korngold, who had written the book on Chinese medicine *Between Heaven and Earth*. They had actually been following the long-cherished Jewish tradition of being able to translate, convey, and develop others' ideas in an engaging way. "That's the thing about Jews. They rise to the top of every religion they are involved with," I was told by Roger Kamenetz, a well-known Jewish writer on Buddhism, after I heard him speak in Chicago. After all, as we have always straddled different cultures through time, we have become experts at interpreting them and extracting from them what we need. Besides, as entertainment experts, the Jews add some Hollywood, some pizzazz, to old ethereal Eastern philosophies. I wanted Lao-tzu meets Louis B. Mayer, the Tao of Samuel Goldwyn and David O. Selznick.

At that time, I recognized that as I waited for that cure or significant reduction in pain to happen, I was gaining some very concrete coping tools through this study of alternative medicine. These made me feel at least a bit more powerful and in control. Instead of always being vulnerable, at the mercy of the weather and other forces, I had some tools at my disposal— yoga, acupuncture, meditation—that sometimes worked as "antitriggers," to raise the pain threshold and bring some sense of peace.

I was still mourning over my new limits in life and the loss of my old self, but now at least I had some insights into the new ones I would build. I knew what I wanted to discard, such as the undercurrent of fear that I associated with my work and the constant negative thoughts and emotions connected to the physical pain. Like the boxes of clothes that I had not worn for years, which I was giving away at that time, I realized that these old attitudes also no longer fit. I knew I could not work for newspapers again, but then again, I no longer had that desire.

One of the highlights of that hopeful period was my visit to California to lecture at a university. On a whim, I decided to stay there in nearby lush Santa Barbara for three weeks to focus completely on working on my health. I knew that my publisher was about to approve the request for a year-long extension, and my schedule was suddenly free. Perhaps also because of the intensive acupuncture I had had before leaving and the very tranquil, unchanging weather, the pain had also been down to record low levels.

I had just seen a movie about Dorothy Parker, who extolled the joys of living in a hotel, and I decided to follow her lead. I found a pay-by-the-week hotel with a bathroom down the hall, which seemed much less seedy to me than it actually was because it was art deco—instead of looking like something cheesy like an old aqua and orange Howard Johnson's from the 1970s. When I had the energy, I spent the days walking miles from beach to beach along the shoreline and against the cliffs and flat mesa above. I also bought a book about walking tours of Santa Barbara and would take a bus somewhere, maybe to an old mission, and just start walking back. At one point, I walked along a path in some kind of nature preserve and came across a stream blocking my way. A woman walking in front of me instinctively turned around and gave me her hand to help me cross.

Unlike in Chicago, it was effortless to eat healthfully in Santa Barbara, where every decent restaurant offered foods like steamed vegetables and brown rice. And I always knew what to order: whatever the always-bountiful crowds of beautiful, thin blond people around me were ordering. For snacks, I ate fruit, like the sweetest strawberries I had ever tasted, from the weekly farmer's market. As a result, I saw that I was finally losing some weight and looking more like my old self, which gave me an added sense of control.

Avoiding the Scientologists set up across the street, I went to the nearby health food store and loaded up on dietary supplements, including fish oil, which I had read was good for headaches. On the way out, I also picked up a postcard with a saying by the renowned and prolific philosopher Thich Nhat Hahn, a Vietnamese Buddhist monk, which read, "There is no way to enlightenment. Enlightenment is the way."

I sat down and started to write a message to a friend on the back of it and then decided to keep it for myself, for inspiration, which I knew I would need. The weather in Santa Barbara was starting to change, bringing violent rains that nearly flooded the streets, and I was about to go home.

10

The Foot Orgasm

○ ○ ○ ○ ○ ○ ○ ○ ○

As 1995 DREW TO A CLOSE, I was over the initial euphoria of learning about inner balance, and functioning much better with a drug-free mind. However, I soberly noticed more that despite my hard work and highly cultivated and sophisticated sense of spiritual enlightenment and self-actualization, I still had my main problem: the Headache. I remained in constant pain. And despite following Bill's advice to sleep more, I continued to battle that mysterious fatigue, typically needing hours to recover from minimal activity.

I was still seeing Dr. Chung and Bill the chiropractor, but through no fault of theirs, the treatments' effectiveness had reached their limits. I realized that I had given Dr. Chung an ample try after his receptionist learned my credit card number by heart. She didn't even have to have me hand it to her anymore to use as reference when she punched in the numbers. The treatments became more painful, as he tried more sensitive spots on the feet and even, precariously, around the eyes. "Don't blink," he said, as I saw the top of the needle get so close that it blurred and seemed to split in my vision.

I asked Bill about why I wasn't getting better, although I was working so hard and was assuming "all the right" thought patterns. He encouraged me to recognize how much I had grown emotionally and spiritually, which was true, and said that I was still in my old goal-oriented mindset. He pointed out that getting well is not a matter of doing X, Y, and Z and said I had to let go of expectations. But the outside world *did* have such expectations. I had deadlines I had to start working to meet.

The good news about alternative medicine was that there were no drugs, and the bad news about alternative medicine was that *there were no drugs*. Without drugs of any kind, even in the form of caffeine from iced tea or the boost of a Tylenol Sinus geltab, I had few options for quick relief during important periods of work. I feared I could never live up to the standards of liver-cleansing purity that Dr. Chung recommended. I was having an especially hard time giving up caffeine, which could provide simple short-term pain relief to help me get through some task I had to accomplish.

Although my most serious depression was lifted, I still was attacked by strong periods of it, especially when I had to struggle to complete what should have been a relatively easy task. In those moments I became most aware of the limits that the Headache was imposing on my life in every possible area. I wouldn't have used the term *disabled*, but that state became increasingly clear and disturbing. I was especially discouraged one afternoon at a pain treatment clinic where I was asked to take part in a research survey. It was about how headache pain may impair mental activity. Part of my challenge was to name illustrations on index cards, which looked like the kind you might find in a kindergarten classroom. Most were very simple, like a car or a chicken. But I still took a while to focus, and then I was stumped at a few that seemed to hark back to rural farm life, such as a thimble, a wooden checkered "trellis" supporting a vine, and a "yoke" worn by oxen. I wondered whether even off drugs, I was still getting dumber by the day, like Charlie from *Flowers for Algernon*. Or maybe this test was just antiquated in its cultural references. What was this, I thought, modern-day Chicago, or *Little House on the Prairie*? I thanked the Lord above that I had taken my SATs before the onset of the Headache, or I don't know what would have become of me.

At about the same time, I got back in touch with my physical therapist friend, Elizabeth, who worked with pain patients, and told her what I was going through.

"Everywhere I turn, I come across more limits," I said.

"Well, at this age, so does everyone else. Everybody has limits. At this age, we all start realizing what ours are, according to physical limits, or how the career path we chose really sucks."

"Yeah, like that British documentary *35 Up*, where they follow those people around through their life. At age thirty-five, the cab driver realizes that he won't be a horse jockey. . . . But this is different. This is a big one, about health. And this is about who I am. I miss my old self."

"So do most people. That's what's hard about getting older."

"But this is very depressing."

"Yes, it is. I agree."

"It's depressing that this is how I'll be the rest of my life," I said. "My uncle had told me that the pain 'eventually burns itself out,' which I tried to believe for a while, but now I'm not so sure."

"Yes, you're right. When pain has been around for a while, then there is a chance that it will never go away. But that's not to say that it still couldn't go down a lot. That's a possibility."

This seemingly depressing conversation ended up soothing me somewhat with the idea that I didn't have to spend all my time rushing around for a cure, that some acceptance would release me to do other things. She also offered some encouragement with a suggestion that I address the pain on multiple levels and in a more coordinated fashion with a "team" approach, an idea that was gaining steam around that time. Besides some form of "energy work," like acupuncture, perhaps physical therapy would help. She additionally advised taking some medication to raise the overall pain threshold, but I was completely against it, now through with conventional M.D.'s for good. I reasoned that the greatest plus of alternative medicine in that past year was precisely that it had *kept me away* from doctors.

As a start, Elizabeth recommended me to a physical therapist at her old workplace, Northwestern University, who might make a good head of my "team." This woman had been trained in cranial-sacral work, which involved her supporting the head in her hands and making very gentle adjustments of the neck. It relieves pressure by manipulating the cerebrospinal fluid between the cranium and the end of the spine in the tailbone area, the sacrum. It was worth a shot.

I saw this physical therapist (who stood out as an unusually beautiful woman), on a very rainy day, when the Headache was going strong. She cradled my head in her hands and pressed with all fingers in varying rhythms, as if she were playing a piano upside down. After the adjustments, as I walked outside into the newly sunny day, I felt the pain greatly diminish. For the first time in more than four years, the pain went down to about nothing, just palpable as a faint pressure. The next day, it remained at about a zero to 1 level out of 10.

I was thrilled and scared at the same time. I marveled at how everything in life was now so incredibly easy with this relief: returning phone calls, doing errands, cleaning up. I remember stopping in the middle of the aisle at the Jewel grocery store and feeling as if I would float away to the paper goods section because of the ease of my movement. But I didn't want to get my hopes up, as I had done with drugs and alternative treatments in the past, when they had worked at first, only to be crushed later. So I suppressed my desire to work nonstop, to make a dent in the always-accumulating chores and correspondence that I had been neglecting. Like a baseball player on a winning streak, I didn't want to change anything and push my luck. I made sure to stay close to home and not deviate from my routine of the past few days.

I could not help but think again about Charlie from *Flowers for Algernon*, who has an operation to improve his intelligence, which works temporarily. Most chilling, his writing quality changes through the story to reflect his intelligence levels going up or down. He writes very poorly in the beginning, becomes hyperliterate in the middle, and then we watch him decline at the end, in some of the most wrenching pages I have ever read in literature.

I imagined myself writing my sex book in this new and improved state of lucidity and then slowly becoming like Charlie, trying to rit down what I think and remembir for the perfessors out there. I would try to talk about the docter I saw who had a white coat like a docter but I don't think he was no docter because he dint tell me to opin my mouth and say ah. He gave me a *raw shok* test that he said would not hirt.

After three days in this state of bliss/fear, a rain front came in and I was back to "normal" in its wake. I was now at the old 3 to 5 pain level, with the old strain just to think straight coming back.

I called the physical therapist to tell her the news but didn't get the supportive reaction I expected. She seemed nervous, admitting that she wasn't sure what she had done and informing me that she was leaving soon for a new office in the far western suburbs, a few hours away. She recommended that I see someone else in Chicago. I tried to argue with her. I told her I'd travel to the ends of the earth for some good adjustments, even if it meant traversing the most precarious suburban sprawl, but it was no use.

Encouraged by the short-lived but terrific results, I began a long quest for the perfect cranial-sacral treatment, which ended up being a very circuitous journey, branching off in many unexpected directions. The fleeing physical therapist referred me to a pain center, which happened to be in a touristy part of Chicago, between the Hard Rock Café and Hooters. She told me that there I would be "seeing the best people" and benefiting from the team approach that I had wanted. I saw the coordinating psychologist there, a man only a few years older than I, to whom I took an immediate dislike. While we talked in his office, the phone rang every few minutes and he answered it and talked at length, still charging me for the full hour.

I also felt oddly and irrationally snobby looking at his Ph.D. diploma from an obscure state college, although I had attended a public university myself. I thought, well, *my* university wasn't the kind with one or more cardinal directions—north, south, east, or west—in the name. It was just plainly and elegantly the University of Illinois, as in the *premium* state school. Recognizing this peculiar snobby attitude of mine, I wondered why so many people have such elitist tendencies of expecting the Ivy League when it comes to their doctors, or to their presidents—wanting them to be smarter than you, or at least have the pretension of being smarter than the average. (Many years later, when I saw this doctor's name on a program for a medical meeting, as presenting some important research on pain, I was riddled with guilt for previously thinking him inadequate.)

But recently, while looking at my chart from him, I understood some of my annoyance—not with him personally, probably, but with doctors in general, who blame the victim. Demonstrating a typical narrow attitude, he made a positive note that I didn't "display any pain behaviors" by not acting as if I was physically in pain, such as by groaning. This was a good thing, in my favor. It did not appear that I was in pain, and therefore, according to psychoanalytic "logic," the chances were that my pain was real. The absurd reasoning was that those who act as if they are in pain have some subconscious emotional attachment to it, seeking a "secondary gain," as Freud called it.

The psychologist did impress me, though, with a systematic "scientific" approach to treatment, after pointing out that I had never been correctly diagnosed. This method, based on my answering a long series of questions on a computer, was based on reason. The diagnostic computer program, which he said was the only one of its kind in operation in the Midwest, spit out a diagnosis of "chronic tension-type headache," which at that time was the only term used for a constant headache in the International Headache Society classifications. The rest of my treatment would follow the protocol for a tension headache.

Before I knew it, I was undergoing twice-weekly physical therapy there, with a young and conscientious former Big Ten cheerleader, Lauren, which had some results at first. Like the other physical therapist from Northwestern, she was incredibly good-looking, solidifying my belief that this is the most undeniably attractive type of health care professional. (I think you must have to pass some kind of beauty screening before they will let you enter this field.) She was also hardworking and conscientious, consulting regularly with the young psychologist, who was just a bit older than she, somewhere in his late twenties or early thirties. Meanwhile, she never failed to forget his higher authority and call him by his first name, to which he would sharply react each time by correcting her: "That's *Dr.* ____," he said. She would apologize and then do the same thing a few minutes later.

Lauren, who did not know cranial-sacral therapy, took out a huge metal arm with a bulb at the end of it. It emitted some kind of electrical current that pummeled away at the very large knot at the base of my shoulders. But after a few weeks, the knot returned, in a slightly different place. Lauren gave me a large blue plastic contraption, resembling a plowing device or shepherd's hook, basically a handle with a hook arm reaching to the back, that I was supposed to use to dig into and loosen that area every day. She also gave me weight-training tips to correct my "extremely forward" posture, such as weight training for the back muscles. At that time, I had almost an epiphany as to the source of the problem, now blaming it on my bad posture, which had been aggravated as I wrote my first book, while hunched over that tiny Mac screen, on a flimsy folding chair in the closet.

She also was kind enough to consult with Bill, to try to make my treatment a coordinated team approach. But when I saw her, she reported, "He was a nice person, and all, but I had no idea what he was talking about. I was talking about your shoulders, and he was saying something about your sharkras [*sic*] and gallbladder channel."

"He means well," I said.

I got fewer results from a series of relaxation sessions at the center, which involved listening to recordings of nature, such as a "snowstorm on an Alpine roof." The point was learning to relax, as I had a "tension" headache, but the power of this practice to aid serious pain may be overstated. I thought about the double standard the medical profession applies to chronic pain patients, for *this* to count as real therapy, especially if it had been my only one. If I had diabetes, a doctor giving me a recording of an ocean tide, before getting to the part about the insulin, would be sued for malpractice.

At one point, the psychologist hooked up my shoulders to a biofeedback machine and had me squeeze them together. Afterward, the tension levels, according to the height of bars of light on the control panel, diminished temporarily. The main finding of this hundred-dollar session: "Squeeze your shoulders as often as possible."

The psychologist then referred me to a leading neurologist at the center. To my relief, that member of the team had gone to Harvard.

Looking at the diagnosis that I had a tension headache and the report from the physical therapist about the tension in my shoulders, the neurologist asked me some new questions. His theory was that my muscles were the culprit, that I had a disorder that made them unnaturally tense. The muscles formed a vice around the neck and shoulders, which led to the headache. To demonstrate, he pressed his hand against my neck. Tight and painful. I responded that yes, I felt pain when pressed. Then against my shoulders. Tight and painful. He moved down to the top of my chest. Tight. He moved down, and as signaled, I unerotically peeled down my sleeveless T-shirt. The chest, also tight and painful.

Now nodding with a look of recognition, he pointed to a diagram on the wall that demonstrated "referral" points in the neck and shoulders, which lead to the point behind the eye where I felt the most pain. The remedy was to continue physical therapy to relax those areas.

But in my view what I needed was a good cranial-sacral therapist. Bill skillfully practiced this kind of therapy on me several times, but it soon wore out in its effectiveness. So I continued my year-long quest for another such practitioner, one with even more experience. At a party, someone told me about a holistic doctor in the suburbs, an osteopath who did such adjustments. I recalled reading about such a doctor in Andrew Weil's best-seller *Spontaneous Healing,* and bells of recognition went off in my mind. In that book, Weil related how this Tucson doctor, Dr. Robert Fulford, had successfully treated his stiff neck with a "percussion hammer," which is basically a very large vibrator with a long power cord. Weil described the instrument, used to manipulate the cerebrospinal fluid, as a "modified dentist's drill motor with a thin round metal disk that vibrated up and down" (26).

I visited the suburban doctor, who I had learned made use of such an instrument in his practice. I expected him to take it out immediately, but then he cautioned that he took a "holistic approach," and the drill was only part of treatment. It wasn't time for that yet. First, I had to be evaluated with a series of very unconventional tests measuring all kinds of toxin levels, to help direct an entire multifaceted regimen of treatment.

"I have already had every type of blood test imaginable," I assured him.

"No," he said decisively, "I doubt you have ever had these types of tests."

I looked over his price sheet and realized I was in for a large investment, over a thousand dollars. My insurance would not cover these tests because of their alternative nature. One of the tests even involved collecting a hair sample from me.

Soon, taking these extensive tests became a part-time job for me. They included some tests I had to do myself for weeks at home—peeing, spitting, and shitting into various collection devices. I spent my leisure time with tests such as the following:

- A Saliva Collection Test. Included in the home test kit were: two caffeine caplets (NoDoz 200 mg each), two Tylenols (325 mg each), two aspirin tablets (325 mg each), and two tubes for saliva specimens. I had to follow complicated directions about when to take the pills, and then I had to pull a cotton roll from the tubes and place it in my mouth until saturated, for about a minute. I then had to put these back in the tube and send them via Airborne Express (approved to ship bodily fluids) to the Great Smokies Diagnostic Laboratory somewhere in North Carolina.

- Comprehensive Digestive Stool Analysis. Included in the test kit were one Cary-Blair tube for return of stool specimen (yellow top), one Formalin tube for return of stool specimen (orange top), one collection cup, one plastic "Biohazard" bag with absorbent pad, disposable gloves, and a prepaid Airborne Lab Pak mailer. (Needless to say, they aren't paying those Airborne Express carriers enough.)

- Temperature Treatment Log. Every morning, I recorded my saliva acidity level, taken with litmus paper, and my temperature, registered with a basal thermometer stuck in my armpit.

But the bulk of the tests were conducted at this guy's office, where blood was the only vital fluid extracted, for a "biochemical profile" and then hormone, allergy, mineral, and digestive testing. I also had a five-hour glucose tolerance test, which involved fasting for hours before and then periodically drinking a sweet substance and getting blood drawn to measure any changes.

At last, a few thousand dollars later, he agreed to give me the long-desired percussion hammer treatment. But before, as I sat on the table waiting, he gave me a long lecture about the science behind it. On the back of my lab sheet, he drew a complicated diagram of the body, with arrows pointing in all directions from head to toe, referring to the thyroid, FSH (follicle-stimulating hormone) levels, and insulin. I didn't understand a word of it. Clutching my head, I thought, "Oh brother. Just give me the damned treatment already! What happened to the good old days of doctors not caring about educating the patient?"

Finally, he agreed to stop the lecture. I lay down, and curiously enough, he worked it on the soles of my bare feet, probably to get energy moving. The

buzzing rattled my entire body, and I had one strong realization: It was possibly the most powerful vibrator in the world.

Very soon, the intense pressure in the soles of my feet seemed to draw the
blood there, the result being an oddly familiar sensation. The pressure built
and built and I suddenly feared the unimaginable. I was about to have a foot
orgasm. In my sex book research, I had read about paralyzed people who had
learned to have orgasms in other parts of their bodies, and I wondered if I
had stumbled upon this highly rarified bodily art. True, this reaction was
highly inappropriate. But on the positive side, I was about to become more
erotically advanced than the most highly cultivated courtesans of Europe. I
would experience what most people could only dream about!

But in an experience echoing the frustration that many women can identify with, the motor suddenly turned off.

"OK, that's enough for today," the doctor announced, and began folding up
the power chord.

"Are you sure?" I said. "I thought it was just getting going there."

"Yes, see how you feel and we'll try it again soon."

"How soon?"

"Next week."

"How about tomorrow?"

"No, that's too soon."

"OK," I conceded, holding back my impulse to ask him how much those
things cost and where I could order one for myself.

Actually, the next visit was the most important one in his opinion, where
we would evaluate the results of the tests. The verdict: I was a mess. The
doctor handed me my own copy of the results, secured in a thick folder by
two metal fasteners drawn through punched holes. He and his wife, who was
in practice with him, then went over them page by page, explaining points I
did not understand. During the visit, I jotted down cryptic notes like "hypera-
drenal," "homeostasis having a terrible time regulating itself," and that I had
"erratic blood sugar typical of entrepreneur on own schedule." From time to
time, the woman quoted the words of Deepak Chopra, the well-known holistic best-selling author (who has written books about interpreting your soul's
codes, as well as a new one about how to improve your golf game). But she
kept pronouncing it as if it were a four-word name—Dee Pack Cho Prah——
—somehow distracting me.

The most depressing result was with the food allergy test, which showed
that I was allergic to, well, about everything: wheat and most other grains,
anything made with corn syrup, milk, eggs, and many odd food groups—like

most so-called yellow vegetables (such as potatoes, squash, eggplant, and mushrooms).

Although the results looked hopeless, the doctor and his wife had a plan. They recommended that I consume a special liquid cleansing diet made of special protein powders. Each drum of the stuff cost a hundred dollars, and I could only buy the product from them. For eating between drinks, I could buy some snack bars. I pointed out that the snack bar they handed me had peanuts in it, prohibited by the food allergy tests. They said that one or two peanuts once in a while would be OK.

I left feeling confused, depressed, and fatigued, and I decided never to go back to these "doctors." But I still wasn't sure I had made the correct decision. Even in cases like this, where the treatments were expensive and seemingly irrational, I still doubted whether I was doing the right thing. What if there was a minute possibility that their toxin theories were correct? What if their recommendations could change my life? I had heard stories from acquaintances and accounts in books about this type of diet doing wonders, but I knew I didn't have the energy and finances to go through with it. Elizabeth reassured me that I was doing the right thing, that the reality was, for better or worse, that I wouldn't be able to find just "one thing" to cure me. As with the rest of her realistic advice, I was unnerved but then calmed down. Though I liked the idea of "one thing" to cure me, giving up on a single cure-all enabled me to ignore something over-the-top, like this liquid diet route.

Meanwhile, as I realized, with alternative medicine, the tables had turned. In the past, with Western medicine, the hidden subtext of the visit was the doctors wondering if I was crazy. Now, I was the one having these doubts about them.

11

Ayurvedic Medicine

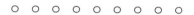

THEN I CONSIDERED AYURVEDIC MEDICINE, the ancient Indian art and discipline of healing, after reading about it in *Glamour Magazine*. Or maybe it was *Natural Health*.

But I couldn't work myself up to try it. I didn't quite understand what it was about, and I had no one personally recommending it to me. And I couldn't relate to any of the three body types or *doshas* described: the bony and mercurial Vata, the orderly but sweaty Pitta, or the lethargic, possessive Kapha. Plus, I learned that it may require purification through vomiting and enemas.

So that is all I have to say about ayurvedic medicine. Time to continue.

1 2

When in Doubt, Blame Milk

o o o o o o o o o

QUITE POSSIBLY, THE MEANEST PLACE ON EARTH is the parking lot of the Whole Foods grocery story on North Avenue in Chicago. This is no reflection on the kind folks who work at the store. I'm talking about the customers, in this upscale yuppie neighborhood of Lincoln Park.

Patience is not a virtue they have learned, despite years of psychotherapy, chakra cleansing, and toxin-purging ninety-five-degree Bikram yoga sessions. When organic food is involved, any semblance of midwestern politeness goes out the window. They want their authentic, multigrain, multitextured, gluten-free, wheat-free, nonhydrogenated foodstuffs, and they want them now.

This attitude is evident in the undersized parking lot, which seems to have been designed as a sadistic experiment in urban engineering. Creeping fearfully in your 1989 Mitsubishi Galant and dodging hurtling vehicles and shopping carts from all directions and at varying speeds, you feel as if you are trapped in the Atari "Asteroids" game you played so many years ago as a child. Watch out for the large black Hummer pulling out suddenly from its parking space without any sort of warning—and there, just as warlike, the large black Lexus SUV and large black Mercedes SUV (the one with the Greenpeace bumper sticker) about to ram head-on into each other, with you caught in between.

Finally, with no other choice, you leave the car off to the side of the road in front of a fire hydrant, with the blinkers on (a crafty move to trick police into thinking that you are not parking illegally). Despite your brisk pace as you walk through the aisles, other shoppers impatiently jam their carts into your ankles, bloodying them a bit. Once you reach the checkout counter, make sure to have your wits about you. This is a critical time. Don't swipe your credit card the wrong way and delay the transaction for a second, because all those people talking on their cell phone headsets behind you may revolt. They will pelt you with pine nuts, scorch you with espresso, and poke you with the toothpicks left from the sample display of aged Spanish Manchego sheeps' milk cheese.

When, at last, you exit the store and run toward your car, an errant hybrid Toyota Prius (next year's model) emerges at full speed from behind a corner. With maximum fuel efficiency, it drives clear over you, leaving your trembling body in the middle of the pickup lane. A fleet of other cars honk angrily as they proceed to run over you and, an even more tragic waste, your $150 bag of groceries. A stream of brownish-white soy milk now mingles with your blood on the pavement. Perhaps one pedestrian, while still seamlessly continuing her cell phone conversation, will have the compassion and grace to unfurl a rubber yoga mat over your now-flattened corpse and then drag your body over to the landscaped edge of the strip mall. There you will reach the apotheosis of your holistic journey, contributing with your body's rich compost to the welfare of our fragile ecosystem, continuing the magical circle of life.

Such a harrowing shopping trip was one of the many hazards I faced venturing into the extreme fringes of alternative medicine. It was a part of an escalating quest to live as healthfully as possible, even if I might die trying.

On this journey, every alternative doctor and healer I had visited in the past year or so had recommended a different class of foods to avoid and new exotic ones to incorporate. Each list of the forbidden was different, but all shared one imperative: When in doubt, avoid milk. My quest to keep up was all a part of a never-ending effort for such purity, which extended to even the most routine and minute areas of life, and which became more and more expensive.

The tests I had undergone with the suburban doctors had left some burning questions in my mind, mainly about food. I had heard stories, perhaps urban legends, about others who had odd health problems, who allegedly were cured when they just avoided certain foods. A lasting question in my mind at that time was whether I could find just one thing to cure the problem, as so many others apparently had.

Specifically, many people I met were suddenly asking me if I had food allergies, a concept now suddenly in vogue, although I had no overt signs of such a problem. I had known about their existence, but only in cases with obvious cause and effect. A person eats the wrong food, such as peanuts or shellfish—and boom! his or her throat swells up and chokes him or her. He or she could even go into some kind of a coma.

But given my new awareness of foods after the tests, I recognized I had experienced allergic symptoms after eating one food: eggs. After I ate them, I would feel strangely spacy and tired, such as after a Sunday brunch of an omelet or when I staggered around in the narrow stacks of the Northwestern Library, after stopping for a chicken sandwich with mayo at a drive-through just before. It wasn't anything life-threatening, but it was a sign to me that maybe these food allergy gurus were onto something. Perhaps their theory that these allergens weaken you over time and cause headaches had some truth to it. Perhaps I had to investigate this further.

For another opinion, I decided to see another holistic M.D. (read: insurance would cover it), whose office happened to be within walking distance of where I lived. I had heard her name from a few people over the years and knew that she was well respected. Following the address on the street, I was led, once again, to a nonoffice building. This was in a century-old apartment building. One buzzer had the name of the doctor and another had the name of her practice. Not thinking, I rang the first one repeatedly and got no response. Finally, I rang the second buzzer and was let in. I climbed the stairs and saw a pile of shoes; taking the cue, I took mine off as well.

This was a stately old apartment, the kind that is vast and kind of echoes and probably was designed to hold servants' quarters in the back. It was also the most sterile, toxin-free environment I had ever experienced. Many rooms featured large black HEPA air cleaners, and the long stretches of wooden floors gleamed. A receptionist stood behind a podium that was set up in the gap between the kitchen and living room. She looked forward, as if she was ready to deliver a speech to those few people sitting on the couch in front of her. She kindly reprimanded me for buzzing the doctor's home apartment, and then I took a seat in the living room. As an encouraging sign, the coffee table book that lay on a wicker platform was *Off the Pedestal* by Michael Greenberg, M.D., a book that criticizes the medical establishment.

I finally saw the doctor, who skimmed through the thick binder of test results I had brought. She asked me questions, mainly about toxins.

"Where did you live when this headache struck? In an old or a new building?"

"Well, I was living in a brand-new building just before it all happened," I answered.

"Aha," she said. "The paints, the building materials, all of those chemicals can have lasting side effects."

"But since then I have lived in very old apartments."

"Interesting," she said. "They have molds that can aggravate illness."

I was thinking about asking her what kinds of apartments do *not* make one sick, but before I could get it out, she handed me a photocopied page. It was from the Sharper Image catalog, showcasing a $600 HEPA air-filtering system. She strongly encouraged me to order it immediately. She also gave me another catalog, of a supply house that provided antiallergy products, including a $138 cotton mattress protector, that is, a large rubberized pillowcase-like covering for the entire mattress, to protect me from allergens lurking inside it. Along with the HEPA system, I also agreed to order special pillowcases and antiallergy cleaning solvents.

The bottom line was to avoid allergens of all kinds. She closed the booklet of my copious test results and said that most of the tests I had taken in the suburbs were useless, except for the one about food. That was real. She advised me to heed its findings, which she also did, basically living on grilled meat, potatoes, rice, and vegetables stir fried in olive oil. Since I was to avoid dairy, one tip was to use organic clarified butter with the milk solids removed (known as ghee in Indian cuisine) made by a company named Purity Farms. Soy sauce, with wheat, was out of the question, so I was to buy a substitute of "liquid aminos" by a company called Bragg.

Despite all this detail, I was still confused. What if I only had a small amount of a forbidden food, such as a dab of soy sauce? Was that alone enough to ruin the entire diet and incite the food allergies in full force and nullify all my previous hard work?

"Just stay away from everything listed," she answered, instructing me to get on the table for an acupuncture treatment. After that was done, she closed the door, turned off the light, and left me there in the dark. As I lay there, I heard her interactions with a few other patients in the adjoining thin-walled rooms. One of them had cancer. I vaguely made out the advice: Buy a HEPA filter and heed food allergy warnings.

Even though she was apparently giving one-size-fits-all advice to her patients, I still wanted to believe in the food part. So, soon after, I first set out across town to the brand-new Whole Foods store on North Avenue, then the only comprehensive local source of the new products recommended by her and others I had seen. And after I had further read books on my own on healthy cooking—such as the useful *The Self-Healing Cookbook* by Kristina Turner, my shopping list became even more extensive. This book, an apparent DIY effort that looked like it had been partly laid out with a typewriter and a ruler, and that resembled a very large ransom note or leftist-sponsored zine, was convincing. I stopped and stared in wonder when I came to the part that listed "recurring headaches" and "migraines" as a prime indication that the body was not in balance and was in an advanced state of disrepair.

In the past, I had wondered what losers used "wheat-free" products, and now I was one of them. I bought a $5 dense bricklike "sprouted bread" in the refrigerator case, a $6 box of wheat-free toaster pastries in the breakfast aisle, and a $7 bottle of tamari (fermented soy beans), another acceptable substitute for wheat-tinged soy sauce. To avoid corn, I stopped buying products made with corn syrup, which included about every processed sweet product at a conventional nonholistic supermarket. This required thinking about the smallest of details. I even got rid of cornstarch to use in cooking, such as with stir-fry thickening, and instead bought a small $8 bag of arrowroot powder. I picked up a handful of $9 bags of sea vegetables—hijiki, kombu, wakame— to be soaked with beans and vegetables for their nutrients and tenderizing qualities. I went to the bins and bought grains with names like quinoa, millet, and amaranth, which seemed so ancient that I supposed that even the pharaohs of Egypt had considered them outdated.

But even in the supposedly pristine Whole Foods store, I encountered myriad types of food I could not have. That sensuous aroma of coffee emanating from Aisle 3? Could I try that? No, the caffeine is bad and, besides, it weakens the liver. The organic fat-free yogurt? That's dairy, phlegm forming, slows down the *chi*. That succulent, shiny organic $5 red pepper from Holland? Nightshade vegetable. That's prohibited by a macrobiotic diet, for some reason. Millet bread? Hmm, it still lists wheat as an ingredient.

Suddenly, I had changed my view of what was "good" or desirable in food. Years before, when someone at a potluck told the group that the lasagna he had made "contained no cheese and no meat," I had half-jokingly asked, "What's the point?" Now I realized that this lack of "real" ingredients had been considered a virtue. And I was now playing along by eating foods that were simulations of others: tofu mayonnaise, a tempeh (fermented soy) cutlet, and twig tea. For a snack, I drank a $4 amasake shake, which resembled a milk shake but was really some kind of rice drink.

Making matters worse, I never knew if I was a fool doing this, if it was helping at all. The Headache's intensity fluctuated from week to week, but then again, it always had. Overall, it seemed to be at the same level. And it turns out that I was probably overdoing it. As I read much later, just in browsing a women's magazine in early 2004, only 40 percent of foods that come out positive on skin-prick allergy tests actually reflect an allergic reaction that will happen when the person eats that food. And although they may seem more "scientific," the blood tests for food allergies that I had taken are thought to be even less accurate than the more standard skin-prick tests. In both cases, tests overestimate allergies because of the highly concentrated nature of the tested foods, in contrast to how foods are consumed in real life.[1]

This is not to dismiss altogether the concept of allergies, which are actually common in chronic headache patients. In rare cases, allergies may be at the root of the problem, if an infection or a structural abnormality exists. Studies have shown that migraine patients—and to an even greater extent, chronic daily headache patients—are more likely to have allergic reactions of all kinds, whether food reactions, hay fever, or bronchitis.[2] But a distinction to make is that allergies are a recognized "comorbidity" with chronic headaches, exacerbating and coexisting with them, but not necessarily *causing* them.[3] And so this means that when approached with some caution and common sense, treating allergies makes sense, as they may exacerbate the existing pain.

These difficult questions about food allergies are an example of the great and endless confusion that exists in treating migraine: Which conditions cause it, and which ones merely coexist with or aggravate it? You may detect a health factor that truly exacerbates the pain, such as an allergy to eggs or to pollen, but that may not be the root cause of the headache. And the numbers of such exacerbating factors or triggers can be endless, providing an infinite source of material to investigate. Plus, you have to figure it all out for yourself because everyone has a different set of aggravating factors.

As I waited for the detoxifying effects of my new pure and virtuous diet to work their magic, I explored yet other options. Because I still felt like I was approaching my overall treatment too idiosyncratically and independently, I continued to pursue the idea of a "team" multidisciplinary approach. Without a comprehensive knowledge of which practitioners were available and who were the best ones, I was feeling my way in the dark. I was like a dog following a bone, just gravitating to anyone with a headache theory who happened to be in my path. I fantasized about someone to systematically coordinate the treatment from a variety of people, not leaving such selections up to me to cobble together randomly.

After my failed experience at the conventional pain clinic, I thought that perhaps the problem was that I needed to go to a center that was more *holistic* and into alternative medicine. Somewhere that would think more innovatively. As was my luck, the local New Age newspaper in Chicago, *Conscious*

Choice, ran a special feature on the new outcropping of such establishments. At that time, I told a friend and her husband about this concept. He related passing such a new center in suburban Evanston, with a sign in front saying it offered acupuncture, reikki, massage, and many other methods. The message he got was that the center should put up another sign: "Hell, we'll try anything."

Skepticism notwithstanding, I made an appointment at a very new holistic center on South Michigan Avenue, in an old skyscraper from the turn of the twentieth century. I walked into the office suite during the middle of the day and found I was the only patient. I quickly filled out some paperwork from the receptionist and went on to reading a *Conscious Choice*, which was laid out on the table. The receptionist then appeared to ask me about my insurance policyholder number, which apparently was not legible in my hurried handwriting. I took out my insurance card and said that I assumed she would make a photocopy of it, as other doctors had. She was oddly perturbed and insisted that her copying the number by hand was as simple as her photocopying the card. Finally, to convince me to give it to her, she admitted that the center had no copy machine.

I was to see an M.D. about my age who had recently graduated from medical school. He would coordinate the rest of my treatment in the center. As I was reading, I looked up and saw him peering at me from the hallway. It seemed that I was the only patient that day, and he had made a special trip in just to see me. He was the one waiting for me.

During that exam, as with that vibrator guy, I longed for the terse and brief sessions of the olden days with a busy neurologist. This doctor had nothing but time on his hands. He asked me every conceivable question about my health, most of which seemed irrelevant to pain and headaches. He even did a full physical, including a breast exam. I thought, "That's not where it hurts."

I left, never to return. Instead, I decided to try a more "established" holistic health center, Whole Health Inc. (not its real name)[4] in Lincoln Park, located inches from the Fullerton stop on the Red Line el stop and above the very unholistic and famous Demon Dogs stand. But my confusion about food allergies only intensified there, when the main coordinating M.D. told me that it wasn't a matter of avoiding foods. The solution was to buy a hundred-dollar collection of dietary supplements there, which would fix the problem.

Immediately, I recognized this place as a parody of the perils of combining supposedly more compassionate and natural alternative medicine with corporate pressures to earn a profit. This large center was obviously an expensive enterprise, newly refurbished in a spare Asian motif, with black-lacquered light fixtures and chairs, and employing dozens of staff members. The good part about an "interdisciplinary" center is that many types of doctors and therapists are available to offer their perspectives. The bad part is they all have to be paid, and the doctor seemed eager to sell products and fill up his colleagues' schedules, as well as his.

And so, in response to these financial pressures, this center strongly focused on publicity. Often I could hardly squeeze into the waiting room because of local television news cameras blocking the entrance. Prompted by the latest university study on a certain herb or vitamin, reporters had taken over the office. One week they interviewed the doctors on how vitamin E was the answer to everything; next week the miracle cure was St. John's wort.

Indeed, Whole Health Inc. never missed an opportunity to charge me, and when I left, I often felt like I had been grabbed by the soles of my Doc Martens and shaken up and down for loose change. The doctor told me he wanted to run another battery of costly tests. I told him I had probably covered everything possible between the Western and alternative doctors I had seen. Every bodily fluid had already been analyzed comprehensively. But he had a convincing reply, that I probably had never had these tests that he was thinking of, which included one for thyroid, which often was an underlying problem with "mysterious" women's ailments (and a comorbidity for chronic headache). And even if I had gotten such a test, those past results might no longer be accurate.

So I came back on a Saturday morning to see a technician, who made small talk with me as she fruitlessly poked about in my arm for a vein. Finally, I agreed to the alternate site on the side of the wrist. Then I fainted, or perhaps I had some kind of seizure, as I had passed out and was shaking on the ground. I then spent three hours in the back of the offices throwing up. The doctor said something about a reaction of the vagus nerve, which apparently is sensitive in younger women (perhaps explaining the "hysterical" fainting reported widely in Victorian times). When I finally felt well enough to leave, the receptionist ran out and stopped me at the front desk. The question: "Visa or Mastercard?" I was happy that at least they had the blood they needed.

That night, still feeling sick, I watched a movie on cable, *The Apprenticeship of Duddy Kravitz*, starring Richard Dreyfuss. Suddenly, at about the part where Duddy goes to work in the bourgeois resort town outside of Montreal, I noticed multiple odd red pinwheels spinning on the periphery of my vision. At last, I had lost my mind, I thought. But after a few minutes, I realized that for the first time, I was experiencing a migraine aura, which is expressed in the form of distorted vision and minor hallucinations, often in the form of geometric patterns and shapes. I lay down and felt a full-fledged migraine descend, with the pain a few levels more severe and gripping than normal. I felt like someone had reached into my head and was squeezing from the far left side to the middle. The more intense pain lasted less than a few hours, but the nausea and feeling of spaciness continued for another day.

That's what I get for going to a holistic center, I thought.

Nevertheless, I returned to the center for follow-up, wondering if they had the solution among their numerous caregivers. After my tests came back negative, through the next months the center's main doctor referred me to about every type of alternative healer that I had not yet seen. In a typical visit, he would fumble through my folder and then ask me the same litany of questions until he came to a method I had not tried.

"Have you tried acupuncture?"

"Yes."

"Cranial-sacral?"

"Yes."

"Massage?"

"Yes."

"A chiropractor?"

"Yes."

"How about a homeopath?"

"Well . . . no."

So, the following week, I started seeing the center's homeopath, who prescribed little white pellets named after their treating substances, such as belladonna and sulfur. However, in homeopathy, any poisons involved have been diluted to the extreme point where they are no longer poisons (and to where scientists would say they are just sugar pills). Some of the rationale behind this process is that the trace elements of substances (which may include poisons, plants, or minerals) may stimulate the body's natural healing processes, in the same way that some through the ages have used bee stings for pain relief. Different poisons set off different antibodies. Although this may seem zany, homeopathy has been popular in Europe for centuries. Even the alternative-medicine skeptic Wendy Kaminer admits in her 1999 book, *Sleeping with Extraterrestrials*, that she practices homeopathy regularly.

One time, I forgot to buy the vial of pellets at the center's store and went instead to an "apothecary," a long-established and charming German-style natural pharmacy in a nearby neighborhood. (With its full stock of European balms, tonics and lotions, it struck me as the kind of place that Eva Braun would have visited after completing her morning calisthenics.) The man behind the counter asked the name of the remedy, and I pulled out a piece of paper from the doctor. He said he recognized the handwriting as that of a long-lost employee of the store. In other words, I was paying $90 an hour for advice that I would have gotten for free at a good health food store, from someone not necessarily wearing a white doctor's smock. I gave him the $5.50 for the vial.

13

The Tired Girls

○ ○ ○ ○ ○ ○ ○ ○ ○

Women, Pain, and Fatigue

I WAS NEVER SURE IF THE HOMEOPATHY WORKED—the pain was still ever-present—and soon discontinued it. But still seeking relief, I became more encouraged when the well-known holistic doctor at Whole Health, Inc. made an entirely different diagnosis of my problem. He pressed down on a sore spot on the top of my thigh, which I had barely noticed. (In any case, I never would have mentioned it because the head pain upstaged every other complaint, and this one was very minor.) When I agreed it was sore, he looked buoyant. He said that was one of the eighteen "tender spots" used to diagnose fibromyalgia, a chronic, widespread musculoskeletal pain disorder that also causes fatigue. He proceeded to press on the rest of the tender points. They were all sore to the touch, and he informed me that this response was very unlikely in someone *without* fibromyalgia.

Under "diagnosis" on the medical form, he wrote "fibromyalgia." And I was strangely relieved to get this label, any label, in fact. If I had a name for what I had, then it must be real. (At that time, I didn't know about "chronic daily headache"—and "tension headache" and "migraine" really never accurately covered me.) I went home to call a friend to tell her the good news, and before I could speak she said, "Let me guess. He sat down and pressed on your thigh. Then he pressed on all eighteen points. Then he had you buy the fibromyalgia supplements and the book *From Fatigued to Fantastic*."

"Uh, yes," I said. I added that after his diagnosis, he had prescribed the muscle relaxant Flexeril, which just made me fall asleep everywhere that I went that involved sitting down—at friends' houses, in movies, and in restaurants.

She discussed her similar diagnosis, complaining that her working-class mother from Grand Rapids didn't understand it, repeatedly calling it "fibro-Malaysia."

A few months later, I met another patient of that same doctor through friends. Before she could tell me more, I predicted the same thing, that the doctor had told her that she had fibromyalgia and had her buy the same stash of useless products. She was amazed by my intuitiveness, just as I had been by my friend's.

Given the number of people I'd met diagnosed with the disease by the same doctor, I was skeptical that fibromyalgia even existed. I suspected it was an all-purpose nonsensical classification for those problem patients whom doctors couldn't cure. But years later, while doing research for this book, I changed my mind. Journals I read described fibromyalgia as a "comorbidity" with chronic headaches and migraines—meaning that the same neurological abnormalities behind headache also could lead to more diffuse pain across the body and fatigue. Although fibromyalgia was once thought to result from muscle malfunction (just as tension headaches were, having been called *muscle contraction headaches*), researchers now also generally characterize fibromyalgia as neurological.

Indeed, fatigue—a hallmark of fibromyalgia—is a common companion of those who suffer chronic headaches, thought to affect 70 percent of migraine patients.[1] Although the causes of such fatigue are not adequately known, fibromyalgia has been specifically implicated in many cases. In one study of 101 chronic daily headache patients, one-third were diagnosed with fibromyalgia.[2] Like chronic daily headache, fibromyalgia is thought to be experienced by about 4 percent of the population, with an even greater percentage—90 percent of the patients—being women.

Likewise, other disorders involving fatigue often overlap with headaches, further indicating common brain chemistry imbalances. As experts in all these areas are now noting, head pain is a common complaint of those with depression, fibromyalgia, and chronic fatigue syndrome. Some researchers even think that fibromyalgia and chronic fatigue and immune deficiency syndrome (CFIDS) are really the same ailments, but with fibromyalgia patients having more pain and CFIDS patients reporting more fever-type symptoms, such as sore throats, swollen lymph glands, and low-grade fevers. They are both classified as "syndromes," as opposed to diseases, without (as yet) a clearly defined cause or course of treatment.

In fact, headache is one of the eight symptoms listed in the international classification for chronic fatigue syndrome. CFIDS patients and migraine

patients also commonly report the same seemingly quirky neurological experience of cutaneous allodynia (CA), characterized by increased scalp sensitivity, which can make even hair brushing and wearing earrings painful. (This is
theorized to be the observable result of the same neurological dysfunction
deep in the brain, central sensitization.) In fact, indicating the importance of
headache in these patients, the topic of headaches was the cover story in a
recent issue of the official CFIDS newsletter.[3]

Although I was wary about my fibromyalgia diagnosis, I did notice parallels
between my experience and that of other women with other invisible and
fatigue-related problems. Like those with chronic fatigue or fibromyalgia, I
seemed to "pay" for everything I did, such as with having to crash the next
day. They also shared my fixation with a limited number of marbles (energy
reserve units) and worked diligently to ration them wisely.

Other patterns slowly emerged. We were all likely to first get these problems in our teens or twenties, often with the trigger of a major stressful event,
which sent us over the edge. We feared rainy weather. None of us were morning people—and sometimes we were not even day or night people.

I started slowly meeting these women and didn't feel quite so alone.

I called them the Tired Girls.

Like me, they were private about their problems, which were poorly
understood and diagnosed by science. Medical professionals—and the public
at large—dismissed their problems as mere "women's complaints." Instead of
fearing that they were "hysterical" because of media hype about their illnesses or some kind of subconscious cry for attention, I saw the opposite: Like
me, they were usually isolated with and shamed by their problems and worried that they were the only ones with them.

Only later, while reading medical literature, I learned to recognize these
problems as one related "women's issue." Chronic fatigue, fibromyalgia, vulvodynia, irritable bowel syndrome—they all have to do with central sensitization. Even though I have been a writer on feminist issues for almost twenty
years, I myself have been slow to identify chronic pain as one of them. I only
very recently have realized that women are more likely to have some of the
same root imbalances in brain chemistry, that make us more prone to such
problems of pain and fatigue, as well as depression. This discovery has also
spurred me to investigate with a whole new lens feminist activist history,
which has long neglected issues of women's pain and fatigue. I now better
understand—and ultimately question—why these topics have been very controversial and have even been seen as roadblocks in the advancement of the
cause of women's rights for more than a century.

Pain as a Women's Issue: Let's Do the Numbers

Only as a researcher working on this book, and not as a patient, have I recognized the magnitude of chronic pain as a long-neglected "women's issue" (although men also are certainly affected by chronic pain). Today, with a little digging, much new scientific information is available to justify this political and medical focus on women:

- In general, women are much more susceptible to chronic pain disorders of all types, constituting a majority of those reporting chronic pain across cultures.[4]

- Women are more likely to report multiple pain sites, intense pain, and frequent pain.[5]

- In addition, women are more likely to have other disorders involving pain and fatigue, including 6 times the rate for men of fibromyalgia.

- About 18 percent of women experience migraine, compared to 6 percent of men. (However, until puberty, the rates of headaches in boys and girls are about even, with boys experiencing slightly more by some accounts.)

- Up to one-third of women between the ages of twenty-five and fifty-five have migraine.

- Like migraine, chronic daily headache is an overwhelmingly female disorder, also typically striking in the reproductive years; doctors estimate it as affecting 10 percent of women over thirty.

- Women are about 50 percent more likely than men to have temporomandibular joint disorders, also known as TMJ, or jaw pain, experienced by 4–12 percent of the population.

- Women are twice as likely as men to suffer from irritable bowel syndrome, experienced by 15–20 percent of the population. (Pain is one aspect of this syndrome, with bowel problems being mainly limiting.)

- They are 2.5 times more likely than men to have rheumatoid arthritis, an autoimmune disorder of 1 percent of the population.

- They are 0.5 to 4 times more likely than men to have osteoarthritis, a disorder typically striking up to 80 percent of the population after age sixty-five.

- And they are 9 times more likely to develop interstitial cystitis, a chronic and often painful inflammation of the bladder, affecting about 0.5 percent of the population.[6]

Of course, these chronic pain disorders, and their relatively high reported rates in women, are not just genetic in origin. They can all be influenced by social and psychological factors. Studies have shown that women may have more "permission" to express their pain and seek treatment, without the pressure to be "manly." Women are more likely to suffer from depression, which can aggravate and often coexist with chronic pain, as a part of the same imbalance of serotonin and other neurotransmitters. Women experience special challenges just because they are women, such as being burdened as single mothers and having to take on multiple roles (and before that, they had the stress of *not* being allowed to take on multiple roles). Their particular occupations, such as factory workers and secretaries, may put them at risk of certain types of repetitive stress disorders.[7] And ironically, even when they may feel more pain biologically, they may still react to it with more "skill" than a man, as they have been shown to have greater coping strategies, such as with expressing feelings and seeking emotional support.[8]

However, studies have also shown that women are biologically more sensitive to pain signals. Though clinical results are mixed and often show minor differences, women generally report more severe levels of pain, more frequent pain, and pain of longer duration than men. The most obvious—and studied—factor is female reproductive hormones, which can influence chemicals that determine pain perception, including the neurotransmitters serotonin and norepinephrine, and the "beta-endorphin systems," or the brain's natural painkillers. "It is hard to imagine any disorder more affected by the female reproductive cycle (spanning the life of women from their early teens to after menopause) than headache, and in particular, migraine," wrote Dr. Leslie Kelman in the journal *Headache* in January 2004.

Hormones are thought to be a factor in creating women's greater overall incidence of central sensitization, of the brain becoming more sensitized to pain signals over time. At the same time, hormones affect blood vessel reactivity, a major source of head pain. (Backing up this claim is one recent study published in the journal *Neurology* about male-to-female transsexuals getting significantly more migraines—at a rate of 26 percent surveyed—after hormone therapy.[9])

In fact, "migraine is a factor in every hormonal event" in a woman's life span, said Dr. Vincent T. Martin, codirector of the Cincinnati Headache Center and professor of clinical medicine, in an interview. I spoke to him at the 2003 meeting of the American Headache Society. He explained that migraines typically come on at puberty with menstruation, subside in the last two trimesters of pregnancy, and then often taper off with menopause.

(Hormone fluctuation has also been found to exacerbate fibromyalgia and irritable bowel syndrome, among others.)[10]

But hormones don't entirely account for women's greater incidence of chronic pain. Other parts of women's biology may be vulnerable. This is simply revealed by the fact that women continue to have more migraines than men after menopause, even past the age of seventy.[11] (In fact, chronic headaches are experienced by 14 percent of postmenopausal women.)[12]

Some established pain researchers describe structural differences in the brain that may help determine how strongly pain signals are felt.[13] Women's immune systems also differ and may be an influence, as autoimmune disorders strike about three times as many women as men. Researchers are looking at the eighty autoimmune disorders—including rheumatoid arthritis, multiple sclerosis, lupus, and Graves' disease (which affects the thyroid)—as part of the same phenomenon of the body attacking itself, often resulting in fatigue and pain. They have also seen autoimmune disorders as "comorbid" or more likely to coexist with headaches than in others in the population, indicating a common underlying mechanism.[14]

Through the years, one Tired Girl after another came out to me in separate situations, making me realize the large numbers all around me. In fact, about everyone has a Tired Girl in his or her family, even without knowing it. I had thought I was a freak, but I was actually part of a huge closeted group, one which I wouldn't have noticed if I hadn't been in a similar situation. And in many cases, despite some signs and foreshadowing, I was very surprised to hear that these people also were living secret lives. In turn, I became offended when I heard others talk negatively about them (who didn't realize I was also a Tired Girl): "Oh, with her, it's always something." They would assume that if someone had multiple problems, then *all* were false—whereas the underlying brain chemistry of one disorder, in fact, indicates the reverse, that is, higher vulnerability to other problems.

Here are some examples of those Tired Girls I began to meet at that time, who reported similar behind-the-scenes struggles with work, relationships, and doctors—all made easier with a sense of humor:

- Instead of Tired Girls, I thought that perhaps I should call them Under the Desk Girls, after I ran into Jane, the sister of a friend, at the acupuncturist's office. She had been diagnosed with a form of multiple sclerosis (MS) years before. But she said she still struggled to hold onto her full-time job, as a graphic designer at a textbook publisher. No one in her office knew about her MS. But she did get relief when the company laid off dozens of workers on the floor above her and moved her there, to work alone. She had the luxury of sleeping or resting under her desk, undetected, as long as she was able to complete her workload.

- Tracy, also a few years older than I was, had what felt like a form of MS, with blurred vision, dizziness, numbness in the extremities, and fatigue—but she did not neatly fit that diagnosis. And that was a major problem in her life, almost as much as the illness itself, as her parents and others thought she was just being dramatic. "I show all the signs of someone who had a stroke, and sometimes I wish I had had one," she told me. "Then people would take me seriously." She still dated lots and lots, with her good looks and sense of humor well intact. But as with the rest of us, this effort was sometimes a comedy of errors. As with many sufferers of chronic fatigue, she had multiple chemical sensitivities and commonly had to mysteriously ask her date to move tables several times in one evening, perhaps when a smoker came too close. When she told one guy what the real reason was, he said he couldn't see her, as his last girlfriend had been a Tired Girl and he was tired of always feeling as if he was "mending the wings of a broken bird."

- I met Rivka on a Listserv for women writers. She was a well-known author, but still struggling to get by on $575 a month in disability payments for her chronic fatigue. ("But really, what does it matter what I have?" she asked me, as we were discussing her specific diagnosis. "They can't cure it anyway.") Luckily, she lived rent-free in her mother's old house. Like the others, she did not let her illness keep her from dating. But she acted in what seemed like an odd manner in not wanting to waste any time, taking any date very seriously, with no marbles to spare. Noting that she was too fatigued to function on the day after a date, she asked a guy on the second date, "Where is this heading," and scared him away. But the last I checked, she had found a new boyfriend. This time the illness wasn't an issue. "We're fine, as long as we stay in bed all the time," she explained.

- I bonded with another Tired Girl, Wendy, who had just moved to Chicago. She also had severe migraines, which were just one of her worries. I knew she had been institutionalized for a nervous breakdown sometime during her first marriage, which happened when she went on Prozac, which probably triggered a manic episode. While there, she kept up her spirits and managed to organize her Princeton class reunion. She also suffered from eating disorders and helped me understand their seriousness. In the past, these things would have been red flags. I now saw these "weaknesses" as a sign that she was someone I could relate to.

- I was getting more interested in the world of Chicago theater and went to a meeting of a women's playwriting group at the apartment of a former advertising executive, Marge. When I asked why she couldn't attend an event, she confided that she had chronic fatigue and was on disability and could not leave her apartment. Years later, she had a play produced and managed to see it only on opening night, telling reporters she had "a form of arthritis" to explain her absence from rehearsals. Afterward, she slept for days.

- While doing research for my sex book, I had stayed with another Tired Girl in DC. A friend had put us in touch. When she moved to Chicago to take a teaching job at a private grade school, she looked me up, although many years had passed. After a few minutes of small talk, she told me why: "I went on a new drug for my epilepsy and gained fifty pounds. The entire time, I was thinking, 'This is what Paula was talking about.' I had to get in touch with you to tell you." We commiserated, and she told me that she was going through a very difficult time, being fired after taking too much time off work for sick leave. Her epilepsy had worsened, and she was constantly fatigued. Just talking on the phone to me now was consuming much of her energy for the day. I was surprised at this limited marble level, as I had just considered epilepsy a problem people deal with episodically, during attacks—which I'm sure many people also assume is always the case with headache sufferers, forgetting the weakness it often creates. She was in the process of suing her school, a lawsuit she eventually won. We shared drug stories, realizing we had been on almost all the same antiseizure medicines (also used for headaches), complaining about how dumb they made us. "Yeah, when I'm on those drugs, it's hard for me to even read magazines at the health club. Even sometimes *Entertainment Weekly* is too much, with its ironic references. I stick to something easy, like *Us*, with paragraph-long articles. That's about at my level," she said.

- But some Tired Girls can be more annoying, even to other Tired Girls. I went to a "state of the women's movement" conference at a university and was picked up at the airport with a few other speakers. One, who was in a wheelchair and was an activist on behalf of people with chron-

ic fatigue syndrome, monopolized the conversation in one long monologue. At one point, the organizer of the conference interrupted to ask
us to come to the event early the next morning, although we both
weren't speaking until later. The chronic fatigue activist declined, basically saying that she was saving her marbles. I chimed in that this was
the case with me, that I had chronic pain—feeling liberated, as this was
the first time I had "come out" professionally. The organizer, while driving the car, rolled her eyes, as if to say, "How could I be so unlucky as to
end up with such lazy neurotic freaks?" But even I was annoyed with
the activist, hearing her complain nonstop for days about her illness:
every pain, every blood test she'd had, the state of every bodily function,
every anti-chronic-fatigue "debunker." I had wanted people to "come
out" with such stigmatized illnesses, and, unfortunately, I got my wish.
But probably the greatest reason for my annoyance was wondering if *I*
personally was *that* irritating and tedious to be around.

- Less off-putting was another Tired Girl, whom I never would have suspected of being a part of those ranks. In 1997, I moved again, after my
old landlord did not renew my lease because he wanted to occupy that
apartment himself. I met and exchanged pleasantries with my neighbor,
Carol, a very fit and charismatic fifty-something blond receptionist, who
was a former actor in local theater. At about that time, I got a newsletter
from Whole Health Inc. Inside was a very personal profile of her as a
success story. She had been worn down to a nonfunctional state by
years of severe alcoholism, prompted by the death of her husband. The
newsletter story told how she had worked to get herself better: with tai
chi, spirituality, a new diet, and, of course, plenty of supplements. I was
surprised by all she had been through, as she was one of the most functional people I had met, with a life chock-full of volunteer work and
socializing. One day, I told her I had seen her in the newsletter and said
I was going to the same place for chronic pain issues. Probably out of a
bit of embarrassment, she hesitated and then invited me in to talk. We
started to look out for each other. When she went on vacation, I watered
the multiple rows of thriving plants in her apartment, noticing all the
twelve-step affirmations all around: "You are a spiritual being having a
human experience," read the flyer on the refrigerator. In the past, I
would have dismissed such clichéd advice as pabulum. I thought how
I regretted that my list of things to make fun of was growing shorter by
the day.

- I was most surprised—and heartbroken—realizing the secret health challenges of another Tired Girl, Gina, a legal secretary who had worked for me on the side as a typist for many years (and transcribed all the interviews done for this book). Always very reliable and conscientious and bright-eyed—with long black hair—she reminded me of myself when I was her age, in my mid-twenties. I appreciated that she seemed so responsible, letting her elderly grandmother live with her. Like me, she occasionally seemed a bit anxious. Sometimes, after I sent her tapes to transcribe, she would call me with great concern if there was just a little more work than estimated. I would reassure her that in that case, I would extend the deadline. No problem. Finally, after yet another such exchange, she said she had to get something out in the open. "I have limited energy because I have fibromyalgia," she said. "This is why I have to make absolutely sure I never overcommit." She explained that her intense widespread physical pain and fatigue had started several years earlier, after her father, to whom she had been very close, had died from MS. She admitted that the reason she lived with her grandma was not to take care of her; the situation was the reverse. "I come home from work every day and just collapse, with pain all over my body," she explained. "My gram cooks for me, cleans for me, does my laundry. I rely on her for everything."

Although chronic pain (and fatigue) is clearly a women's issue, activism has been slow to address it, to build awareness and tap money for research. Ironically, the women's health movement (a separate branch of feminism that emerged in the 1970s) generally has been apathetic, if not resistant, to the issue of pain and fatigue. In their efforts to counter enemies portraying women as essentially "hysterical," feminist thinkers have gone too far to the opposite extreme in denying chronic pain's reality, portraying it as mainly a tool of propaganda against us, a social construct. No wonder the Tired Girls of today still find it hard to "come out," partly because of the legacy of these deep-rooted political fears.

After all, we have been fighting the idea of women as "the weaker sex" for centuries. This view of women as biologically inferior, and hence inferior overall, has been used against us to justify widespread discrimination in everything from voting rights to attending college and being able to work in "male" careers. So, instead of addressing women's chronic pain as biologically based, many feminist intellectuals continue to support a seemingly more "enlightened" view: Chronic pain and fatigue are the result of patriarchy (and maybe American capitalism and globalism, too). This view incorporates the Freudian concept that women's professed chronic pain represents "subconscious political resistance." Along these lines, the women's health movement has addressed pain created or magnified by sexism, such as from domestic violence, sexual abuse, and menial backbreaking and/or repetitive jobs. Although social pressures certainly play a part in the development and exacerbation of chronic pain, the overall denial of chronic pain as also being biological has taken its toll on these patients (the majority of whom are women)—in further isolating us and discouraging medical treatment.

After all, to acknowledge the truth that women are biologically more prone to pain disorders, one would risk sounding as condescending as the famously paternalistic Dr. Silas Weir Mitchell, the influential pain doctor and strenuous opponent of admitting women to higher education. In a notorious observation from his nineteenth-century "classic" book-length essay, *Doctor and Patient*, he blamed women's greater levels of pain on their "thinner blood":

> As I look from my window, on the lawn below are girls at play,—gay, vigorous, wholesome; they laugh, they run, and are never weary. How far from them and their abounding health, seem the possibilities of such torment as nature somewhere in life reserves for most of us. As women, their lives are likely, nay, certain, to bring them a variety of physical discomforts, and perhaps pain in its gravest forms. For men, pain is accidental, and depends much on the chances of life. (83)

Yes, he was saying basically the same thing that I am, that women are more vulnerable to developing chronic pain. (But instead of because of thinner blood, I talk in terms of neurology.) Indeed, through at least the past century, any feminist making such a statement would be controversial—seeming to share a platform with the staunchest adversaries of women's rights. But instead of using such information to limit women, I argue the importance of discussing "weaknesses," in order to address them and then move on.

In response to their most virulent enemies through time, during the "Second Wave" of feminism in the 1970s, feminists generally denied women's greater physical pain was at all biologically based. Much of the focus of the women's health movement of the 1970s was gynecology, focusing on how women's bodies are essentially healthy and how childbirth is a natural process. Activists argued how doctors had needlessly "medicalized" it, making it into a type of pathological problem that had to be heavily mediated and controlled. (As a result, women's experiences of childbirth have been

Neurology Versus "The New Woman"

Discussing women's weaknesses has long been controversial. During the first wave of American feminism in the late nineteenth century, activists protested the label of *hysteria* as totally lacking in biological merit, as being used to keep intellectual and ambitious women "in their place." Even today, scholars take note of the power that medical "science" had during that time to combat women's rights; women attending college was a major source of concern. Writing in the magazine the *New Statesman* in 2000 about female intellectuals, author Karen Armstrong recalled the threats to women when universities in Great Britain first opened their doors to them in the 1800s. She cited one of many protest letters to Emily Davis, the founder of Girton College (the first college established for women, at Cambridge University, in 1869) about women's neurological differences: "[Women's] brains are light, their foreheads too small, their reasoning powers too defective, their emotions too easily worked upon to make good students."

In her 1985 book *The Female Malady*, feminist Princeton professor Elaine Showalter convincingly documented cases in which progressives—identified as "New Women"—were condemned to insane asylums. She demonstrated that this was a real method of political control of women activists and intellectuals in the late nineteenth and early twentieth centuries. She also gave accounts of women claiming to be sick, or being driven to it, as the only socially acceptable way to "break down" and escape insufferable responsibilities and circumstances. It's a logical reaction to an impossible situation.

Backing up that case is literature of that time by women like activist Charlotte Perkins Gilman. In Gilman's 1892 story "The Yellow Wallpaper," a woman who has recently given birth hallucinates from her forced "sick bed." With symbolism that is not very hard to interpret, she reports seeing another woman being stifled behind the wallpaper, "just as if she wanted to get out." In response to her unhappiness, her doctor husband blames "hysterical tendencies" and points to the lack of visible physical illness as proof. "He knows that there is no reason to suffer, and that satisfies him," she says.

revolutionized because they have much more say in the process, including the types of anesthetics taken.) In fact, the two main issues addressed by the women's health movement have been reproductive rights and eating disorders. Both of these are clearly affected by expectations of and limitations imposed by society at large. In the 1970s, women's sports, which emphasized women's physical vigor, were also central to politics. One of the high points of feminism at that time was the highly promoted tennis match between Bobby Riggs and Billie Jean King. The fact that King won was a major victory for the movement, to prove that women are not "inferior," as had been assumed.

At that time, when women were trying to enter traditionally male careers and universities, bringing up their invisible chronic illnesses, to say the least, would have seemed to be counterproductive. Then, activists were denying that hormones, often used to belittle women, had a role in making them less reliable. They also argued against the reality of women's more common experiences of having multiple types of pain, which sounded a little too much like the psychosomatic "somatization disorder," that had also been used to put women down in the past. They also were not eager to acknowledge that women were in any way neurologically different, as that also had been an excuse to keep them subservient. Tying all these efforts together, a famous dictum of the women's movement, denying that biology is destiny, came from writer Simone de Beauvoir in the 1952 *The Second Sex:* "One is not born a woman but rather becomes one." In other words, the "take home" message of the women's movement of the 1970s was "I am woman, hear me roar," not "I am woman hear me kvetch."

An example of how women's "weaknesses" were addressed in the 1970s, and still continue to be seen today within the feminist movement, is Phyllis Chesler's classic 1972 best-seller *Women and Madness,* which portrays such conflicts as subconscious political "resistance" against the patriarchy. At the time, this was a revolutionary and empowering argument, defending the allegedly misfit and "odd" behavior of women who challenged traditional roles and fought for social change.

Literature specifically on women and chronic pain was very sparse in the 1970s and 1980s. One of the rare articles was Dorothea Z. Lack's 1982 essay "Women and Pain: Another Feminist Issue," in the journal *Women and Therapy.* Like other feminists at that time, Lack did not address pain as more common in women. Instead she critiqued how women are mistreated as pain patients. Her arguments still apply today. For example, she noted differences in the terminology used in the medical records of female and male patients. In the typical female patient's record, she found, observations about chronic pain were often fixed on marital status, appearance, and sexual attractiveness. Further, a doctor might say a woman patient "claimed" to have pain, while stating that a male patient was "experiencing" pain.

Although they had the best intentions, some feminists in the 1970s and 1980s acted as adversaries of women pain patients, denying their realities as valid. I have noticed this only after experiencing pain myself, when I have recently reread authors I had previously never questioned. For example, one of my most dog-eared books is the 1978 *For Her Own Good: 150 Years of Doctors' Medical Advice to Women*, by pioneers in the women's health movement Barbara Ehrenreich and Deirdre English. They critiqued the medical system and its treatment of women. Central to this book is a description of the real meaning of women's "hysteria" from the nineteenth century as a form of social protest or resistance. The description starts with accounts of some of the most prominent figures of that time, including Jane Addams, Margaret Sanger, and Charlotte Perkins Gilman, who all fell mysteriously ill in their twenties. Ehrenreich and English confidently described this illness as the subconscious reaction of these ambitious and talented women to recognizing the limits on their opportunities. Although discrimination may have been a contributing factor, it is also true that disorders of pain and fatigue typically first occur when women are in their twenties.

I also question a similar interpretation in an equally provocative 1982 volume, *The Female Malady* by Freudian Elaine Showalter. In fact, she portrayed the basic elements of "hysteria," such as pain and weakness, as purely cultural in nature. She even explained the phenomenon of male "hysteria" experienced by numerous soldiers returning from World War I as a subconscious expression of their "female" selves, which had been suppressed during the extremely "manly" experience of war. At the end, she was even doubtful about the validity of the medical label of *depression*, which was gathering steam in the early 1980s, and which she also saw as a way to clinically classify (and dismiss) the results of women's oppression.

With the publication of her controversial 1997 book *Hystories,* Showalter went on to "debunk" the label of "chronic fatigue syndrome," blaming it on "*fin de siècle* anxiety" (4) and media hype, classifying it in the same dubious category as UFO sightings and "Satanic ritual abuse." Ironically, this feminist critic, whose ideas about sickness as a cultural expression were invigorating and validating in the 1980s, acts today as one of the greatest adversaries of those with chronic fatigue syndrome, who are mainly women. In contrast, I have always seen the purpose of feminism as voicing women's truths, not prescribing what they should and should not feel, as we have faulted our enemies with doing for centuries. The same argument that seemed validating to "healthy," ambitious women twenty-five years ago—to women not having biologically rooted chronic pain—seems invalidating to women suffering real and disabling invisible health problems today.

Today, as a member of the next generation (the "Third Wave" of feminism), I naturally have fewer doubts in openly addressing this oddly controversial issue of women's pain and fatigue. I don't fear weakening women's political case for equality with this topic. One reason is that we are at a more advantaged point, forty years after the start of the modern-day women's movement, when women found themselves in a much more vulnerable political position to prove themselves equals. Still, I understand the greater sensitiveness of the political climate back then. After all, to go from a second-class to a first-class citizen, one must emphasize strengths, not weaknesses. An activist faces limits in being able to tell people only what they are ready to hear.

In her 1996 book *The Rejected Body*, chronic fatigue sufferer and feminist professor Susan Wendell sought to bring long-overdue attention to these biological weaknesses, what she called the "rejected" or the "negative" aspects of the body, to finally address them adequately. "One thing is clear," she wrote. "We cannot speak only of reducing our alienation from our bodies, becoming more aware of them, and celebrating strengths and pleasures; we must also talk about how to live with the suffering body, with that which cannot be noticed without pain, and that which cannot be celebrated without ambivalence" (179).

She commented that her greatest struggle with chronic fatigue syndrome was with her own guilt about her limits, which went against how she had defined being an activist since the 1970s: "Adding to the difficulty, the subculture of feminists of my generation is one of self-sacrifice. Good feminists, like good women everywhere, are supposed to give 'til it hurts: everyone is supposed to feel exhausted and overworked, so why should I be the exception? 'We' don't have time to be ill, to coddle ourselves" (4).

But today, thanks to the contribution of earlier activists, we've already proven ourselves, that we can indeed compete with the guys. This is true in the case of other women's issues, such as in younger generations of women (or at least the more affluent ones) now feeling more secure to request family leave or to leave a job to raise a family. We also have more permission to talk about depression during or after pregnancy, which affects 10–15 percent of mothers. And we are less defensive about addressing PMS, which is suffered by 40–50 percent of women, and even PMDD (premenstrual dysphoric disorder), a more intense form of it, experienced by an estimated 3–10 percent of women. (Both are associated with high rates of migraine and have been

used as excuses to prove women's supposed unreliability.) And not incidentally, we have the benefit of very recent biological research on women and pain,
which actually didn't gain momentum until the late 1990s, after women had
at last been included as subjects in drug research (as a result of feminist
activism).

A valid remaining challenge to medical research on these problems may be
activist suspicion of pharmaceutical companies. This trepidation justifiably
lingers from the 1970s, a time when activists exposed the fact that the original birth control pill had been poorly tested before going on the market and
was overly potent. With this history in mind, feminist activists have been justifiably suspicious of supposedly "new" terms for old problems. A common
current feminist argument, for example, against brand-new drugs for the
newly coined "female sexual dysfunction" is that they encourage women to
deny the problem's social roots—for example, an abusive relationship. Many
feminists are arguing that such medication discourages questions about why
a woman *really* isn't turned on. Today, "chronic daily headache" may also
sound to many like a marketing ploy used to medically classify a woman's natural experience as "sick."

But I am not comparing the disabling chronic daily headache problem to
those other new "diseases" that have been coined and promoted largely to sell
products, like deodorant for "Body Odor" or mouthwash for "Halitosis."
Instead, I relate fighting chronic pain to feminists' fighting against other realities they have dared to name, such as sexual harassment and sexual abuse.
In the beginning, these struggles also sounded highly suspect, and even
absurd, to the greater society. Feminists were daring to name problems that
had previously been accepted as "just life," as Gloria Steinem has quipped.
Although a new name for an old problem may raise red flags of suspicion, we
have to realize that in every era, the naming and classification of diseases has
been political and will only continue to be so.

Another basic response of mine to feminist fears of women coming out
about pain is to acknowledge the great variation among us. Just being a
woman is by no means an indicator that one will be tortured by chronic pain;
in fact, more variation is present among individual women than between
women and men as a whole. "Quantitative differences between sexes are
smaller than differences within each sex," noted Dr. Roger Fillingim, a noted
scholar on gender and pain, in a presentation at the annual American Pain
Society medical meeting in Chicago in 2003. I add that I know about this
variation well, as I have somewhat of a stuttering problem, which is typically
known as a "male" affliction.

Is It Just a "Sexual Hang-Up": The Confusion over Abuse

One long-held stereotype that women pain patients face is that their pain is "all a result of abuse." The risk, when this view becomes the operating assumption, is that *all* women with chronic pain have been victims of abuse, especially sexual abuse. The resulting danger is withholding medical treatment and instead recommending only psychotherapy. A belittling attitude also often results that says this is just "a sexual hang-up," creating guilt for the patient.

But reality is more complicated. The connection between abuse and pain relates to both psychology and neurology. Indeed, our neurochemistry can be shaped by traumatic life events. As brain researchers have documented, abuse can definitely make pain worse or trigger its onset. And this issue is very significant because abuse does happens to a great number of women, with one in four reporting it in her history.

The effects seem clear. Many studies show that female patients who have been abused as children, or who report current abuse, report more frequent and severe pain. And they also show that women with more constant head pain are more likely than episodic migraine sufferers to report abuse in their history. This effect has also been studied with face pain, fibromyalgia, and TMJ disorders.[15]

The reason for this link between abuse and pain seems to be genetic. In general, women are more wired than men to have their nervous systems put out of whack by traumatic experiences. (But men do also experience this, especially when they have had periods of sustained trauma, such as returning from war "shell shocked" or with posttraumatic stress disorder.)

Another often-glossed-over point in this discussion is that doctors and therapists have tended to single out "sexual abuse" above all other kinds of abuse as triggering pain. But in contrast to Freudian dogma through the past century, the act of sex itself does not have any special connection to pain; women's genitals and brains are not embroiled in a special mystical battle with each other. In reality, any type of trauma, especially in childhood as the brain is developing, can cause this neurological reaction. Someone who suffers a severe ongoing trauma (whether it is related to sexual abuse or not) basically becomes at risk by being in "fight or flight" mode for long periods of time, always anxious about another attack and unable to "relax" and let down her or his guard.

When discussing this issue of abuse, more conscientious researchers go beyond sexual abuse and also study the possible involvement of emotional and nonsexual physical abuse and parental alcoholism.[16] And doctors and therapists should make the topic of abuse a priority in their evaluations, while also explaining the neurological link. Patients should know

(continues)

(continued)

that doctors bringing this up is *not* merely an effort to invalidate their pain as "psychosomatic," but to put it in the proper context as a stressor.

In reality, like no other issue. This dynamic of how sexual abuse can contribute to chronic pain illuminates the complex origins of pain. It tells us much about the neurobiology of chronic pain, that it is a product of preexisting genetics but also can be modulated by the environment. The influence of sexual abuse in triggering chronic pain supports *both* feminist claims that the environment can shape neurology, *and* biological evidence that women are indeed wired to be more vulnerable to the experience of pain, especially after trauma.

Also, perhaps as another contrast to feminist fears of "coming out" from past decades, I do not interpret women's greater incidence of chronic pain and headaches as evidence that we are inferior. I recognize that men have their share of problems, also rooted in genetic differences (and varying social forces). For example, they are much more likely to have cluster headaches, alcoholism, autism, criminal histories, schizophrenia, and suicidal tendencies. But somehow, our culture has not used these facts against them to keep them out of public life, as they have with "women's" illnesses. The reasoning through the ages has been that it's not more a risk to hire a man, even if he is more likely to go on a workplace shooting spree, than a woman, who is more likely to have a headache at that time of the month.

Yet, hopefully, more activists will expose these myths, both old and relatively new, about women, agreeing that women are not totally weak (as the patriarchy has said) or totally strong (as old-school feminists have said in reaction to the patriarchy). I'm still waiting for the main goal of the women's movement to be achieved, for everyone to acknowledge women as flawed humans, just like men—yet still deserving of equal rights. Like men's bodies, women's bodies have *both* strengths and weaknesses. This is no longer a radical concept, but one whose time has come.

1 4

Mind-Wallet Connection

○ ○ ○ ○ ○ ○ ○ ○ ○

I FOLLOWED THE ADVICE in my latest self-help book, *Fatigued to Fantastic* (1996) by Jacob Teitelbaum, but despite this effort, I never got to fantastic.

Although I had given up on Whole Health Inc., many options were still open to me. Although I had been trying what had seemed like every possible aspect of alternative medicine for months, I still had far from exhausted the possibilities. As alternative medicine was becoming hugely popular at that time, no longer a fringe practice, I never ran out of choices.

And herein lies the problem: There was absolutely no end to it.

Conventional doctors had a limited number of medications. But with an alternative doctor, if one herb didn't work, you could always try another of the dozens of brands, since the FDA does not regulate them, and they are all different. If one acupuncturist wasn't effective, you could see an endless variety of others, who all had different techniques and tried a different array of points. Your shiatsu massage didn't work? Why not try reflexology, Swedish massage, Thai massage, or soft-tissue manipulation?

Just following what my—again, very-well-meaning—mom advised was a full-time job. She would call me weekly with remedies suggested by random people she had met in the grocery line or at the health club. One said that I should put a banana peel on my forehead. Another day she recommended drinking tomato juice without ice three times a day, a practice that had "cured" the daughter of an acquaintance. She also called me saying that she had talked to the husband of her friend's daughter, who said I had "comorbid." (Clearly, something was lost in the translation.)

Meanwhile, I felt like I was being pillaged of all traces of cash. Insurance rarely covered these treatments, and my father refused to help at all with alternative medicine, seeing it as a huge waste of money. The expense of alternative medicine was the most common cause of tension between us involving the chronic pain. It wasn't that he doubted the legitimacy of my problem. Knowing how I had been before, he always believed that my pain wasn't all in my head. When I suffered, he seemed to suffer, saying he "would take it for me" if he could. His biggest frustration, he said, was just standing there powerless on the sidelines. And despite his getting his Ph.D. in psychology in the 1950s, at the height of the cultural popularity of psychoanalysis, he roundly discounted Freudian theories that explain pain as psychosomatic. (My dad told me he remembered that he and his classmates called Freud "Sigmund Fraud.") Though licensed as a clinical psychologist by the state of Illinois, he couldn't stomach this field. Instead, he worked as a senior research psychologist for the Department of Defense, a researcher for private business, and then a business professor at Indiana University. As an officer in the American Psychological Association, he continued to rail against the proliferation of "fraud artists and pretenders."

And so, always trying to be logical, over and over again he would rant to me about how I was being duped.

"These are all witch doctors!" he exclaimed. "It's like throwing money down the toilet."

I railed back, feeling insulted. "Sometimes it helps," I said. "Don't think I'm just carelessly throwing away money, that I'm so easily fooled!"

"Oh, it helps 'sometimes'? Are you even sure of that? These things go up and down on their own. There are natural *fluctuations*. If you just left it alone, you'd have the same result."

My mom, as was often the case, tried to argue for me. "But a lot of people do alternative medicine. They swear by it. There are testimonials."

"There are testimonials about fucking Lourdes, too," he said.

Sometimes I found this view humorous, and other times I did not. True, I did recognize that this pursuit of alternative medicine to an extreme was a comedic situation. But the absurdity wasn't that these "cures" were alternative and increasingly offbeat. It was that, in my desperation and hope for a magic bullet, I would almost always try them, no matter how irrational they became. I feared that if I passed one up, that would be the *one thing* that would have changed my life.

To convey the variety and endless supply of alternative methods and the typical desperation of someone in pain to "try everything," here is an abridged list of those from my "late-alternative medicine" period from 1996 to 1998, which further drained my meager resources:

- Energy Work at the Book Expo: In the summer of 1996, I was sitting in the audience of a reading at Chicago's Printer's Row Book Fair when I was confronted by a vision of pure ethereal godliness. An earthy older woman from Southern California, draped in white layers of gauze, turned to me. She asked me if I knew where she could find the annual American Booksellers' Association expo, which she had heard was in town that weekend. She was a healer and wanted to go there to try to sell her book idea on energy work. I told her that it was at McCormick Place, on the Near South Side.

  Before I knew it, the next afternoon I was driving the woman, who was dressed in another wispy white dress, to the book expo in exchange for some on-site energy work. (Like all desperate people, I never knew when such an unusual person's suddenly appearing in my life was a sign of something important and life-changing and when it was just another random goose chase.) I used a nametag pass from a friend who worked for one of the show's French producers, and the healer scored one from a guy, conveniently named Kim, in the parking lot.

  After we made it through security, we found a place to sit, and for her to go to work: a table in the very public food concessions area, which had just emptied out after the lunch rush. With the fevered inspiration of scientist John Nash sketching theories on a glass-paneled door in the film A Beautiful Mind, she drew circles on a piece of paper, swung a pendulum she had worn around her neck over these circles, and then frenetically started doing mathematical equations and shading in parts of the circles on the paper. I'm not sure if I felt any energy shifts at the time. I was too worried at that moment about running into my editor from New York, whom I had assured I was hard at work writing the sex book, with the newest deadline approaching. When we parted, the healer's advice was to wear more white, "the color of healing."

- Pummeling from a Russian: I later was treated by a husky Russian woman, an expert in "reflexotherapy," whom I met during her day job as a clerk in one of Chicago's leading health food stores. I had asked her about feverfew and other herbal supplements, and she shook her head and waved her arms in exasperation. "None of these work! A total waste of money!" she exclaimed. She explained that she had been an expert in Russia in acupressure, which taps into the same points as acupuncture but reportedly can be much more successful in clearing blocks. She had learned the technique from a Siberian monk. To demonstrate, she hooked a muscular finger into the top curve of my eye socket and pulled up forcefully, in that one motion almost raising my entire body. Her grip was that strong. Although this hurt, I had some trust in her because it turned out we knew some of the same people through my Russian roommate from college, Anna. (She was curious about Anna as a potential match for her newly divorced son and later asked me for her number.) Brimming with confidence and charisma, she bragged about her unusual abilities in curing everyone who saw her: She had developed a reputation so strong that even a doctor from the Chicago Headache Clinic had called her begging for her secret.

At the first session in her small one-room Gold Coast office, she had me lie naked on a table with a sheet over me, wrapped my shoulders in hot towels, and proceeded to *beat the living crap out of me*. Using all her strength, she pressed fiercely on different "trigger points" in my shoulders, neck, and face, which I thought were going to cave in from the pressure. On the days after the first few sessions, I could hardly move. I felt as if I had been run over by a truck. A friend then told me that this is a common response; strong massages can release toxins in the body and cause fatigue the next day. (This is a basic part of experiencing such "body work" that no one had ever warned me about.) I kept going to the fifty-dollar-an-hour sessions, feeling some improvement two days afterward, which I hoped would become cumulative. But at the last session, the final one of twenty, she looked at me and suddenly the great confidence she had possessed for the past two months melted away. She handed me a vial of "cleansing" herbs, including milk thistle and dandelion, and said that the problem was probably with my liver.

At least Anna got something out of it. She and the Russian's son had started dating.

- Light Therapy: The holistic toxin-oriented M.D., the one who had recommended the HEPA filter and mattress case, suggested light therapy or "photron-applied light technology." This was done in a small room off the office kitchen, which had probably been some kind of pantry area in the office's past life. After paging through the material provided, including the new, highly annotated book *Light Years Ahead* (1996, published in Berkeley), I realized the chances of this approach's succeeding were slight. For the first time in my journey, I was trying a remedy out of pure curiosity and adventure. (The other exception was when I allowed a friend to douse me with "holy water," which his late Lithuanian mother had had specially blessed by a priest.)

My light therapy session involved looking into a Viewmaster-like peephole in the front of a large black metal box. The equipment featured an array of blinking lights, lenses, knobs, and levers, reminiscent of the control panel on the front of a robotic pal from *Land of the Lost*. The doctor periodically inserted different single-colored films in the back, making the machine internally resemble a particularly dull kaleidoscope. After the insertion of each film, she had me raise my right arm and asked me to resist her as she tried to pull it down. Noting my particular apparent weakness after I viewed the color orange, the doctor told me to wear more of that color. (So, I reasoned, if the wearing of orange and white didn't cure me, I could always get a job as a Creamsicle spokesmodel.)

- Immersion in Lavender: Another suddenly ubiquitous trend was "movement therapy," of which there are many schools, including Pilates and Feldenkreis. A purpose is to retrain the body away from movement that may cause pain. Again, in *Conscious Choice*, I read about a practitioner who taught the Alexander Technique, which was invented in the 1880s by Australian F. M. Alexander. In the 1920s and 1930s, it attracted such forward-thinking supporters as Aldous Huxley and John Dewey. This method is also currently popular among actors, to help them gain awareness of their bodies, as I saw by the steady stream of them coming in and out of the practitioner's home office in Ravenswood.

  This treatment basically involved advice about how to become more aware of my posture in regular life. The therapist also had me lie down, with my head poised on a stack of paperback books, while she adjusted my legs from a straight to a bent position to "release the musculature" and provide "a context for release." This didn't do anything for my headache, but she actually did come up with a remedy in side conversation that was worth the sixty-dollar-an-hour investment. She told me, "*Immerse* yourself in lavender!" I was to apply and inhale the oil, a natural muscle relaxant, at every opportunity: sprinkle it in lotion and rub it on three times a day, inhale it as I slept from a ceramic essential-oil diffuser (sort of a tiny fondue pot heated with a votive candle), put it in my bath, and so on. In other words, I was to develop an obsessive-compulsive lavender habit.

I had tried lavender oil before, but with no results. She explained that I had bought the cheap Body Shop stuff and needed the purer grade. She also advised mixing it with peppermint oil for a synergistic effect. I returned to the apothecary and bought a premium German peppermint oil, the Euminz brand, which is widely sold in Europe to treat headaches. Reflecting this use, the bottle has a rollerlike tip, for easy spreading on the temples, in the same way that you would apply deodorant. I poured out half of it into an empty glass bottle and then filled it to the top with a high grade of lavender oil. I rubbed it on my temples, and surprisingly, the pain diminished strongly, at least for a short time. As with other types of alternative medicine, the effect was irregular, but overall, it worked more effectively than any over-the-counter drug, and with no side effects.

Later, in 2003, at the annual meeting of the American Pain Society (a real group, not a 1980s heavy metal band) in Chicago, I attended a panel on alternative medicine at which Dr. Serge Marchand explained that scents go right to the primitive limbic nervous system, the part of the brain responsible for emotional states and pain. Curiously, his work has revealed this effect only in women, not men—and only with "pleasant scents," such as roses and almonds.[1] Whether he is right or this is just a case of the placebo effect, I'll take it, gladly.

- Figs: Another, more experimental, cure was from a member of my parents' synagogue. Reading the Bible one day, this older man had an epiphany about the curing power of figs. Not missing a beat, he immediately started making his own fig tea—which he claimed had cured everyone to come in contact with it—and selling it in health food stores.

  After being approached by him several times, my mom dragged me to his house, and he sang the unique praises of figs to me while he cut out rows of Xeroxed jar labels with a razor blade from sheets of white contact paper, using a ruler as a straight-edge. He insisted on drizzling some of the tea into my left eye, from where much of my pain radiates. But this action irritated my weirdly sensitive nerves, giving me the added sensation of glass on the surface of my eye for the next three days. My increased pain, however, did not diminish his fervor for the fig tea, and he went on evangelizing its effectiveness for every type of ailment.

- Vibrating Hat: As the truest testimony to my growing level of desperation, I ordered a massaging hat, the Skalpi, from one of those cheaply made infomercials broadcast in the middle of the night. Cost: $99.80, with shipping and handling. I had just lectured in Columbia, Missouri, and turned on the television, too hyped up on adrenaline to sleep. I was moved by interviews of people who had used this hat, which was equipped with two motors that vibrated to massage the temples. Suddenly defying the staged feel of such commercials, one woman looked deeply into the camera and sincerely declared, "I can't tell you how good it feels to get my life back." She should have won an Oscar. When I got the hat in the mail and tried it on, I found out that the tiny massaging motors were so crude that they really didn't massage; they just drummed harshly against the head and created a worse headache. The good news was that at least the promise of a "money-back guarantee" was accurate.

- Magnets: I also bought a more famous product from late-night TV, which has become a must in the wardrobe of the American pain sufferer: the sixty-dollar "ionized bracelet," from Q-Ray. The commercial echoed that for the Skalpi, with people given the bracelet at a trade show suddenly feeling their pain vanish and getting their lives back. The bracelet, resembling one of Wonder Woman's bullet deflectors, was also advertised in the brochure as being worn by Bill Kazmaier, "The World's Strongest Man" (1980, 1981, 1982). (It also adds that this bracelet is not magnetic, but "ionized.")

But my biggest product investment of all was a magnetic pillow, blanket, and mattress, ordered from a local distributor of Nikken, a Japanese-based company, that works with local representatives in the same way that Amway and Mary Kay do. (This cost so much, just over a thousand dollars, that I contemplated taking out mattress insurance. When e-Bay later emerged, I hesitated to visit it, for fear of finding that same set on sale for eight dollars.)

At first, magnets do sound like the most obvious type of snake oil—and have been exposed as such for hundreds of years. The "science" of magnets was popularized by the controversial eighteenth-century Viennese doctor Franz Anton Mesmer, who became a great celebrity in his day. His claims of an underlying magnetic body coexisting with the physical one were quickly investigated by a royal commission, which ultimately concluded that "this fluid without existence is consequently without utility."[2]

But other signs were more positive. I had just clipped out an article from the December 9, 1997, *New York Times* about a new study at

Baylor University which claimed that the use of magnets offered some short-term pain relief. After all, although magnets as therapeutic tools have been debunked for hundreds of years, others have sung their praises for at least that long, I thought. The scientific-sounding theory was that they reduced pain through increased blood flow, by attracting the iron-carrying hemoglobin in red blood cells.

I had learned about Nikken after passing a sign in the window of a chiropractor in my neighborhood. Immediately afterward, I called the number, and an independent distributor was soon visiting my house. She was striking, with the leathery, wrinkled face of a lifelong sun worshiper her age (late fifties), but her tight jeans displayed the nubile body of a teenager. Long, feathered blond hair completed the discordant effect. She gave me a magnetized mattress pad to use for a few days as a trial, and I did feel better on those days. I asked a physical therapist (very good-looking, like the others of his profession) I was visiting at the time about this company. He said that it was highly regarded and pulled out from under his desk a Nikken pad that he used regularly.

With that advice, and because I needed a new mattress anyway, I decided to buy the products. But like other alternative methods and drugs, it pooped out without any noticeable effects. I also wasn't sure if this was purely me being neurotic, but the force of the magnets may have been too strong. I couldn't sleep, feeling oddly wired. I called the sales rep, who paused and then said her son had the same complaint with his mattress; she advised me to use the magnetized blanket as a mattress pad to minimize the mattress's effects, which I did.

On a positive note, I had a new career opportunity. To get a discount on the goods, I signed up to become an official distributor for Nikken, which sent me a large box of sales materials. Can I interest you in some magnets?

- Leopold and Loeb Neighbor: Besides magnets, another area that I had read and heard much about was healing visualizations. This tool, basically known as *guided imagery*, is rooted firmly in the "mind-body" connection, directly using the mind to heal the body. One might, for example, visualize the pain as a pool of light and then shrink it. Or imagine the pain as a band around one's cranium and then loosen it.

    I met a therapist who specialized in this type of work in an unlikely place, a high-rise lawyers' office downtown. A friend had been working on a political campaign in the southeast side of Chicago, and he asked me to help him out for a few hours by calling voters before the election on behalf of his progressive candidate. I would also be paid a few shekels for my trouble. I arrived in the late morning on a rainy day and was immediately depressed to realize that I could hardly accomplish this basic work. An elderly, red-haired, and energetic woman nearby, resembling Ruth Gordon in the film *Harold and Maude*, asked me what was wrong, and I told her a bit. She gave me her business card, which looked antique, with neither an area code for the phone number nor a zip code. I made an appointment to visit her at her home office in Kenwood, just north of the Hyde Park neighborhood.

I was surprised to arrive at the 4800 block of South Ellis Street and find a mansion, by a famous architect, Charles Sumner Frost, who had designed many well-known railroad stations, the Newberry Library, and buildings at Navy Pier in Chicago. The woman, Betty, told me that across the street was a vacant lot where formerly stood the house of either Leopold or Loeb, the infamous pair of the 1920s, who had murdered another neighbor, fourteen-year old Bobbie Franks, as a sort of intellectual challenge. One block south was the mansion of Julius Rosenwald, a founder of Sears Roebuck. And she had at least one famous living neighbor, Louis Farrakan, who owned a mosquelike yellow brick mansion complete with guards from the Nation of Islam out in front. (He was probably the one person in Chicago left whom I had not already consulted about the Headache.)

Like many crumbling mansions in this area, which had its heyday in the early part of the twentieth century, Betty's house had seen better days. Inside, it looked like a boarding house. She was renting to a couple living in the basement and to a family of hippies who resided on the third floor. The elaborate woodwork was all painted butter yellow, and she commented that the house had been built a hundred years ago, when wood seemed plentiful and painting over it wasn't considered a waste. In the cavernous living room, which looked like a train-station waiting room, were only a large overgrown fern, with a peace sign sticker adorning its pot, and a few pieces of furniture, including a huge piano and a futon, which had been used by Betty's nurse. She explained that she had advanced cancer and untied the colorful scarf around her neck to reveal some crude-looking black stitches, which had been well covered in the downtown office by a turtleneck sweater.

I followed her up the back stairs to the spacious one-room fourth floor, which was her meditation room. On the way, we passed postcards adorning the walls and rows of shoes left outside the door to the third floor by the hippie family. Then we reached a sanctuary. Windows on all four sides looked out to the foggy green foliage and budding spring flowers outside in the yard. The echoing room was completely empty, except for five broken tiles from her roof spread out on the wooden floor. These tiles held the text of a poem she had written, with a couplet written on each. As I had left my purse (with its notepad) downstairs, I only got to write one down on paper from memory, which read, "In solitude I sit/ Thinking where the pieces fit."

I liked Betty, so I didn't mind when the visualizations we did afterward did not touch my pain. But they were relaxing. I couldn't argue against that. They mainly involved me closing my eyes and imagining "walking down a plush carpet barefoot" downstairs and then journeying to different relaxing memories in my life. I thought of a hill in the middle of a field in Urbana, in college, where some friends and I had biked and then lay down to see the stars. In the winter, we had sledded there using cafeteria trays.

After I paid her twenty-five dollars, I dropped her off at her telemarketing job downtown. I did not see her again, but in 2003, I passed that house and saw it had been completely renovated and was for sale.

- Brainwave Biofeedback: At first, this approach seemed more scientific, as it had to me in 1979 in my sixth-grade report. Since then, I had read about three kinds of biofeedback: the traditional kind (electromyographic, or EMG, biofeedback) that measures muscle tension, another type that helps you regulate the temperature in your fingertips, and the rarer type that helps you monitor and regulate your brainwaves, also called *neurofeedback* or *neurotherapy*. I had tried the first kind at various places, but not the third, which seemed promising. (I decided to table the second kind.) An acquaintance told me about his brother's girlfriend's mother, who was a specialist in it. She worked at one of the hundreds of brainwave biofeedback clinics in the United States. Like the other forms of biofeedback, neurofeedback was a result of a behavioral psychology movement in the 1970s, to control a person's pain with behavior change.

  Apparently, this woman had some success with headaches at her northwest Chicago clinic, which was across the street from a fast-food stand with a huge smiling hotdog on the front lawn. When I found out the price on the phone, a thousand dollars for twenty sessions (fifty dollars each), I told the woman that was impossible. But then she said if I didn't have success, she would give me the money back. I thought I couldn't lose either way: If it didn't work, I wouldn't be set back financially. If it did work, I would be thrilled to pay her anything she wanted.

But before we began the treatment, she gave me hours of tests to measure brain activity. These required me to insert multishaped pegs into their proper holes on a wooden board while being timed. As she mainly treated children in her practice, I sat hunched on a tiny chair at a miniature table.

She also gave me a test for attention deficit disorder (ADD) (a specialty of brainwave biofeedback, explaining the child-centered focus), which involved pressing a computer button as soon as I heard a beep through my headphones. As in a typing test, the score depended on my speed, with points deducted for errors (such as pressing the button mistakenly, revealing a too-active mind). After a series of missteps, I realized that the computer would try to trick the person taking the test by suddenly changing patterns. It would transmit a series of four beeps in a row, many times over. Then suddenly, it would follow with a quick series of three beeps, misleading the person to impulsively press the button for the missing fourth one. But I caught on too late: I failed the test miserably.

In the headache therapy that followed, she hooked me up to a computer via dime-sized sensors lubricated with some kind of conducting goo affixed to my scalp. For many sessions, I sat in front of a computer screen with a Pac Man game. Through the wires fastened to my head, I actually controlled, through my concentration, the activity of the Pac Man and his feeding frenzy through the maze. This was a form of intense meditation, forcing me to focus my attention on one thing and ignore all errant thoughts. During the sessions, she experimented with different settings of the monitors, which made the game more or less difficult, and sometimes I did feel slight relief.

When the sessions ended, she insisted on repeating the brain tests, including the one diagnosing ADD. However, despite some fluctuations through the week, overall my pain had not diminished. I then asked for my money back, and she refused. "Well, according to these tests," she said, sorting through my folder and adjusting her bifocals, "we have cured your ADD."

As a last gasp, she sent me home with an audiotape featuring a scientific panel singing the praises of a new vitamin supplement she was selling, which was supposed to deliver the nutrients of several servings of vegetables with every pill.

Actually, I would have kept trying brainwave biofeedback, as I had felt it maybe had worked somewhat, but time was scarce. I needed all my marbles to make the last and utterly unappealable deadline on my sex book. And the coffers were completely empty, with no room for any further financial risk.

• Pulling My Arm: The last straw was seeing an osteopath, a Filippina doctor on Michigan Avenue downtown, who another acquaintance had insisted had cured her mysterious health problems. Like some other healers I had met, her main diagnostic tool was not scientific; it was based on arm resistance, which is actually a common tool of "naturopathic medicine," the result of a nineteenth-century European and American health movement rooted in "the healing power of nature."[3] Just like the holistic M.D. who treated me with light therapy, she had me raise my arm, asked a question about my health, and then asked me to resist her as she tried to push my arm down. If my arm became "weak" and I couldn't fight her, then the answer to her question was affirmative.

But I couldn't get the hang of the action. My arm, strengthened from weight lifting, resisted her pressure every time. Then she called in a large Polish nurse to assist in pushing down my arm. She would hold my other still hand, to create a circuit between us.

"Is the problem pollution?" she asked my body, inquiring as to the source of my headache.

I resisted the pressure of the nurse on my raised left arm.

"No," she said. "Then is it biological?"

Same lack of response.

"No. Then is it food?"

The nurse rammed my arm down and the doctor had me raise it again.

"Interesting. Then it is food, and nothing else?" she said, looking astonished.

The arm was forced down again.

She asked what I ate, and I mentioned the numerous food groups I had excluded because of the food allergy tests. But as with everyone else, it was time for her own tests. She extracted vials of different foods from a drawer and had me hold each in my right hand. Then she asked me to resist the nurse's pressure again with my left arm. According to when my arm went down, those were the foods I was allergic to. She came up with an entirely different set: soy, turkey, rice, carrot, potato, fish, and chicken.

The solution was for me to come for more visits so she could "densensitize" me to each of these foods, one by one, with energy work.

Afterward, she asked me if I "wanted to receive the light of God."

"That depends," I said. "How much will it cost me?"

My level of disbelief had grown too large to continue suspending, and I wasn't even trying to force myself to go along with the treatment. The irrationalities had become too great to ignore.

She summoned another large Filippina woman, who told me to clap two times with her and bow three times. They sang a prayer to my face and then had me turn around so they could sing it directly into my kidneys, liver, and then ovaries.

On the way out, the receptionist gave me a bill for two hundred dollars for the first visit, the "consultation." Although the doctor was an M.D., I knew that insurance would not cover this amount, and I felt it was overblown in any case. I asked about a sliding scale, as I was only "an office temp" of modest means. She agreed to a reduced price of fifty dollars.

The most alarming part of this visit was the doctor's certainty. She seemed absolutely sure that she could cure me, as long as I followed her advice. I realized this was a definite sign of a quack, someone who thought she could easily fix a complex problem. At such times, I looked into the person's eyes, trying to find hints of wavering and wondering if this was a deliberate scam. But then I concluded, probably giving them the benefit of the doubt, that most of these overly confident practitioners did believe what they preached. Yet this was not reassuring. I would prefer someone who consciously knows that he or she is ripping me off over someone who is self-deluded, who may be more dangerous in the end, not being able to distinguish reason from fantasy, nor dangerous practices from safe ones.

I was also facing other limits with alternative medicine. I realized that most of the alternative medicine work of any kind was so subtle that it wouldn't work if I wasn't totally relaxed when treated. That was a challenge in modern city life, even in simply getting to an appointment. I started to skip yoga, realizing that I would be more stressed out overall by trying to get there in rush-hour traffic and parking, or by taking two forms of public transportation to get there. Once, massage therapy failed to relax me because the therapist had had her wallet stolen in the bus on the way there and was obviously preoccupied and tense. Another time, I laid my head down in the face cradle and almost gagged because of the strong glue that had been used to repair it earlier that day. For the next day, I had the taste of it in my mouth. Oh my God, toxins, I thought.

Some foibles were purely my own. On the advice of one healer, I put geranium oil on my forehead; it was supposed to lift me to a "happier" vibration, but then I applied too much and it dripped into and stung my eyes, inflaming the pain. One night, I repeatedly woke up to the sounds of munching coming from my closet, which I convinced myself I was neurotically imagining. The next morning, in a pain-addled state, I opened the closet door, got on my knees, and found in the back the now-empty white case of my U-shaped buckwheat pillow. It was supposed to relieve muscle tension after being heated in a microwave and then set on my shoulders. I had barely used it. At least the mice had gotten some joy out of it.

In addition, I was becoming turned off by what I saw as a lackadaisical attitude on the part of many healers. They had all the time in the world to follow "the mystical course of nature." Just as no neurologist had ever admitted to me, "I don't know," none of them had said, "Well, you've given this enough of a try. You can stop with these twice-weekly sixty-dollar visits." If I didn't stop these sessions, they would go on indefinitely, and we would grow old together.

And the more providers I saw and the more prohibitions they gave me, the more resentful I became about fearing the modern outside world. I felt overly fragile and sensitive, constantly shutting things out, including processed foods, stress, and the mildest over-the-counter medications. Someone would present me with something innocent, like a piece of birthday cake, and I would recoil in horror: "Wheat, sugar, dairy, gluten! Are you trying to kill me, for God's sake?"

I was also tired of the drudgery of constantly going to appointments, of turning down so many foods that I wasn't even sure had been harming me, of trying to always think positively and fight the natural feelings of distress and anxiety that often accompany pain, even as a part of the same neurological circuitry. I was also sick of thinking about the problem. In giving it so much attention, I had let it take over my life.

In contrast, Western medicine had asked nothing of me and had let me off the hook. Just take this pill and remain your old shitty self, it said.

I also realized that some patients I was meeting who claimed to be cured by alternative medicine over the long term really were also involved with other modern "modalities" (drugs). A friend of a friend recommended an eccentric chiropractor, working in the back of an Allstate Insurance office in suburban Skokie, who focused on only the top vertebrae as the cause of all imbalances. Although this person claimed this chiropractor had cured her constant headaches, she later casually remarked that she had started at the same time taking Paxil, which affects the neurotransmitter serotonin (involved in chronic headaches).

In one e-mail, my friend Wendy described a therapeutic touch (TT) session she had just had, which seemed to work wonders: "She [the therapist] supposedly made everything [the energy] go in one direction, by moving her hands above the fields and then 'unruffling' them and then moving her hands over the fields and then 'modulating' the energy. Unfortunately, it failed to get rid of my migraine and I had to take narcotics to get through the treatment."

A man that I met at a party put me in touch with a friend he had met at his tai chi studio—who had allegedly been cured by an acupuncturist there. She had suffered constant pain that sounded a lot like mine. I called her and she said what had made the headaches taper off in her case was menopause, which sometimes has that effect. I started to eagerly await that change of life, just as I'd imagine a young child ticking off the days to Christmas in an Advent calendar.

Then I realized that the only real hysteria in my life was from absorbing the overblown promises of alternative medicine, the idea that I could honestly cure myself through positive thinking.

Visits to questionable providers led to an increasingly common feeling that I was a sap, that I was being duped, that thanks to that thing called hope, a headache patient and her money are soon parted. I was in no better a position than Dr. Thomas Willis's famous chronic daily headache patient in the seventeenth century, who went on an epic and fruitless "tryal" across nations to see "both the Learned and the unlearned, from Quacks and old women."[4]

Besides, I was sick of myself. All these alternative medicine techniques emphasized healing through self-knowledge. In addition to being tired of analyzing my personality and figuring out the demands of my "true self" and my "soul's code," I was also bored by my body. In yoga sessions, when the instructor asked us to spend forty-five minutes observing our left and right thighs, I would think, "Isn't my life bad enough? Why do I have to subject myself to this further tedium?"[5]

I had been trying hard to "listen" to my body and interpret its meaningful physical signals. Then I realized that instead of being wise, my body was a village idiot. I was trying to follow the advice of a chatterbox that mindlessly repeated the same pain signals for no reason at all—not for any type of useful warning, as is the case with acute pain, like the sting from touching a hot stove.

Three years earlier, these concepts of alternative healing—to achieve purity and balance—had sounded good on paper. As I said, they were exciting, independent, and invigorating punk rock. But it turned out that they also shared some of the banalities of punk rock, with highly varying quality and few external regulating standards. At the most, even after devoting an entire day to alternative healing—with meditation, exercise, acupuncture, and other techniques—I could expect only a short-term result, if that.

Further, I recognized that all the testimonials I had read in books and magazines included no follow-ups over the long term. Whether it was drugs or alternative medicine, everything was uncritically heralded as "the wonder cure." (See the sidebar.) Certainly, alternative techniques worked for a lot of people, but there was never any discussion of when they didn't.

Like someone falling off the wagon of a too-restrictive weight-loss diet, I started binging on my old habits. I reverted to my old nonstrategies of denial and distraction, devoting all my marbles to my work. And reacting to the suggestions of those around me, I wondered whether the Headache would disappear after I finished the book. Relief after meeting the deadline might cure me. That made about as much sense as anything else I had heard, and so I lunged forward, appreciating the new engagement with messy current events and the outside world, toxins and all.

Inflated Promises: Mind over Matter as "Science"

The propaganda that makes unrealistic promises about the mind-body connection is not just limited to self-help books. Every academic history of chronic pain includes provocative discoveries of how the mind influences the body—which are often exaggerated in their practical application to controlling pain in everyday life.

A prime example is David Morris's overly optimistic profile of the novelist Reynolds Price in his 1998 cultural treatise *Illness and Culture in the Postmodern Age*. Morris used Price's case to argue that pain is ultimately controlled by the mind. He discussed how Price used biofeedback to mentally separate himself from his pain, "allowing him to escape a drug-fogged underworld of constant pain and to begin creating a life he calls not only new, but . . . whole" (117).[6]

But in a seeming contradiction, four years after the publication of Morris's book, Price appeared on NPR's *All Things Considered* (on March 13, 2002) to deliver a commentary about the "nonstop assault on [his] mind" by his pained nerves. A theme was his helplessness. Nothing, including any drug, helped his pain "more than 20 percent." Although he did mention that biofeedback had worked to give him "welcome degrees of self-possession," he concluded that he, like millions of Americans, had not been able to transcend the physical agony. "Can there be no resolve?" he asked in the end.

Some overstated reports of mind over matter are actually based on some good science, which has become exaggerated through the years. A well-known breakthrough study about pain and the mind-body connection—included in every text on the subject—was conducted by Lieutenant Colonel Henry Beecher, an anesthesiologist in the army during World War II. He interviewed 215 soldiers at a combat hospital within thirteen hours of their typically severe injuries. He was surprised that only a minority wanted morphine and that "75 percent of these terribly wounded soldiers reported that their pain was not just tolerable but insignificant," reported Dr. Scott Fishman in *The War on Pain* (109). He quoted Beecher's explanation that the relief they felt from not being able to fight anymore had trumped the physical sensation from their injuries: "Pain is an experience subject to modification by many factors: wounds received during strenuous physical exercise, during the excitement of games, often go unnoticed. The same is true of wounds received during the fighting, during anger. Strong emotions can block pain."

This was a radical concept at the time, a challenge to past theories framing pain as purely a proportional reaction to physical stimuli, with nothing modulating it. But as a result of this work and much more to come, doctors often apply a double standard to pain patients, expecting

(continues)

(continued)

them to accomplish superhuman feats with the mere power of the mind. The misguided assumption is that since the mind can truly affect the body, it has the power to overcome it.

"The idea that I can make my body do anything I really want it to do, such as making the pain go away completely, is a form of the myth of control, a childish belief in the omnipotence of what I want," astutely observed philosopher (and chronic fatigue syndrome patient) Susan Wendell in *The Rejected Body*. "It is a failure to admit that the human mind is much bigger than our egos, and, even more obviously, that the rest of nature is bigger than our egos (facts about which we should be thankful, in my opinion)" (103).

In reality, there are limits to how the mind can influence pain, with mental distractions and emotional cues sometimes working temporarily, but not able to endure over long periods of time. The truth is that distraction and emotion can help relieve *any* problem in the short term, not just pain. A soldier on the front lines can temporarily forget about his divorce or financial problems or gonorrhea—at least while a hand grenade is being lobbed in his direction. In less life-threatening scenarios, many of us have witnessed actors onstage giving rousing performances, despite being collapsed with flu during the day. That performance is not necessarily "faked"; the actor can give a genuinely good performance. And in the winter we see news reports of "polar bear" clubs, people who go out to swim in icy waters. That doesn't mean that we should expect all people to go naked through the winter, and that the mind is powerful enough to override such hardship over time. With enough willpower, anyone can be thin: Just eat about twelve hundred calories a day until you get there. But then, needless to say, most people cannot keep this up over the long run.

Scientists who talk in the media about the power of distraction also commonly fail to differentiate between severe and moderate chronic pain. Through the headache ordeal, I have also experienced other types of pain that are more "ordinary," such as pain in the elbow from typing, which I rarely mention to anyone else and which has sometimes awakened me in the middle of the night. But unlike head pain, it is not at the core of my being. In my case, this hand and arm pain also fluctuated greatly, appearing more rarely and being more easily "tuned out."

Part Four:

THE VERDICT

15

The Nose Doorknob

○ ○ ○ ○ ○ ○ ○ ○ ○

SLOWLY, MY LIFE GOT BUSIER, more like that of a "normal" person. I resurfaced from the Valley of the Ill to finish the first draft of my sex book, just in time for the newest deadline—and five years past the original one. But instead of getting better, after that longtime pressure was lifted to perform mentally (despite pain, drugs, and financial worries), the pain and fatigue worsened. Part of it was that I always felt worse *after* a period of stress than during it, when I was able to let my guard down. Also, as the weeks had gone on, my previously sustaining discipline of meditating, eating entirely health-fully, and exercising had diminished to nothing and I was back to my old pre-alternative-medicine ways.

In addition, my publisher rejected the manuscript, partly because of its extreme lateness. But surprisingly, that part of my life ended well. After emerging from an almost catatonic depression a week later, I was able to sell the book myself soon after to another publisher, an energetic and irreverent, relatively small press with a genuine enthusiasm for the project, which, in turn, made me much more excited about it. Instead of seeing the book as a burden, I started to view it with my old idealistic eyes as an opportunity to speak out about important issues and once again engage with the world. (At that point, I finally understood what Dr. Chung had meant years earlier, that I never had control over such matters to begin with. And that wasn't necessarily a bad thing.)

Even with this new enthusiasm, I needed to increase my energy and decrease the pain to a more reasonable level in order to continue the months of rewrites that such a research-intensive book requires. At this time, now the end of 1998, a friend made a suggestion. She told me about her amazing experience seeing a very sharp otolaryngologist (known in lay terms as an ear, nose, and throat doctor or doctor of the head holes), who stood out from others because of his common sense. She had been suffering from an odd ear problem, a blockage that affected her hearing, for which another doctor had wanted to do surgery. This doctor gave her a decongestant, and that cured the problem. She was saved from going under the knife. Perhaps there was some simple sinus connection to my problem also?

I agreed that this made sense. I had always been one of those nasally people who always seemed a bit "stuffed up." And over the past few years, I had also discovered that sometimes the most effective painkiller for me was a decongestant, something simple, like Tavist D or Tylenol Sinus. I started buying these over-the-counter decongestants after going on a trip earlier that year to Colorado and meeting a hippie potter, a friend of the friend I was visiting. She gave me some fresh-brewed herbal "Mormon tea," and I was astounded that it tamed the broken glass feeling in my eye, which had been activated by a robust local allergy season. Even potent drugs rarely had that effect. I had asked her what Mormon tea was exactly and vowed to give those Latter Day Saints a chance. She explained that this tea was from the herb ephedra.

I later tried to buy the herb in capsule form but realized that it was about to be banned by the FDA as dangerous, so I settled for teas and pills infused with its chemical derivative, pseudoephedrine. The decongestants also gave me a good boost of energy at pivotal times, such as when I had to be "on" and give a lecture. (But like all other painkillers, it was the most effective when I did not take it very often, and overuse would cause additional "rebound" headaches and insomnia.) In any case, it was at least one more available tool in my growing bag of tricks to get by, along with the lavender and peppermint combo.

When I finally saw the ear, nose, and throat (ENT) doctor for an appointment, he looked in my nose and gasped with excitement. He said he had most likely found the source of the headaches: a deviated septum. The top of the septum, the bone bisecting the nose, veered very severely toward my left eye and possibly had been crushing the nerves in that area.

As a "diagnostic test," he put an anesthetic at the end of a greatly elongated Q-Tip and stuck it all the way into my nose. If that worked to mute the pain, it would show that this was the source of the problem. However, my own ebullience was deflated immediately afterward: Even though it was an anesthetic, the chemical inflamed the eye pain tenfold. It responded to any kind of irritant, even one that was meant to numb it. The doctor seemed unfazed by my increased pain. He told me he was referring me to a second ENT doctor, one who did these types of surgeries. The second ENT guy would give me a better diagnostic test, a more advanced nerve block in that area, to see if I was a candidate for surgery. I was intrigued because I had wondered for years if sinus problems were a root cause of the Headache.

But the irritation from the Q-Tip remained, not letting up for several days. I was unable to work and kept calling the ENT doctor's office for advice. I never got a call back. Finally, his exasperated nurse told me that the second doctor would answer all my questions and I was now *his* patient.

A week later, as that extra pain was starting to fade, I went to the office of the new ENT doctor. My parents came with me, as they had in the past, as an extra set of eyes and ears to relate my now complex story to the doctor. We found the office in a sleek skyscraper in the Gold Coast neighborhood. I was overwhelmed by its grandeur. Its splendor and luxury resembled that of a high-roller penthouse in Vegas.

As I approached the office suite, I spotted the panel of glass doors. They made a statement, even from many feet away. Their huge brass doorknobs each represented half of a giant nose, almost comparable in my mind in size to the cloned body part of the "Leader" in Woody Allen's science fiction comedy *Sleeper*. My dad became infuriated when he reached inside one of the nostrils to open the door and cut his hand. For the next hour, in front of the others in the waiting room, he openly swore and ranted against what he already considered an overpriced doctor.

"Well," I told him, "think on the bright side. At least this wasn't a gynecologist's office."

Inside the office, the receptionists, who were petite, fashionable, and attractive enough to be models for Ortho Tri-Cyclen ads, sat in a space surrounded by a black marble countertop ring. On the countertops were three-foot sculptures of ducks. A large, narrow aquarium filled with tropical fish bisected the waiting room. And the clientele, mostly women, were, by far, the best groomed I had seen, with lots of form-fitting black outfits, black leather jackets, high-heeled black boots, and what looked like *real* Kate Spade bags (not the ones you buy on Canal Street in New York City). It was as if I had entered Donna Karan's cerebellum.

This fashion-forward appearance contrasted dramatically with the clientele of other recent "doctors" I had visited. And after I'd seen so many alternative doctors who did not practice out of "real" offices, this office suite seemed safely antiseptic and professional. It contrasted starkly with the crumbling wooden Victorian home office of my last practitioner, a naturopath, in Madison, Wisconsin, and the back of a grocery store in Chinatown, where an old acupuncturist practiced in a room that smelled like a combination of ginger and kitty litter. I bet that they wouldn't even make me pay in cash. I recalled the brain-imaging center we had visited periodically in northwest Indiana, where everyone—men, women, children, and even babies—had mullets.

But now I felt suddenly thrust from the Stone Age into the futuristic glory of the twenty-first century. When I got in to see the doctor, a tall and confident man, he also had the goods. He threaded a long, tapered plastic tube up my nose with a tiny camera on the end of it, to show me the extent of the obstruction and the dysfunction of my swollen turbinates. These are membranelike growths in the nasal cavity, he explained. Mine was a concha bullosa, or one resembling a small balloon that was filled with air. Out of the corner of my eye, I watched a staggeringly close shot broadcast on the video monitor, with the nose hairs blown up to the size of redwoods alongside each other in a surreal nasal fairyland space-scape. Immediately afterward, he gave me a Polaroid-type photo of four round turbinates, colored with swirls of faded pink and beige, resembling any of the thirty-one moons of Saturn.

Yes, I thought, modern technology, the men of the hallowed halls of science, will save me after all!

Finally, the Enlightenment resumes, I thought, after years wasted in my naive detour, mired in superstition and ignorance. Give me microchips, lasers, test tubes, double-blind control groups!

Modern progress is not the enemy; it is the savior of us all! Forget the meandering "enlightened path" of Lao-tzu and Thich Nhat Hahn. Give me the goal-oriented life and instant gratification!!!

No more tedious self-examination and trying to change the core of my personality; I was off the hook!

I could rejoin mainstream, processed, nonorganic, noncontrarian modern society again and become a part of the rest of the world, no longer fearing it but embracing it!

And best of all, I could start drinking coffee again!

So long, suckers!

After my extreme close-up, I asked the doctor if he wanted to do the diagnostic test that the first ENT man had mentioned, the nerve block. If that anesthetic applied to the area of the septum stopped the headache, then we would know for sure that this was the source of the pain. But he said it wasn't necessary. And he made some logical sense. After all, the pain was continuous. That meant there had to be some kind of a physical cause, he said. In response, I argued that meditation sometimes helped, revealing that the pain must be the result of some kind of a brain chemistry problem. He countered that meditation would have the same soothing effect on someone suffering *any* pain, like someone who just had a boulder roll over her toe. He added that if I really had migraines and brain chemistry was the problem, one of those medications would surely have worked on me. And the truth was that the pain was strictly on the left side, the same side as the deviation of the septum. Later, an encounter in the waiting room further boosted his arguments in my mind: I talked to a chipper young woman who had just had the septum surgery, telling me that she slept better and had more energy. It looked as if I was headed for the OR.

But as a precaution, he said that before scheduling the surgery he would take some other standard diagnostic steps. He ordered a CT scan of the sinuses and prescribed a round of antibiotics; we needed to rule out the possibility of a sinus infection causing the headaches. He also had me take another round of special RASTs(radioallergosorbent tests). These blood tests to determine allergies cost an astounding twenty-five hundred dollars. When we hesitated, suspecting correctly that this would be too much for insurance to cover, he assured me that these tests were cutting-edge and, if they turned up an allergy, would spare me surgery. Not surprisingly, like the results of the tests I had had in Oak Park, these results revealed allergies to about every organic substance found on the planet, both plants and foods. And so he signed me up to come to his office once a week for allergy shots, which my insurance would cover.

The antibiotics and shots didn't work to relieve my pain, but this doctor was optimistic about the surgery—in his opinion, now my final therapeutic alternative. He gave me more information about the surgery in a slick dark-green folder, imprinted in gold lettering with Psalm 103, the one about God "who heals all your diseases." Inside was a catalog from an antiallergy supply house, as well as other "point of sale" (my dad's marketing terminology) information about the allergy tests.

But my uncle and parents were extremely skeptical, and their doubts led me to delay the surgery. My CT scan had come back showing perfect sinuses. "No evidence of sinusitis," rather nonambiguously stated the report. And the Gold Coast doctor's prices were extreme: The surgery on turbinates, sinuses, and the deviated septum would approach twenty-five thousand dollars. We doubted the insurance would cover this amount, which was hardly "reasonable and customary." Even though the receptionist assured us that they would later adjust the price to allow for what my insurance paid, we thought this ask-questions-later plan sounded risky.

Indeed, increasingly perturbed, my dad noted that the asking price was higher than the median price of open-heart surgery. He also pointed out that the doctor was cashing in on my deep-pockets private insurance, which was a rare *non*prenegotiated HMO. (My private insurance plan didn't have any pre-existing deal to limit doctors' charges.) The sky was the limit on what the doctor could charge. And so, this doctor's plan evidently was to charge as much as possible and then see what the insurance would cover. The bill for the first visit alone was three thousand dollars, which included more than five hundred dollars for the two-minute videocamera procedure.

The more my father thought about this, the more incensed he became. He even eventually wrote an op-ed piece about the skewed economics of the experience (the piece was accepted by the *Chicago Tribune*, but then he declined to have it published in order to protect my privacy, which I guess now is a nonissue). In this article, my dad called this doctor's method "souk pricing," named after African or Middle Eastern open-air markets, where the seller tries to push for as much as possible until curbed.

Despite my father's cynicism, I tried to believe that this doctor was not a crook, partly because I saw this as my only chance to relieve the pain and reenter mainstream life. I also decided to give him the benefit of the doubt because when I called his office and was put on hold, a recorded track quoted the Gospels—surely a sign of his piety. As I waited to make appointments, I would hear an ebullient male voice reciting something like "And lo, in the tenth year, in the tenth month, on the twelfth day of the month, Matthew said to Luke, heed the teachings of thy Lord . . . " And then, mid-verse, the recitation would be abruptly cut off by "Hello. Nasal and sinus. May I help you?"

Still, my dad had a point, and I agreed that it was time for another opinion. I saw a highly respected suburban ENT man. He told me that the sinuses were fine, and that surgery on them would be foolish, but that the deviated septum was indeed the likely source of my pain. He had seen this many times before, as in a patient whom he had recently cured. In return, he said, the patient had given him a bottle of Chivas Royal scotch.

So, considering this doctor would charge more than twenty thousand dollars less than the one in the Gold Coast part of town and actually had more impressive medical credentials as a surgeon, we decided to go with him.

Actually, my insurance would cover the cost—at least, barring the possibility of investigation by the insurance company. After all, I was probably the only thirty-one-year-old Jewish female ever to *legitimately* get an operation to fix a deviated septum.

It was November 1998, and I felt rushed to schedule the surgery. If I acted by the end of the year, the insurance would cover the procedure completely, as I had already met my hefty deductible, which was the size of the average GDP of a small rural state. But I still also decided to get another opinion, from a highly regarded Loop ENT doctor, who, like the Gold Coast guy, was also a plastic surgeon, with a waiting room full of rhinoplasty brochures.

I was discouraged by this third opinion. He told me that while surgery might work, there was some danger of making the pain worse. But then I also realized he was the doctor who had actually recommended needless ear surgery on my friend—the same one who had gotten me started seeing ENT specialists. He had certainly steered her wrong.

But he said that if I still wanted to go ahead with the surgery, he would write a letter to the suburban doctor about his concerns. That way, at least the risks would be on the table.

With this warning in mind, I again pondered the risks, of both going ahead and not going ahead with the surgery. And I decided that *not* doing it was the greater risk. I knew that if I declined, I would wonder every day for the rest of my pain-addled life if I had passed on the "one true cure."

In the days and moments leading up to the surgery, now scheduled to take place on the second-to-last day of December, I decided to think positively. So, on the morning of the surgery, a few minutes before going under, I did not flinch when my mom summoned the anesthesiologist to ask him a question concerning something she'd read in a women's magazine about a dangerous type of anesthetic that she hoped he wasn't using. In response, he muttered something defensive at her, not really understandable because of a heavy Indian accent, and walked off shaking his head. I changed into the blue cloth dress, put my clothes and purse into the locker they gave me, and lay down on the gurney, ready to be wheeled in for surgery.

And here, according to conventional self-help book and memoir formulas, is where my journey should end:

And then I found the miracle drug/surgery and lived happily ever after. It had been literally right under my nose all along! The best part is that I married the kind doctor who had cured me, the one who reached out to me selflessly with hours of personal care and attention, treating both my body and my spirit. And what's more, soon after, I went on to win the Tour de France!

But unfortunately, chronic pain often refuses to stick to scripts and inspire others with miraculous cures.

Immediately after waking, I began to vomit blood. I felt the old headache still present, but with an additional sharp dot of pain on the inside of the left eye, where the crooked septum used to end. I asked the doctor about it, and he said, "That means we got it."

After I became less focused on the nausea and went home, I felt the true intensity of the new, and not improved, Headache. This pain was so severe, the worst of my life, that I hardly felt the pain of the broken septum (about the level of pain people feel with a nose job or a broken nose). The surgery, along with the cotton packing now lodged in the sinus, had truly stirred up the nerves behind and in the eye to their maximum fury. The old broken-glass sensation was back, but with a new intensity. Even though I was not crying, the tears flowed from my eyes nonstop. I was panicking, afraid that the doctor had done nerve damage (as the last medical consultant had warned).

A few days later, we drove through a blizzard to see the doctor to remove the packing. Feeling terror, I asked him if the surgery could have done any nerve damage. He was shocked and very defensive, suddenly turning from friendly to hostile.

"None of my other patients have ever said this," he said. "Do you have mental problems?"

My dad, who had just stepped into the room, stood there silently, surprised by this accusation. He looked at me with sympathy and helplessness. Even I was taken aback. Though I had been through the ringer with doctors, I was still (naively) surprised that the doctor was so defensive, that he seemed more interested in protecting himself legally and shrugging me off than in helping me at that most vulnerable point in my life. I had returned to Western medicine, confronting the Ego once more. Once again, this was about him, not me.

"I was just referring to the letter," I said softly, trying to explain myself, remembering the one written by the last ENT doctor to warn him about such risks.

"What letter?" he asked.

I never knew if he had even gotten it. When I tried to request my records from this doctor who did the surgery, to use as background for this chapter, they were all missing.

I know the letter was sent, as I later found it in the records of the doctor who wrote it. But I was very surprised that, in fact, he did not include any warnings. Instead, his letter backed the choice to have surgery.

After a few minutes, the surgeon regained some composure and told me that the pain would subside soon, when the agitated nerves calmed down from the trauma of surgery. But over the next few weeks, the intensity of the pain budged only slightly, and I settled into the worst depression I could imagine, fearing my life was over. I thought of a friend's description of depression as entering a series of rooms, each one dimmer and smaller than the last. "You think it can't get any darker, and then, it is, a darker room," he said.

During that time, while making a zombified trip in the middle of the night to the bathroom, I happened to look up into the mirror and was jolted completely awake by my reflection: The white parts of my left eyeball were now colored red, now mixed with blood. Around the eye was an odd swelling, as if something was about to burst.

I had a mini panic attack a few nights later reading a biography of Michael O'Donoghue, a groundbreaking writer in black comedy who had been on the staff of the early *Saturday Night Live*. He died at the age of fifty-four in 1994 after a massive brain hemorrhage, which ironically mirrored his longtime SNL routine of getting long steel needles plunged into his eye. With horror, I read an excerpt in the book from his *Village Voice* obituary, about the last moments of his life, when he

awoke with what he believed was another of the migraines that had tormented him throughout his life. He got out of bed, went to his bathroom and took some medication to relieve the pain. Later, he awoke a second time and exclaimed, "OH MY GOD!!" His wife . . . reported that his eyes were the color of blood and that she could see bolts of "lightning" flash behind his eyeballs.[1]

Putting down the book, I considered looking in the mirror again at my bloody eye but was afraid of seeing lightning bolts. I thought that this pain was too great to just be benign. Even though the doctor later told me that this bloody eye was a common reaction to such surgery, I was worried that it was building up to some horrible type of stroke, to which some migraine patients are more vulnerable.

In the days that followed, I read other more uplifting books, for short ten-minute periods, all that I could handle. I also tried to keep running my transcription business and keep some "normality" in my life. But I could barely do this rudimentary management work and feared I would never be able to do the rewrites on the book, which the new publisher wanted in a few months.

In search of relief, and a better diagnosis, I asked the ENT surgeon if my problem could have been trigeminal neuralgia, a condition I had read about through the years. It is typified by severe pain after even the most minor physical contact with the nerves in the face. Even a strong wind can set it off. The doctor said he didn't know, but to calm the nerves down, he prescribed the neuralgia drug of choice, Tegretol (carbamazepine), a drug I had not taken before then because of its potential harm to the liver. But now I was desperate, liver be damned. Sadly, it had no effect beyond making it difficult to urinate; I would sit there and realize I'd forgotten how to do it. After we discontinued the drug, thankfully, that skill returned in full.

With the surgeon still acting defensively, I felt I had nowhere to turn. I wasn't even appeased by words of encouragement from my uncle, who told me how Cole Porter wrote some of the best songs of his career after failed surgeries for knee pain.

I had little hope of even operating at a diminished level. With such an outrageous level of pain, no amount of good "management" skills could make a difference. I meditated, did visualizations, slept the right amount, exercised, and so on, and still, nothing changed. In that first month, after a few hours of money-earning work with my business in the afternoon, I took some strong narcotics, Lortabs and Lorcets, which only slightly dulled the pain. But they did provide relief in that they knocked me out, and I floated for hours watching television or napping in a vegetative state. This is how life will be from now on, I thought, just like the lives of other chronic pain sufferers I had heard about: Take drugs, watch TV, and stay in bed. For years, I had fought to stay out of their ranks, but now the struggle was just too great.

Specifically, the painkillers provided relief by getting rid of one nagging thing: my ambition. I realized that the pain didn't matter much—as long as there was nothing else I really cared to do. The drugs fully squelched that burning desire, which has been with me ever since I can remember: To not just sit there, to do more (in true "wood" fashion). Otherwise, one of the worst parts of having pain is thinking about all the things I would rather be— and should be—doing. A friend who had suffered from both depression and cluster headaches recently described to me this special frustration with severe pain. When he was depressed, he lost the will to do anything. But with the cluster headaches, he retained his will but lost his physical ability to act, being constantly engaged in a struggle with himself to break free.

As another positive, being without ambition meant that I could not even muster the will to follow through on any dark thoughts, which were increasingly occupying my brain. But at the same time I had these visions, I knew I was not capable of suicide anyway. After all, I reasoned, I didn't even have the nerve to cut my own bangs, for fear of making a mistake.

Nevertheless, I couldn't help but think these thoughts, especially over the next month, when I was further alarmed by a new pain, now also on the right side of my head. The Headache, which before had been limited to the left side, was now seeking fresh real estate. This new right-sided pain was not continuous, but it became more and more common as the days passed. Behind the right eye and in the right temple, I now had a headache that mirrored the original. From this surgery, a twin had hatched.

16

Down the Rabbit Hole

○ ○ ○ ○ ○ ○ ○ ○ ○

IN THE ORIGINAL *Alice's Adventures in Wonderland* and *Through the Looking-Glass* of the late nineteenth century (as well as in the Disney cartoon version, which I am more familiar with), the characters face many absurdities and illusions. Not the least of which is headache.

After reading the *Wonderland* book, no one would be surprised to learn that the author, Lewis Carroll, was a migraine sufferer. In one chapter, the Queen of Hearts complains of a "forehead ache," and in another Tweedledee comments, "Generally I am very brave . . . only today I happen to have a headache."

Yet, other parts of Alice's journey down the rabbit hole and through the looking glass—which do not specifically address this ailment—also serve well to illustrate the generally confusing and topsy-turvy nature of the chronic headache experience.

Likewise, the world of headache treatment is one of doublespeak and doubt: a world where decisions made by the authorities around you seem arbitrary, where you suddenly find yourself on trial when no crime has been committed, where sentences (or courses of action) are decided well before any sound verdicts or diagnoses are handed down, where one mysterious potion begging, "Drink me," unexpectedly turns your life upside down, and where, worst of all, you cannot trust the logic of your own senses to guide you through it all.

"Alice felt dreadfully puzzled," Carroll wrote, describing her reaction to the Mad Hatter at the tea party, a comment that could, in my view, describe a patient's state of mind after a typically brief conversation with a high-level medical specialist: "The Hatter's remark seemed to her to have no sort of meaning in it, and yet it was certainly English" (62).

Indeed, the world of chronic pain and headache is essentially one of illusion. Here, not only does one appear crazy but also commonly privately wonders if he or she has reached that point.

In fact, as I learned only years later, the migraine experience, which takes on endless types of forms and symptoms, is often hard-wired for such a seemingly crazy trip.

This "trippy-ness" may characterize all stages of the attack. Before the pain sets in, many patients experience a variety of bizarre neurological events, which doctors actually refer to as the *Alice in Wonderland phenomenon*, and which at first may seem like hints of a nervous breakdown. About 20–70 percent of migraine patients have *prodrome*, or *premonitory phenomena*, hours and even days before the migraine attack. A prodrome may include extremes of elation or depression, strong food cravings, and insomnia.

Then, when the migraine phase hits, distortions may intensify. Besides the terrible pain, complaints may include oversensitivity to light, sounds, and smells; difficulty in integrating mental activities, such as speaking or reading or writing; nausea and vomiting; feelings of fear and delirium; numbness in the extremities; widespread pain; and a sense of being detached from one's surroundings. For this reason, migraine has historically been labeled *sick headache*; General Ulysses S. Grant famously reported suffering one before Lee surrendered to him in the Civil War.

Some of Alice's most seemingly idiosyncratic adventures illustrate other very specific neurological effects. The patient may feel too big for his or her surroundings, as in Alice's experience of almost bursting a small cottage after drinking one of her tonics. She also describes tunnel vision and vertigo, which migraine sufferers may also experience.

For about 20–60 percent of migraine sufferers, a visual aura appears in the hour before the pain descends. (This type of headache is now, rather plainly, classified as *migraine with aura* and was formerly called *classic migraine*. It contrasts to *migraine without aura*, formerly called *common migraine*.) This aura, which either disappears with the onset of the pain or accompanies it, typically goes on for less than an hour, but it sometimes reappears for days.

In about 20 percent of these cases of aura, no pain follows the aura at all. This aura experience without pain mainly happens to children and also describes twilight states involved in other neurological problems, such as epilepsy, Epstein-Barr virus, and schizophrenia. In fact, this aura trip strongly resembles what one would see with certain hallucinogens, such as

LSD and those funny little mushrooms. This aura all happens within the brain, as a result of brainwave changes. The phenomenon does not result from changes taking place in the eyes themselves. And this light show varies greatly from person to person, and even from attack to attack. During an aura, the internal brain can broadcast to itself a festival of twinkling stars, called *phosphenes*. Some shapes are bigger blobs called *scotomas*—also referred to as *negative scotomas*—which may actually act as blind spots and blot out what you see before you, the effect being like that of a hole in a movie screen. Patients have reported their visual fields broken up by honeycomb patterns, bizarre tiltings, and cubistlike mosaic visions—the type of special effects that you would expect to see in a psychedelic 1960s video with The Doors music in the background.

Some auras feature particular types of zigzag shapes, called *fortifications*. A term also used is *teichopsia*, which is Greek for "town wall" and "vision." In reality, these shapes really do resemble, from an aerial view, the protective, fortifying battlements around medieval towns. (Driving home this point, the migraine textbook, *Headache in Clinical Practice*, actually gives a photo of the walled city of Palmanova, Italy, to illustrate a "migraine with aura" [72].[1]) To use a more modern metaphor, these structures resemble a ring or horseshoe made of Legos, or an aerial view of an urban mid-twentieth-century courtyard apartment building, the kind that my grandmother lived in.)

Although typical episodic migraine attacks of all types may last less than a day, often under two hours, some may go on for days and/or occur many times a week, blurring the line with, and even evolving into, chronic daily headache. Afterward, as is typical of drug trips, some patients feel refreshed and euphoric, and others are depressed and fatigued. (See the sidebar.)

In my particular case, at the beginning of 1999, after my surgery, I felt as if I had been under the spell of other types of illusions. I was troubled, especially because of my personal complicity in this surgery, by how strong my powers of self-delusion could be. Again, I had seen what I had wanted to see. I realized that when I was dealing with pain, even the "concrete" was really not concrete. This nasal obstruction of the septum that I could feel and see (with a brain scan), which physically dug right into the site of pain behind my eye, was just a red herring. I was as confused as Alice at the tea party.

Finally, about a month and a half after the surgery, the blood in my eye slowly faded away. The intense broken-glass feeling in the left eye subsided, and I happily stopped taking those fog-inducing Lortabs and Lorcets. I was left with a headache slightly worse than the one I had started out with. What was also distressing, I was even more confused about the source of the

The Aura Experience: Totally Awesome?

Some famous migraine sufferers throughout history have managed to find some meaning in the seemingly mystical nature of the drug aura. These include religious figures. Some neurologists believe that St. Paul's thorn in his flesh on the road to Damascus, which resulted in his conversion to Christianity, was actually a migraine that met the current criteria of the International Headache Society.[2] In the twelfth century, Abbess Hildegard of Bingen (1098–1180) wrote in awe about her auras, characterizing them as fantastic visions from God:

> The visions which I saw I beheld neither in sleep, nor in dreams, nor in madness, nor with my carnal eyes, nor with the ears of the flesh, nor in hidden places; but wakeful, alert, and with the eyes of the spirit and the inward ears, I perceived them in open view and according to the will of God. . . .
> I saw a great star, most splendid and beautiful, and with it an exceeding multitude of falling sparks, with which the star followed southward . . . and suddenly they were all annihilated, being turned into black coals . . . and cast into the abyss so that I could see them no more.[3]

Even many medical researchers have appreciated this mystical-seeming phenomenon as a source of intrigue. In medical tests, the prodrome part of the migraine, or the phase leading up to it, has been widely described as a real type of "premonition," a concept I had previously thought was limited to psychics. Writing about the aura in his book *Migraine*, Oliver Sacks observed, "It is in this sense, finally, that migraine is enthralling; for it shows us, in the form of a hallucinatory display, not only an elemental activity of the cerebral cortex, but an entire self-organising system, a universal behaviour, at work. It shows us not only the secrets of neuronal organisation, but the creative heart of Nature herself" (297).

pain. I had followed a trail of seemingly stunning clues that all turned out to be dead ends.

Like many patients, I was still having trouble distinguishing common *symptoms* of migraine (such as neck pain and allergy) from the original causes. I also was confused by how structural abnormalities (like a deviated septum) might not necessarily cause the pain. "Indeed," commented Oliver Sacks, in his book *Migraine*, "there is probably no field in medicine so strewn with the debris of misdiagnosis and mistreatment, and of well-intentioned but wholly mistaken medical and surgical intervention" (49, 50).

After recognizing how strongly external stimuli triggered the pain, as the surgery had ignited it to kingdom come, I continued to wonder about recent diagnoses, for example, if this condition was really neuralgia. To get an answer, I saw a prominent pain specialist, one whom my mother happened to spot on the cover of *Chicago Magazine*, who was billed as one of the best doctors in the city. I considered myself lucky to get an appointment. Telling me that my pain was too constant to qualify as neuralgia, he presented another seemingly rational question: Was it from stenosis?

After giving me some MRIs of the neck and brain, the only irregularity he found was a mild stenosis (a spinal narrowing) at the base of the neck. As a treatment, he wanted to do a "bilateral facet nerve block" injection of an anesthetic into the spinal cord at the point of the stenosis. This was a diagnostic tool. If the injection got rid of the pain, the stenosis was the source of the problem and I could have some radiofrequency work done to more permanently sever the nerve at that point. But I declined. I didn't have the stamina to undergo any more invasive procedures involving doctors wielding large and sharp objects near my head and spine—no matter how stellar their qualifications seemed. And my uncle, along with other doctors I would see later, said that stenosis that low in the spine would lead to shoulder or arm pain, not headache pain. My uncle observed that most people have some irregularities in the spine, but they are not all a source of pain. Still, I felt wracked with doubt that I was leaving a major clue unexplored.

At that time, I did not know the basic medical information that I now have—about why so many false clues exist, and about why chronic headache is so prone to misdiagnosis and needless and even harmful procedures. Once again, as with the widespread confusion about headaches as psychosomatic, its inherently invisible *neurological basis* is the culprit. The pain is easily triggered by external and internal forces, such as stress, which are often mistakenly labeled the root cause. All this confusion is further compounded by the multiple forms that migraine takes, all theoretically originating from one basic problem: *a neurological dysfunction in the brain stem.*

As Dr. Scott Fishman wrote in his insightful book *The War on Pain*, a point of origin of all these seeming illusions is thought to be the thalamus, the command center of the brain for controlling pain and emotion. In some people who are genetically predisposed, the thalamus overinterprets even the most minor triggers, internal and external—hormones, the weather, stress, chemicals in food, and so on. When stimulated, the thalamus sends a cascade of signals throughout the brain. Some of these are neurological and are associated with classic migraine, such as nausea; loss of appetite; oversensitivity to light, sound, and smell; visual aura; and numbness in the body.

In addition, this cascade of activity sparked by the thalamus may create muscle tension in the neck and shoulders, which is often mistaken for the root cause of headache pain—as I had experienced with physical therapy and massage therapists. Along with these processes, blood vessels on the periphery of the brain expanded can also trigger sinus pain.

In reality, as many patients and doctors never realize, these sinus problems can be a *result* of the migraine's neurological chain of events, not a cause of it. Specifically, this reaction irritates the trigeminal nerve, which supplies sensation to the face and head. The long trigeminal nerve has branches that also go into the sinuses and the nasal cavities. This process may also stimulate sinus problems, which accompany an estimated 45 percent of migraine attacks. A recent study revealed that nine out of ten patients who had been diagnosed with sinus headaches really had migraines.[4]

The connection between the inflamed trigeminal nerve and sinus symptoms also explains the connection between migraine and sinus medications. Migraine sufferers have found that triptans, such as Imitrex, can relieve their sinus problems. Many of us have also found that inflammation-shrinking decongestants, such as the Tavist D that I have relied on, can help relieve headache pain. A resulting and often false assumption is that if sinus medication helps the headache, the headache is based in sinus problems.

Another major mix-up in treating chronic headache is in blaming stress as the root cause of chronic pain, instead of a trigger.

In truth, a person has to have a genetic predisposition to chronic headaches to have them. After all, saying stress causes a headache is like saying cold weather causes a flu or a smoky room causes asthma. A person has these vulnerabilities to begin with. As Susan Sontag wrote in *Illness as Metaphor*: "Needless to say, the hypothesis that distress can affect immunological responsiveness (and, in some circumstances, lower immunity to disease) is hardly the same as—or constitutes evidence for—the view that emotions cause diseases, much less for the belief that specific emotions can produce specific diseases" (54).

This distinction can be more confusing for those patients for whom stress is the major trigger. Stress is more morally charged than other triggers, such as certain foods and weather changes. Stress is less "legitimate" because it involves emotions, which anyone with proper discipline is expected to control. And so, this factor of emotion—equated for decades with "hysteria"—

becomes the most visible culprit, *rather than* a person's neurobiological pre-disposition.

In fact, confusion also arises because stress is the most commonly report-ed trigger for all types of headaches, between one-third and two-thirds of patients reporting it as an influence. It invariably rates high on the list, even above foods and hormones. But many people have chronic headaches with *no* identifiable triggers, either internal or external.[5] And stress is also a factor in every other illness. Stress can worsen, merely accompany, or result from dia-betes, cancer, hypertension, Parkinson's disease, and so on.

Not that trying to reduce and manage stress is a bad idea. Reducing stress's impact as a trigger may also raise the threshold for getting a headache (or a worse headache, for those who have it constantly). In most people, trig-gers are considered "additive," each one making a difference only when many pile up. These triggers all work together to raise a person's vulnerability to the migraine attack. I've heard this dynamic described as each trigger contribut-ing to lighting a part of the fuse, which varies in length among individuals. (And people with chronic headaches have unusually short fuses.) In other words, a person may not get a headache from lack of sleep, hormone fluctua-tion, or Parmesan cheese, but when all are experienced at once, the oppor-tunistic pain breaks through.

In reality, another reason why stress is *not* the root cause of chronic pain, although it is definitely a trigger, is that stress is a fact of life for just about everyone. It's true that we can learn to manage it better, but it's hard to stop major and minor stressful events from happening in the first place, while we are still trying to live in the real world—and not in some kind of plastic bub-ble. Blaming pain on stress could be compared to blaming hormones for causing a woman's depression. Every woman of reproductive age has fluctu-ating hormones, but not every woman gets depressed as a result. The more fundamental culprit is individual brain chemistry, which determines a woman's neurological response to hormones, not the hormones themselves.

One neurologist I interviewed in 2003, Dr. Vincent Martin, also a headache sufferer, explained the concept of triggers to me in another way, by calling an overly sensitive nervous system the main problem: "So you've got this nervous system that's overreactive to both your internal and your external environment. So all these triggers are floating around out there. Internally, there are the hormonal changes. Then another trigger would be stress. The more stress you have, the more headaches you get. You might eat the wrong foods; you might drink too much coffee and develop caffeine-withdrawal headaches. Weather changes might bother you. So it's as if in this particular nervous system every change in the environment actually provokes a headache. And that's a system that you live with and I live with, and it's just a very sensitive type of nervous system.

"So everything provokes a headache. I have heard that so often from chronic daily headache patients: 'Dr. Martin, everything provokes a headache. I mean, if I eat, if I sleep too much or sleep too little, if I get, you know, get a little distressed, if I have a beer . . . 'And they just feel frustrated because they feel that everything they potentially do or all the good things in life are going to provoke a headache."

As with other types of confusion, the media have played a large part in this widespread misunderstanding of the role of triggers, by not reporting the distinctions. You can just skim the headlines of major stories about chronic headaches to get the drift. A story in the July 14, 2003, *Los Angeles Times* explained why "That Raging Headache May be Anger Based."[6] It reported research from St. Louis University finding that headache sufferers are more likely to hold in anger. That may be true, but the article does not explain that this anger is a trigger, not a root cause. An article in the February 2004 issue of *Redbook* informs you "Why You've Got That Headache," listing "six surprising causes," which range from holding in anger to changing sleeping patterns on the weekends.[7] Although the article itself refers to these provocations as "triggers," it does not talk about a genetic predisposition to having headaches in the first place. Although helpful, because they encourage good anger and stress management, reports such as these also compound the guilt that headache sufferers feel because they suspect they are essentially bringing headaches on themselves and are emotionally disturbed.

Furthermore, this complex and invisible neurological process leads to another source of confusion, a misdiagnosis of the *type* of headache suffered: Is it migraine, tension headache, chronic daily headache, or trigeminal neuralgia, I have asked myself at different times, while in pursuit of different courses of treatment. But as some doctors now theorize, these may all be different manifestations of the *same* problem, a basic stimuli-processing dysfunction in the thalamus.

Compounding problems is many pain practitioners' lack of understanding of these neurological processes. As a result, practitioners see what they want to see, the headache functioning as one big inkblot test (or as Charlie from *Flowers for Algnernon* would say, "*ror shak* test"). Massage therapists see muscle tension as the root of headaches; ENT specialists diagnose sinus problems; and chiropractors blame spinal deformities. Some of this prejudice is human nature. Indeed, "when the only tool you own is a hammer, every problem begins to resemble a nail" goes the famous quote from Abraham Maslow. (A friend's retina-surgeon husband cited this to me after my surgery.)

Even so, paying attention to the symptoms of chronic headache is important. Addressing them can be a step toward at least raising the body's resistance to pain. Just like treating sinus problems, treating the muscle pain resulting from a migraine may, at least temporarily, help relieve the headache. The challenge is to attack the headache at any point along the chain of events, from the thalamus (with antiepileptic drugs) to trigger points on the shoulders (with massage). I have heard of some people getting relief with a dental guard at night that prevents them from clenching their jaw, which could contribute to exacerbating the pain (but may not necessarily be the root cause).[8]

Symptom chasing should be done realistically and responsibly. At best, relieving these problems might reduce headache pain, raising one's resistance to headaches in the first place. But at worst, aggressively treating what turns out to be a false lead, as in the case of my surgery, can make the pain worse.

Unfortunately, as I found out only recently, I was not alone in having surgery for no reason—for confusing a symptom (sinus problems) with the cause. In his 2002 guide *Heal Your Headache*, Dr. David Buchholz reported that surgeries on the sinuses and other structural areas of the head, such as on a deviated septum "pressing against something," are common among chronic headache patients. He even profiled one patient who had six such surgeries before seeing him. He added that he has personally treated six women who had previously had breast reduction surgery to cure their migraines, in an effort to reduce stress on nerves, it such as from bra straps straining the shoulders. These surgeries also failed.

Surgical efforts to relieve pain are notoriously risky and generally ineffective. Doctors through history have discovered this after severing irritated nerves, only to see the pain return in another part of the body, and more severely. Much of the programming of pain is seated in the thalamus, and no matter which nerves are severed in the body, the aberrant signals from the thalamus persist. As in my case, brain scans fail to show the definitive source of pain and are all open to interpretation. Even a structural irregularity, such as a deviated septum or a stenosis of the spinal cord, may be red herrings, typical even in people who have no pain.[9]

I discovered another disturbing risk while attending the annual meeting of the American Pain Society in March 2003: Many invasive procedures have not been adequately tested. "Proper research is rarely undertaken and typically comes late, often 10 to 20 years after the first invention of the procedure," said Dr. Nikolai Bogduk, a prominent Australian pain researcher and authority on evidence-based medicine (or that tiny part of medicine that has been scientifically "proven"). "This is opposite to the way scientists behave in other disciplines, where if the results are negative, that should lead to cessation of the procedure. This never happens. Once it's established, despite the evidence, invasive procedures keep being perpetuated."[10]

Dr. Bogduk warned that doctors often skip important precautionary steps for the sake of convenience, even with procedures that have been proven to work. (In my case, the ENT surgeon didn't give me any kind of control nerve block near the deviated septum, to confirm that this was the culprit.) This failure commonly occurs with nerve blocks themselves, used to relieve pain. Dr. Bogduk said that giving the patient a saline (saltwater) block in addition to one with real anesthesia can easily demonstrate if the procedure has a placebo effect. This precaution can reduce the expense and danger of follow-up surgery to actually sever the suspected nerve.

At that same conference, in a major speech to the hundreds assembled, Dr. John D. Loeser warned that the same problem in using "off-label" drugs exists with "off-label" surgery. A procedure, such as a type of nerve block, may be approved by the FDA for one problem but not for a host of others, for which it eventually may become routine. He said that doctors too often resort to such "quick fixes" instead of spending the time to get to know the patient and treat pain in other ways. "It is not that I am opposed to interventions, for I earn my living as a neurosurgeon," he said. "I do recognize, however, that every needle has a sharp end that goes into the patient and a blunt end that is attached to a provider. And every scalpel has a blade that encroaches upon the patient and a handle that attaches to a surgeon. Anyone who thinks that all the action occurs at the sharp end does not understand either health care or human behavior."

But doctors tend to communicate poorly with patients about the complexities of surgery. Needless to say, the media further contribute to this poor understanding and may unrealistically fan the hopes of patients. As when promoting "wonder drugs," the media often follow a formula that points to technology as a "quick fix." Features often focus on those who are helped but neglect to cover those who aren't. Or they might ignore possible major and likely side effects.

A flaw in statistics adds confusion. Negative results of off-label uses are rarely or never, and positive results (fudged or not) are always, published. Out of 1,000 studies, by chance 50 will show significant improvement at the 95

Usually No Better than a Hole in the Head: A Short History of Surgery for Pain

As long as people have complained about headache pain, doctors have misguidedly longed to cut into it and carve it out.

In a process practiced in ancient times, and still used by some African tribes, surgeons cut holes in the skulls of headache sufferers with special tools. This procedure is called *trepanation*. Archaeologists have unearthed prehistoric skulls, dating back as far as 7000 B.C., with such marks, noting by subsequent wear and aging that many of these patients actually survived these procedures. Trepanation was practiced in Europe until the mid-seventeenth century. A theory behind trepanation was that it released the invisible imps or demons causing the pain. Other cultures have practiced similar methods. Ancient Peruvian Indians cut a slit between the victim's eyebrows to provide an escape hatch for the evil spirits, which were allegedly washed away by the subsequently flowing blood.

Through the eighteenth century, common European practices included bloodletting, also to release the offending spirits and humors. A related practice was cupping, in which a physician made incisions in the head and then covered them with heated glass globes, to draw the blood out. Cupping was also used with incisions to draw the blood to the surface of the skin. (Today, many acupuncturists, including one I tried, continue this cupping practice, minus the incisions.) Some doctors recommended opening up the skull, which Thomas Willis, the famed seventeenth-century brain anatomist, was already decrying as backward. "I think opening of the skull will profit little or nothing," he wisely wrote, in response to a suggestion by the physician William Harvey to his patient, a noble "Lady of great quality" who had a "terrible and inveterate Head-ach" for twenty years.[11]

But doctors, up to the present time, have continued using surgery to sever nerves, often with the terrible results of aggravated pain and severe numbness in some parts of the face. This practice of surgery for head pain picked up steam in the early twentieth century when morphine and other opiates became more strictly regulated, so the options were limited to either psychotherapy or surgery for pain.[12] In his book *Why We Hurt*, surgeon Frank Vertosick recalled the early days of his training: "We still commonly tried heating the nerve using a needle electrode. Twenty years have passed and I can still hear the patients screaming. We would stuff blankets around the doors to muffle their anguished cries so that patients in other operating rooms wouldn't be disturbed" (76).

percent confidence level, leading the talking heads on 10 P.M. newscasts to proclaim, "New hope for sufferers." The other 950 studies will never appear on a printed page or on the air.[13]

On one level, of course, journalistic coverage of surgical alternatives can be helpful, to give patients more options to consider and bring up with their doctors. But the typically narrow and totally uncritical coverage often does more of a disservice in the long run, as it lacks a realistic assessment of the complexities and risks of such surgery. The news peg is that the surgery worked for this one person here and therefore can work for *you*. But the stories fail to convey the bigger picture.

Another motivation contributing to pursuit of the hazard-strewn path of surgery for chronic pain is more craven: financial.

Invasive procedures and surgeries are a major method of making money from headache patients. Some of this work can be done in less than an hour and earn the practitioner thousands of dollars, with the endorsement of insurance companies, which trust surgery to be a "real" treatment. In contrast, the other ways that doctors treat pain, through getting to know the patient, are not so remunerative.

Typically, a neurologist or internist will see a pain patient infrequently, for a relatively small office-visit fee (such as seventy-five to a hundred dollars), and then that patient will eat up her or his time with phone calls about medications and changing symptoms. As an example of the time required to treat such patients, in his textbook for doctors about pain medications, *Management of Headache and Headache Medications,* Dr. Lawrence Robbins outlines typical case studies that require dozens of phone calls back and forth. One example is given in his two-plus-page (small-type) summary of his months-long treatment of Sally, a forty-five-year-old woman with "frequent migraine plus severe Chronic Daily Headache and menstrual migraine" (80–83). After her initial office visit, her treatment involved constant phone calls to adjust the dosages and types of her three kinds of medication: abortive (to stem a migraine at its beginning), preventive (to take daily to increase her pain threshold), and palliative (just to ease the pain). He also noted her other health limits (e.g., a stomach that couldn't tolerate many anti-inflammatory drugs), the influence of comorbidities (insomnia, depression, anxiety), and the constantly changing side effects. By the end of the case study, Sally's headaches were better, but she was still working to balance side effects and relief. Despite all these months of work, her case remained a work in progress. Needless to say, paying such attention to the patient—

necessary for adequate headache care with medications—is not the ideal way to drive up revenue. In contrast, a surgeon could cut into Sally's head and—in one hour—make a hundred times more profit. In that case, he or she would hardly have to bother to talk to Sally. The choices for many doctors, therefore, become very clear, whereas the patient continues to operate under the delusion that her best interests are being kept in mind—and that at long last, the medical world is about to come to its senses.

17

The Hangman's Noose

○ ○ ○ ○ ○ ○ ○ ○ ○

IT WAS EARLY 1999, and now reminded of doctors' limits in helping me, I wondered what tools I *did* have left to try. This was a time of reflection. I thought back over the past eight years. I had been drugged up, spaced out, injected, psychoanalyzed, cross-examined, humiliated, cut up, felt up, and swindled. But had *anything* helped me? What could I return to?

With any positive experience I had had of relieving pain, I realized that *simplicity* seemed to be a key. And as in other areas of life, satisfaction was generally linked to low expectations. As long as I was seeking temporary relief—not long-term relief and not a cure—alternative medicine had some value. I remembered the lavender-peppermint mixture from the Alexander Method therapist and stashed away three bottles of it. Now I would always have one within arm's reach: in my purse, at my desk, and beside my bed, for easy access. I added to my arsenal the Tavist D (formulated with the pharmaceutical equivalent of ephedra), and a type of green tea potion, Alvita Migrafew. I stocked the freezer with blue ice packs, including the newfangled ones that wrap snugly around the forehead and are fastened with Velcro.

I pledged to rest and take things at a slower pace and with more breaks, a simple way to conserve marbles while still being productive. I was making progress in rewriting my book—slow progress, to be sure—but it was still progress. I would just pretend that I was European, working no more than six hours a day and taking off a week every few months or so. After all, in another culture, I wouldn't be considered a slacker. I would just be, well, maybe, Swedish.

The Time-Honored Tradition of the Band Around the Head

Also as a low-tech option, I occasionally started to use an elastic band around my forehead, which sometimes gives temporary relief by physically restricting blood flow. I ordered the TheraP band by Biomedics, which is adjustable with a Velcro fastener. It came with magnets, but I think the real source of the relief is just the plain old elastic band.

In fact, besides opium, acupuncture, and trepanation, this is probably one of the most ancient headache remedies in recorded history. The Sumerian prescription for headaches of 4000 B.C. was

Take the hair of a virgin kid. Let a wise woman spin it on the right side and double it on the left, and tie twice seven knots. Perform the incantation of Eridu. Bind therewith the head of the sick man. . . . Cast therewith the water of incantation over him, that the headache may ascend to heaven.

An Egyptian papyrus of 2500 B.C. recounts the bandaging of a clay effigy of a crocodile to the forehead of a headache sufferer, followed by praying. This procedure, according to the neurological theories of the time, worked to release the evil headache spirit (actually named Tiu in Mesopotamia). But it probably succeeded just as a compressor of blood vessels. Later on, St. Gregory, Bishop of Tours in the sixth century, was described curing his severe headache by pressing his head against the side of St. Martin's tomb, utilizing these same principles of applying pressure.

Shakespeare, in at least two plays, made reference to head binding for migraine. In *King John* (Act IV, Scene 1), Arthur says:

When your head did but ache
I knit my handkerchief about your brows
(The best I had, a princess wrought it me)
And I did never ask it you again.
And with my hand, at midnight held your head.

Shakespeare also portrayed this practice in *Othello* (Act III, Scene 3):

DESDEMONA: Why do you speak so faintly? Are you not well?
OTHELLO: I have a pain upon my forehead here.
DESDEMONA: Faith, that's with watching: twill away again. Let me but bind it hard, within this hour. It will be well.

Into the twentieth century, the Europeans also used this method, tying on a hangman's noose.[1] (That was in the days before Velcro.)

In the months following my surgery, I also revisited some of the best alternative healers, with their equally commonsense techniques—and emotional support. I got chiropractic and "energy" adjustments from Bill, therapy from Lisa, and a few acupuncture treatments. I decided that I would not throw out the baby with the bathwater—that is, get rid of *all* alternative medicine—just because some of it was snake oil.

There is no way to enlightenment. Enlightenment is the way.

But the emotional and physical pain did not diminish to presurgery "manageable" levels until I consulted someone new, Suzen, a myofacial therapist working at Whole Health Inc. As a characteristically attractive physical-therapist type, she was glowing with strength and energy. During my recovery from the surgery, I had read on the Internet about this type of "trigger-point" therapy for neuralgia problems. It is similar to the kind of knot-reducing work I had had with the Russian "reflexotherapist," physical therapists, and massage therapists, but more concentrated.

Suzen followed a type of philosophy practiced most famously in the 1960s by Dr. Janet Travell, an internist and pharmacologist who gained fame working on a famous closeted chronic pain patient, President John Fitzgerald Kennedy. (In fact, she was at the center of a scandal when thieves broke into her office during the highly contentious 1960 presidential campaign to obtain Kennedy's medical records—a crime that is thought to have been linked to his opponent, Richard M. Nixon.)[2] Travell used trigger-point injection therapy, numbing the area with agents like procaine, but her famous disciple, Bonnie Pruden, has used and promoted chemical-free firm muscle-release work that applies physical pressure with the hands or a special cane.

Like Pruden's, Suzen's work involved very firm and strong pressing into multiple trigger points, along the head, neck, shoulders, and back. This pressing would last several seconds, the pain growing and then diminishing. Then she would press on the same spot again for shorter intervals. After the first visit, I was amazed that the head pain was nearly gone and I had absolutely no tension in my shoulders. This relief lasted for about a day, for which I was grateful. But over time, like everything else I had tried, the treatments became less effective. Suzen tried to teach me to do her therapy to myself, but I hesitated to plunge into these sore spots for large amounts of time and was confused about exactly where they were. Without medical training, I was scared to fool around with the sensitive points along the front of the neck, for fear of giving myself a Ninja death lock.

But even those episodes of temporary relief were valuable. They seemed to remind my body and my spirit of what it was like to be without pain, and my mood improved. But Suzen, who was only several years older than I, probably helped me mostly just through conversations we had as she worked.

One day, I told her the source of much of my anguish over the pain, my guilt for causing this problem myself. I had been foolhardy in putting so much pressure on myself years ago to finish that first book without any real break for months. She paused and looked down at me on the table.

"Then I should blame myself for what happened to me. When I got sick, I was working in a holistic health center. If anyone should have been aware enough to avoid such a problem, it would have been me."

"What do you mean?"

"Several years ago, in a matter of a month or two, my house burned down, with all my possessions. Just before that, my seven-year relationship had ended. After that, I was hit with extreme pain and fatigue, to the point where I could hardly walk and certainly couldn't work."

But she had very slowly regained much of her strength through a careful regimen of three kinds of therapy: myofacial release, acupuncture, and chiropractics. Now she was back to working full time.

"It doesn't matter which types of these methods you follow specifically—like you can do another kind of energy work instead of acupuncture—but it's important to have all three of these types of therapy," she said.

"You have to be a Capricorn about it," she continued, pressing her middle three fingers into a space beneath my shoulder blade." That meant, she explained, that you have to keep plugging away, and that small efforts eventually pile up.

Over the next few years, I took this Capricorn's advice and settled into a routine. When the myofacial treatment lost effectiveness, I decided to substitute cheaper and twice-monthly massage, which ended up working just as well to at least take the edge off and was much less painful. I also went out and bought a special Battle Creek brand Thermofore heating pad that Suzen had told me about; it draws moisture from the air when you press a lever. It created soothing moist heat to help loosen the grip of the shoulders and back muscles, referring pain to the head. With the additional help of the elastic head band, ice packs for the neck and head, sweet-smelling bottles of lavender and peppermint, over-the-counter decongestant, and proper pacing, I got by. At last, I finished the final drafts of my book and prepared for its publication.

There is no way to enlightenment. Enlightenment is the way.

18

High Anxiety

○ ○ ○ ○ ○ ○ ○ ○ ○

AFTER ALMOST A DECADE OF THE HEADACHE, the time of reckoning had come. Despite the power of my growing management skills, and after my exhaustive search for a cure, I finally realized the worst had come true: I had done all I could to get rid of that motherfucker, and I'd lost.

The odds were that there was no cure and there would never be one.

I had been looking for something that did not exist.

Even with the best possible resources, I had come up empty. After all, although I wasn't rich, I knew I had been in a more privileged position than most others forced to take such a journey: princely private health insurance, a pain specialist uncle, a psychologist father, a therapist mother, plenty of doctor relatives to consult around the Thanksgiving table, a flexible schedule, and a history of both investigative journalism and studying the women's health movement.

I had spent tens of thousands of dollars to try more than forty types of prescription medications and more than fifty types of herbal and vitamin supplements. I saw:

- seven neurologists
- one brain surgeon
- five acupuncturists
- four physical therapists
- three ENT specialists
- one neuro-ophthalmologist

- three osteopaths
- four chiropractors
- four general practice physicians
- four shrinks
- countless massage and "body work" therapists
- one shaman

In other words, I had explored every possible option, at least once (except colonic irrigation, Jews for Jesus, Scientology, nerve blocks to my spine—and oh yeah, ayurvedic medicine). Alternative medicine did help—but unpredictably and with a high financial cost. And medical doctors overall could not come up with a remedy that wasn't worse than my original problem. Instead, they had cured other problems that I had neither known about nor cared about. The acupuncturist was delighted to have rid me of the white coating on my tongue. Thanks to the physical therapy, I had graceful gazelle-like posture. The brainwave biofeedback had cured my alleged attention deficit disorder. My voice was slightly more resonant because of my new slide-rule-straight septum.

Logically speaking, this was the time to stop struggling, to make peace with the pain, to finally accept it and learn how to live with it. But I had experienced life without pain and with pain—and *without pain* was definitely better. The pain still added struggle to every interaction, uncertainty to every plan made, and guilt for every promise broken.

Yes, I now had much more empathy for all kinds of people, including: the fat, the poor, the dependent, the depressed, the fatigued, and the superstitious. But I would have preferred to be an insensitive, ignorant non-self-aware cretin than what I had become: a more enlightened and almost ridiculously self-aware person with the almost continuous sensation of forks twisting into various trigeminal-nerve endings behind my eyes, as if they were trying to spear and wind up spaghetti.

I had learned from the Headache, but I knew that I would have learned from *any* negative experience. After all, if I had gotten hit by a bus instead, I might have become even more empathetic and enlightened about the eternal mysteries and meanings of life.

I was now in my early thirties, and the limits of the future were becoming clearer. I had survived the years of wedding showers and now was in the thick of a wave of baby showers. They made me think: I could barely make it out of bed by noon; how could I ever take care of a child, as I had vaguely imagined

I someday would? In just a few days of serotonin-denying sleeplessness, I would go crazy from the increased pain and perhaps become one of those awful mothers you see on television who eventually abandons the kid at McDonald's with a twenty-dollar bill and an orange soda.

Even the significant hard-won accomplishment of having my book published, the one on sex and young women, brought some disappointments. Many people had assured me that the pain would diminish upon publication, in reaction to my emotional relief, but it didn't. Unfortunately, this pain was apparently *not* psychosomatic resistance to writing and mental activity. If only it were, I thought.

And no matter how new and improved my attitude had become, I still was human, and an undercurrent of anxiety rattled me, to an even greater extent than before. I still felt isolated, and even freakish, as the only person in the United States who apparently hadn't been cured by Western or alternative medicine.

With an ailment that defied mainstream classification, I remained on the margins, beyond the pale. I was still confused about whether it was neurological, psychological, the result of food allergies or fibromyalgia (whatever that was), a spinal narrowing problem, and so on. I dismissed *all* doctors as vulnerable to the old "if you have a hammer, everything looks like a nail" problem: If you study one discipline, then that's how you view the origin of all the problems you encounter. As a result, I didn't take any one theory seriously. (See the sidebar.)

But one new source of consolation was the growing realization that I was not alone with this crazy particular ailment of chronic daily headache. Others were starting to emerge who, on their own, described very similar symptoms, which they had feared had been unique to them. They also had taken similar twisting journeys, encountering similar doubts and obstacles that they had thought they were alone in experiencing.

True, I had met other daily headache patients in waiting rooms and other Tired Girls on my own through the years. But I still felt isolated. I didn't get to know the headache patients with any depth, and most of the Tired Girls had other types of problems.

Then, in 2000, I met my first friend with this ludicrous daily headache problem. She provided valuable corroboration for the legitimacy of my case. In a print interview about my sex book, when asked about the topic of my next project, I had "come out" about having chronic pain. A graduate student in political science at Indiana University, Janet Johnson, e-mailed me in response: "I was intrigued because I have been battling headaches for five

Personality/Headache Diagnosis Test:
Take It Now!

The credo of "you see what you know" (as Goethe commented) extends to non-doctors. It turned out that everyone, including myself, was judging the source of chronic pain through a delusionally narrow lens, perhaps as a defense mechanism against the overwhelming complexities of the modern world.

As a sort of a game, I found that I could turn the tables and diagnose a person's personality by what they pegged as the source of my headaches. To me, the following guide, accumulated through years of experience, works more effectively than a Myers-Briggs personality test, horoscope, or Chinese chart of the elements to tell me what I'm all about:

Your Opinion	*Your Personality*
1) I'm nuts.	**Cold, unfeeling**
2) My subconscious reaction to "resist" limits of patriarchy, capitalism.	**Second-wave feminist**
3) An expression of social malaise in modern times, responding to media hype promoting "dubious illnesses." Or response to dominating mother.	**Cultural anthropologist (Ivy League school)**
4) Suppression of my natural female side in favor of a career, causing my body to rebel.	**Disciple of capitalist patriarchy, Marilyn Quayle**
5) Pollution, nuclear radiation, milk, technology, bad fruit.	**Earthy**
6) Too many metals, food allergies, blocked chi.	**Trendy**
7) Overwork.	**Lazy**
8) "You need to just work harder. There's nothing you can't push through."	**Over 75/The Greatest Generation**
9) My fierce, abundant intelligence is too much for my mere mortal body to handle.	**Extremely perceptive**

years, and if the headaches aren't bad enough to do me in, my doctors (and other miscellaneous personnel) are. It would all be rather funny if it weren't so sad."

She went on to explain:

My dissertation adviser told me that graduate school was supposed to give me headaches. The first doctor I saw (a male GP) thought I was just depressed because I was crying while describing the terrible, never-ending pain. I survived the first year by taking barbiturates with codeine. The next doctor (a male neurologist) suggested (somewhat in jest) that I get pregnant. [She was referring to the theory that pregnancy helps stabilize hormones.] A third doctor (a female biofeedback therapist) thought this experience was good for me (perhaps, helping me learn to relax?). A (female) pain management physician wrote in my file that I needed to exercise more (after I told her that one of the things I do is teach fitness classes at the university athletic center).

Indeed, a few months later when I met Janet, a petite blond, in person, I saw that she was a fitness expert. In an industrious effort to relieve her headaches, she had even become a yoga teacher, in addition to teaching her regular load of fitness classes. Although I was disappointed that this didn't help her pain much, I was also personally relieved: I had felt guilty for years thinking that if I just practiced more yoga, all my problems would be gone. It was just a question of my being too undisciplined to do it. I was now off the hook with boring-as-hell yoga, at last.

Like me, Janet often clashed with her doctors. Part of this may have been generational. We both felt entitled to be a "partner" with the doctor as a fellow "professional." In an effort to help one doctor, the same one I had seen at Chicago Headache Clinic, Janet had made up a long spreadsheet—using a "logit model" of statistical analysis. The model charted her headaches and the typical correlations between the pain level and other variables in her life (lack of sleep, period, exercise, etc.). She did not find that any single variable was triggering the pain. But she recognized that the pain was worse on days when she had anxiety. Also exacerbating pain, apparently, was wearing T-back sports bras, which seemed to put more stress on her upper back muscles than the regular ones.

"That's impossible," the doctor had said in response. Not interested in any of this information, or in asking any further questions, he prescribed her a one-size-fits-all drug regimen.

"He just said I had that headache personality," she said. "He had met with me for, like, five minutes. And my 'headache personality' made me want to hit him."

In response to this and other incidents, Janet wrote a letter of complaint to the Chicago Headache Clinic. But now she realized that her new doctor there, whom she liked, had a copy of it in her permanent file, and she worried that the doctor would view her as just "difficult." She brought up the *Seinfeld* episode in which Elaine is labeled in her file as a "problem patient," which she can never overcome with future doctors. But for patients like us, this risk was not just the stuff of comedy; such a letter could become a real threat to our health care.

Like me, Janet had faced difficult decisions about surgery. Another doctor had a recommendation that Janet was nervous about trying. Her most recent MRI revealed one irregularity at the base of the head, an Arnold-Chiari malformation (named after the doctor who discovered it, Arnold Chiari). This new neurologist, who was at one of the most prestigious neurosurgery centers in the world (the same one that had targeted my stenosis as the source of my problems), wanted to do surgery. But Janet also wondered if that irregularity was a red herring, if she would be undergoing risk without strong evidence of cause and effect.

She did mention one positive outcome of the recommendation for surgery. Now she had a label—an Arnold-Chiari malformation—to legitimize her headaches to others, and it was dire enough to warrant surgery, she reported back to all others in her life. "That's serious. This is real," she said.

I had also felt such a quick fix (surgery) was tempting—as a way to get rid of medications. Over the past five years, Janet had tried twenty-five different drugs, which, at best, worked marginally but were not tolerable anyway because of high side effects. She rang another strong bell of recognition in my mind when she told me that she now couldn't afford to try any new medications, because the process would very likely cost her two or more months of work, considering the side effects and then the exacerbated symptoms of withdrawal.

Janet's worst experience with drugs had come the year before, while she was in Russia for nine months doing research for her dissertation. At first, she blamed her state of lethargy—of walking around in a "tunnel" while she was there—on trouble adjusting to a foreign country. But she later realized her problem was the Klonopin, a tranquilizer and anticonvulsant, and Trazodone, a type of antidepressant that her doctor had "sent" with her. Both are very common preventive medications for chronic daily headache. "I was sitting in bed all day reading, and then sleeping twelve hours a day. But not really sleeping because the drugs would keep me from sleeping. I was having very vivid dreams, so I wasn't sleeping. I wasn't getting the type of sleep that I needed," she explained.

She saw a Russian neurologist and had an MRI at the Central Neurological Clinic, a visit that made her appreciate some more uniform aspects of American hospitals. "I was, like, 'There are cats in this hospital.' And they were, like, 'If we didn't have cats, we would have mice.'"

The Russian neurologist said he couldn't help her—a statement that she appreciated for its unusual candor. But then she did find some relief there from an osteopath. In a new type of managed-care arrangement, he gave her free osteopathic adjustments in return for her arranging to get his book published by someone with whom she worked. When she returned home to Indiana, she did find another osteopath who continued to help her take the edge off with his regular forty-five-minute treatments.

But despite this help, she was still getting headaches regularly, typically after 4 P.M., when her day would grind to a halt. Now, as a result, she was very worried about fulfilling her obligations in a teaching job she had just taken. In filling out the required paperwork for it, she had been asked if she was disabled. She was still pondering that question. Ideally, she would "come out" about the headaches, to get a more flexible schedule—and even better lighting in her office—to make work easier. She said that even getting a regular office, as opposed to a cubicle, would make a difference, by enabling her to lie down when she needed to. But she still felt hesitant about taking the bold step of talking about her headaches to any employer, especially a new one, and especially in a difficult job market.

Then she asked me a question that caught me off guard: "Do you consider yourself disabled?"

I couldn't answer. I had never pictured myself that way. It was just a headache, after all.

My friend Wendy, another Tired Girl, was going through this same ongoing confusion in dealing with doctors for her frequent migraines, along with a wider constellation of problems, including bipolar disorder. Our dialogue back and forth via e-mail was mostly medical. "I have lost all faith in Western medicine," she said, describing her choice to now see an acupuncturist. "I think if I keep seeing traditional Western doctors, I will eventually die or get permanently disabled."

She had just fallen unconscious after starting an antiseizure medication, Trileptal, and had fired her psychopharmacologist after he had insisted she merely had a "pseduoseizure" and should continue the drug. Her response was to give up on Western doctors. She had now embarked on an intense mission to research the roots of her problem and treat it herself. She was e-mailing me daily with pages of results of her research, reading medical abstracts on Medline. The live chats online also helped her.

"My investigation has taken a new twist: I have started chatting with doctors on some of these medical web sites using various medical aliases, including as a foreign middle-aged male doctor. I've gotten some useful information with the doctor aliases (each with their own e-mail account) and continue these e-mail correspondences. It will be interesting to see how the reactions vary. With the foreign-doctor alias, I even earned continuing medical education credit after passing one of their online tests. I earned a certificate suitable for framing."

Like mine, her frustrations over having so many unpredictable periods of dysfunction were growing. "I am having a bad day," she wrote me. "I realize that the past three years have been totally lost and the past ten years have been straight from hell. It seems like the smallest things throw me into disequilibrium. I am very depressed and exhausted."

Like many chronic pain patients, Wendy and I were realizing that our journeys for relief would never really end. As a result, managing the accompanying anxiety about the pain and its disruption of our lives was a major issue. Although I had thought I had experienced the worst pain and depression with the surgery, some of my greatest challenges remained ahead. As I continued to push for relief and continued to run up against more and more obstacles, internal and external, it became harder and harder to figure out what was and was not all in my head.

In 1995, I had renounced Western medicine, but five years later, I wondered if that was now too extreme a position to take. Should I be totally on my own without any kind of medical help, when brand-new things exist to possibly make life easier? Was I being a martyr needlessly? Would the pain eventually drive me crazier than any drug would? If I couldn't get cured, would I be able at least to get some relief, to make life more tolerable?

I was starting to realize that drugs had evolved during my self-imposed exile from them, and I decided to be more open-minded about them. At a party, a pleasant young man, a political strategist, told me how Celexa, a new antidepressant I had not known about, had relieved his year of constant head pain in just a few weeks. I remembered the words of a holistic doctor that *both* supplements and drugs tax the body, that your liver also has to work to process herbal supplements from the health food store. I had been avoiding prescription drugs partly because I had thought they were weakening my body (and resistance to pain), but I still shoveled down tons of herbal capsules without further thought.

In the spirit of moderation, I decided to resume seeing a neurologist. The choice was clearly Dr. Scott Smith (no, not his real name), a renowned headache specialist in the suburbs. I had seen Dr. Smith only briefly in the mid-1990s, and after my period of reviewing my history after the surgery, I realized that he had been more straightforward and less heavy-handed than the rest, never making any false promises. Most impressively, he himself had headaches.

But the most encouraging sign of his humanity came from a flyer posted on the wall, which he also handed out:

TODAY I HAVE A HEADACHE,
NOT BECAUSE I AM A BAD OR EVIL PERSON,
NOT BECAUSE I HATE MY FAMILY,
NOR BECAUSE I AM ANGRY,
NOT BECAUSE I AM A PERFECTIONIST,
AND NOT BECAUSE I HAVE SCREWED UP,
I HAVE A HEADACHE BECAUSE MY BODY HAS THIS DISORDER.

Every six months or so, I visited him, and he prescribed the newest off-label "wonder drug" for migraine or chronic headache. These included some newer antidepressants, which still gave me insomnia like the old ones, and the antiepileptic Neurontin, introduced in 1994 and since used off-label for many types of pain. But it didn't do much more than just make me sleep very late. I was very surprised by my torpor on Neurontin, as it was being heavily promoted as a low-side-effect alternative to older medications of its kind. (See the sidebar.)

Throughout my visits to Dr. Smith, I was careful not to complain, trying to seem as positive (and sane) as possible, so that the doctor would continue to take me seriously as a patient. Despite my new resolve to have more realistic expectations about pain relief, I commonly came home from the neurologist feeling deflated of hope. A major reason was that he kept bringing up a new mental problem that he also thought I had.

At one visit, Dr. Smith asked me about my experience of insomnia, and I told him that I often was being kept awake by my mind racing, especially when I was in a writing mode.

The Big Crazy Business of Off-Label Drugs for Pain

The use of the "blockbuster" drug Neurontin for chronic headache prevention is an object lesson in the pitfalls, and increasingly huge business of off-label prescribing. As of 1999, the year of a large Duke University study for the federal government on the subject, only one study had been done about its use in migraine prevention, but a very small one, of only sixteen patients. It was dismissed as having "very limited data."[1] And years after I took it off-label for headaches, an Australian study published in late 2003 revealed that Neurontin was less effective than originally thought in the prevention of daily headaches.[2]

Neurontin also illustrates just how massive the business of off-label prescribing has become. In fact, the top two off-label drugs in 2003 in the United States were Neurontin and Topamax (another anticonvulsant), which have been widely prescribed for the unapproved uses of prevention of chronic headaches and many other types of chronic pain. (In 2004, Topamax was finally approved by the FDA for migraine prevention.) According to a newspaper report, 90 percent of the prescriptions for Neurontin in 2003 were off-label, totaling $1.8 billion in off-label sales, making it one of manufacturer Pfizer's top sellers, a bona fide "blockbuster" drug. About 80 percent of prescriptions for Topamax in 2003 were off-label, adding up to $643 million in sales, much of it for pain relief.[3]

The drawbacks of rampant off-label prescribing are a well-known part of a patient's chronic pain experience. A 2003 medication guide from the American Chronic Pain Association cautions patients about common frustrations in trying to get an off-label drug approved by their insurance companies. "Try not to lose your temper or get angry as this only increases chronic pain problems," it warns.[4] Besides wasting time and money, patients have more to risk with off-label prescribing. If something goes wrong, they have much less of a legal leg to stand on because pharmaceutical companies have never officially "sold" this use in the first place. And off-label use poses more of a physical risk with newer (read: highly promoted) drugs, which haven't had the benefit of years of trial and error on their side.

In a 2003 speech to the American Pain Society, Dr. John Loeser elaborated on this threat of off-label prescribing in actually reducing incentives for further research. "Once a drug or device is FDA-approved, there is little incentive to learn more about it," he explained. "Off-label prescribing by physicians means that science can be abandoned and even more drugs or devices can be sold on the chance that something good might happen. It must be seen as bizarre that physicians can apply treatments, drugs, and operations to patients only with the hope that something of benefit to the patient will accrue."

Dr. Loeser went on to explain how pharmaceutical companies pull this off, actually getting around legal restrictions against advertising a medication for an off-label use. One tactic is to sponsor supplemental sections of medical journals featuring articles by doctors, whom these companies have funded, with their own studies on off-label uses. And the studies featured in these publications are generally less rigorous than FDA-approved studies. And the chances of publishing studies that show no or negative effects are near zero. "There is no mandatory record keeping, sharing of outcomes data, or standards for evaluating outcomes," Loeser explained.[5] (Ironically, illustrating how deeply pharmaceutical company marketing efforts are embedded in the everyday lives of doctors, the advertisement below Dr. Loeser's reprinted speech in the American Pain Society newsletter features a thanks to commercial sponsors, including AstraZeneca, Merck, Pfizer, and Ortho-McNeil.)

But sometimes they go ahead anyway, regardless of the law, and directly advertise or promote these off-label uses to doctors. The makers of the major new preventive drugs used for chronic headaches in the past several years—Neurontin, Topamax, and Botox—have all gotten into different degrees of legal trouble with allegations of this practice.[6]

"Well, you're probably bipolar," he said, making a note in my folder.

I froze. "What do you mean?"

"It's very common among chronic headache sufferers. About 8.6 percent of chronic headache patients are bipolar, about twice the rate of the general population."

I sank into my chair, devastated that I had to deal with another major stigmatized neurological problem.

"Well," he said, "there are actually looser definitions now of who is bipolar. I would probably call you 'light bipolar.'"

In other words, I was not regular bipolar, but "bipolar-curious."

I was not comforted by these words. Instead, I drove home from the suburbs with my (bipolar) mind racing: "I'm bipolar. I can't believe it. I am more of a basket case than even *I* had ever imagined."

Later, my sadness and confusion turned a bit to resentment. Dr. Smith had made this diagnosis without any kind of diagnostic written test, such as the Beck Depression Inventory, which measures depression with a series of standardized questions. He apparently based his diagnosis on my offhanded comment that I had a racing mind. That didn't necessarily mean I was bipolar; that meant I was a writer. And besides, appearances can be deceiving. What if I had been just going through a bad period in my personal life, such as a divorce, and showed up to his office visibly agitated? Then would he assume I was bipolar or a depressive? And I certainly did not have the two stereotypical classic bipolar problems: being out of control with casual sex and shopping. Probably the most deviant thing I had done in that area, I thought, was spend a few hundred dollars too much on the J. Jill mail-order catalog in a single fiscal year.

This attention to other problems besides the headache—such as depression, sleep disorders, fibromyalgia, anxiety, and bipolarity—reflected a major wave of research in neurology at the time, and continuing today, on comorbidities. (Again, these are related neurological problems that commonly coexist with a certain disorder, at too large a rate to be a coincidence.) But back then, I did not understand why on earth these mental issues were relevant. Why was he discussing them so prominently, if not to label the headaches psychosomatic? I had argued for years that the pain was not "all in my head," and now he seemed to intimate that it was, after all.

But considering Dr. Smith's unusual medical knowledge and hospitable manner, I stuck with him, still checking in a few times a year about the newest rollout from Big Pharma. A remaining fantasy was to find a drug with few side effects that would not cost a lot and would require minimal treatments.

But at that time, such a hope did emerge from the wilderness. In fact, a great messiah was arriving on the medical scene—with signs and wonders and an outstretched arm—and of course, plenty of free pens, notepads, and refrigerator magnets. And there was great rejoicing through the land.

Yet this elixir, this pharmaceutical manna, emerged not from man's noblest desire to heal, but from a more base desire, the care and maintenance of trophy wives. In the 1990s, a prophetic Los Angeles plastic surgeon had begun popularizing this substance, Botox, for use on headaches after noticing this desirable side effect of head pain relief in his patients. (See the sidebar.)

I had first read about Botox as a headache remedy in the January-February 1999 issue of the National Headache Foundation newsletter, which I had picked up in Dr. Smith' office. At the time, I couldn't believe the absurdity and barbarism of such a treatment, of injecting poison into the face. That was somewhere in the range of sophistication between trepanation and bloodletting. At

Botox: A Star Is Born

Botox is the trade name of botulinum toxin, derived from the most deadly substance known to humankind. In the past century, it has been used for both good and evil. A single gram of the bacteria from which the toxin is derived, they say, is enough to kill more than one million people, cutting off their ability to breathe and swallow.

For some, this could be good news. During World War II, the U.S. military pioneered research into isolating botulinum toxin from its parent bacteria—which had first been identified by a German doctor in the 1820s as a culprit in food poisoning—in a pure form to use in chemical warfare. Saddam Hussein made major use of it in his arsenal of weapons during the 1991 Gulf War.

But in the 1970s, doctors started experimenting with the toxin for medical purposes, mainly to fix droopy eyes and cross-eyed vision. Then, hitting the mother lode, sometime in the 1980s, doctors noticed it was also fixing their patients' wrinkles by paralyzing muscles in the face. In 1991, the company Allergan acquired the U.S. Army's old supply of the toxin and then began manufacturing its own in 1997.

Between 1989 and 2002, the FDA approved Botox for smoothing out vertical lines between the eyes, as well as for controlling eye problems, uncontrollable blinking, and head and neck spasms. By 2003, 500,000 Americans had used Botox as a wrinkle treatment, and yearly sales totaled more than $400 million. Allergan, which had started out as a low-profile eye-droop and acne-treatment company, was now turning into one of "corporate America's glitziest success stories," as the Los Angeles Times described it.[7]

Word spread quickly about the additional multiple off-label uses for Botox, which ranged from treating clubfoot in infants to treating obesity, by paralyzing a part of the stomach. Soon, headaches became Allergan's top goal for a new use of Botox, and it started funding studies and promotions galore. At the 2002 annual meeting of the American Headache Society (AHS), researchers presented thirteen studies involving 650 patients on this use. As with many treatments, doctors still are not exactly sure how Botox works to relieve headaches, but they think it has to do with weakened muscles in the face being less irritable to nerves, and with Botox affecting neurotransmitters in the brain that affect pain.

At the 2003 meeting of the AHS, which I attended, Botox was again a major topic of discussion. At a "satellite" session-reception for doctors funded by Allergan, a prominent neurologist emphasized the skill involved

(continues)

(continued)

as a Botox "injector," that doctors really can't be effective until they have done at least 100 patients. "It takes ten patients before you stop shaking, and twenty before you know what you're doing. It's the technique," he said. "It's like baseball. You can learn to play the game but not bat a thousand." I winced a bit, as if I had just seen sausage being made, now knowing too much about the reality of patients as guinea pigs. It turns out that this fear I had for years of taking off-label drugs—and procedures—wasn't just paranoia, as I had hoped it was.

least the homeopaths had the good sense to dilute their poisons a few trillion times first, before giving them to people.

But when Dr. Smith suggested Botox to me at the end of 2000, I gave it new consideration. He told me that in his recent initial experience with it, many patients had improved, and without side effects. The expense—four hundred dollars—although significant, was actually less than that involved in taking most drugs, which have to be refilled every month. And my insurance would probably cover it.

Well, I thought, if the Headache was going to respond to something, it might well be the by-product of the deadliest substance on earth, one capable of wiping out entire populations by the capful. Perhaps relieving my pain would take no less a weapon than that. I made the appointment, which happened to be for November 8, the day after the 2000 presidential election.

As the day came nearer, I got more nervous, thinking of my past horrific experience with the surgery. At that time, the prognosis for relief had also looked good, and I had believed there would be no serious repercussions. Yet that surgery had stirred up and inflamed my oversensitive nerves. So why wouldn't the Botox do that? And perhaps it would do worse, just lingering for months in my face, never letting up on the nerves. Any irritant could set off the nerves, even one that was supposed to anesthetize them. At a party, someone further flustered me with the half-baked notion that Botox could cause botulism. I felt my throat starting to close up.

I also was stymied by a markedly less rational influence. One of the most scandalous admissions to undermine all credibility that I can make in this book is that sometime in the mid-1990s, on the advice of my unconventional "psychospiritual" therapist, Lisa, I started following my astrological forecast, that of Aries. At that time, *Mademoiselle* also had an influence. Before then, I had not given the matter even a thought. But in April 1995, I read on the magazine's horoscope page a recounting of the myth of Zeus giving birth to Athena, when she had emerged from his split head. Athena was the "patron goddess" of Aries. This article made some new, provocative connections: "As in the myth, the sign Aries rules the head, and Arians suffer headaches when their creativity, goals, or independence are thwarted." I did not quite believe that statement, but—as with anything that offered even a scintilla of insight into my problem—I had a new interest.

Some insight came with ironic detachment; some did not. I had sympathetically observed people making fun of astrology, such as when Nancy Reagan used it to help direct White House policy during her husband's presidency. But I later thought, she had actually brilliantly navigated their tenure—and seemed to personally serve as the most notable endorsement of astrology ever made. Lasting two terms and purportedly winning the Cold War. Not too shabby.

With a mixture of skepticism and desperation, I read my forecast for the month of November 2000 on astrologyzone.com. It was generally upbeat, but then it changed abruptly—when it got to November 8. The forecast remarked how on that day poor Aries was at a "tough angle" with Uranus, which is the planet of surprises and unusual occurrences. That planet also rules electricity and technology.

Being an impulsive, impatient Aries, I decided to do more research. I called Susan's astrologer in Arizona and asked her about my forecast. She went onto her computer and said that the tough angle mentioned might not relate to the procedure. The stars indicated the stomach, not the head, as the day's more vulnerable area. So she said that I shouldn't be alarmed, that I just might have some nausea or something like that.

The night before the procedure, my choice to watch the presidential election returns was a mistake. It seemed that they were about to announce the definitive winner but never did. As an aside, according to the newscasters, Al Gore had some stomach problems that day but was now fine.

Then I suddenly had a realization: Gore was also an Aries. (When in a health food store, I had browsed through a massive astrology book, *The Secret Language of Birthdays*, and looked up my good friend's birthday and read it was on the same day as his. My birthday was labeled as "The Day of Excess," only reinforcing my belief in astrology.) Noting this new link between Gore and me, of our fates being hinged on Uranus's vagaries, I stayed up all night, rooting for his fortunes to improve. If he could overcome bad luck and prevail, despite this negative forecast, perhaps so could I. His fate was entwined with mine, and I looked to him as a barometer of my own personal fortune.

I arrived at the doctor's office the next afternoon in a state of confusion, feeling roiled by the twists and turns of the news coverage of the past fourteen hours. I also felt uneasy because I had had an odd lunch, some probably too-old cold cuts and some leftover salad with blue cheese on it. But despite some visible nervousness, I decided to put on a good face and remain calm. Needless to say, I did not mention the various aspects of that day's astrological forecast.

I got on the table and Dr. Smith started to inject my forehead with a moderately large needle. Not horrible—it was like an especially cumbersome acupuncture session—but still substantial enough so that I knew I was getting a real procedure done. The only shift in head pain was short-lived, lasting a few seconds, when a current of numbness shot from the core of my brain to the surface of my left eye, retracing and negating the exact path of the pain. Dr. Smith said that was a good sign. Meanwhile, I tried to ignore my growing waves of nausea. But in mid-sentence, after the first injection, I ran to the bathroom and barfed. I came back and asked him to continue. Then, when it was all done, I finished throwing up in a plastic bag they had provided for me. He gave me a Xanax and I soon felt more normal.

Well, I thought, so much for appearing sane in his presence. Now he would consider me a crazy person for sure because of this overreaction. I tried, but I really couldn't explain the fear I felt that this Botox would make me worse, that I would repeat my painful experience from the surgery. I was paranoid, but I had been driven to it.

I concentrated to see if I felt any change in pain levels. I was basically the same, but a little flushed from the chemical. I was disappointed, thinking I would have gotten results immediately if it was going to work.

"Well," he said, "you don't always know right away. It could take up to about six weeks to make a difference."

So, like fellow Arian Al Gore, I was left that day with a mostly dismal forecast, but with some faint glimmers of hope. We would have to wait this one out; that was all we could do. For the next six weeks, I followed the headlines with a new passion, noting how his fluctuations seemed to match mine:

On November 11, the *New York Times* headline read: "Democrats' Eyes on Recounts and Courts."

Yes, there is hope, I thought.

November 14: "U.S. Judge Refuses to Block Hand Recount of Ballots."

Yes, a good sign. They would recount the ballots and find that he had really won.

November 15: "Bush Lead at 300: GOP Official Demands Written Justification for Further Tallies."

Well, at least we're gaining on the bastard, coming a few hundred votes closer. No pain relief yet, but there's still hope.

November 16: "Uncounted Overseas Votes Carrying a Bush Profile."

Well, it may not mean much.

November 18: "Florida Court Bars Naming a Winner."

Have patience. It's only been a little more than a week.

November 23: "In Blow to Gore, Recount Halts in Miami-Dade."

November 27: "Bush is Certified as the Winner in Florida, but Gore Says He Will Contest the Results."

Keep hope alive.

December 5: "A Victory for Bush: Judge Finds a Failure to Show Probability in Change in Vote."

It's not over yet.

December 13: "BUSH PREVAILS: BY SINGLE VOTE, JUSTICES RECOUNT, BLOCKING GORE AFTER 5-WEEK STRUGGLE."

December 14: "Bush, Newly Victorious, Pledges to Be the President of 'One Nation,' Not One Party."

January 6: "Over Some Objections, Congress Certifies Electoral Vote."

Defeat, on all levels.

By that time, with the pain in my head at status quo, I was probably as upset by Al Gore's fate as he was. However, by looking at me, you could never tell. Because of the Botox, the area above my eyes was frozen into an expression of neutrality and peace. This had not been a goal, but my forehead was now lusciously velvety smooth (while, as I was only thirty-three years old, it had been merely a normal smooth before that). I was "cured" of another problem I never knew I had.

19

The Yellow Wallpaper

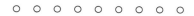

AFTER SUCH A LONG HAUL, some people might have suggested a more convenient and long-honored option: heavy drug abuse.

Unfortunately, even casual recreational drug use has never had much of an appeal to me. This has always been the case but probably had been reinforced most strongly in high school. The best drug prevention message for me was always just to look at the folks that were doing drugs. That was enough of a turnoff.

After all, the last people on earth I wanted to emulate were those who were heavy pot users, like those scary girls who hung out smoking between periods in the bathroom. They were sociopaths, as they demonstrated on that one morning when they destroyed my lunch. I had left it behind by accident in the bathroom and then returned an hour later, after class ended, to retrieve it. The food was wildly scattered around the room, as if the lunch bag had exploded. The bread was torn apart into shreds in one corner. The turkey was in another. The chips were spread all over the room. On the mirror was written a personal message for me in lipstick: "Paula Kamen, thanks for the lunch! It was delicous [sic]!" (My mom, who had made the lunch, had written my name on it, an embarrassing practice I would soon call to a halt.)

When I was a freshman in college, other miscreant drug users whom I observed served to further endorse my straight-and-narrow path. Because of a complex set of circumstances, I had found myself living in a private dorm, on the same floor as some satire-ready members of the richest, most beautiful, and most shallow sorority, in the years before they moved into their house. They were going through a heavy period of experimenting with little white lines they arranged carefully on my roommate's Old Style-logo-imprinted mirror. One night, one joined me in the elevator and confided to me that she had been up all night vomiting foam, after an hours-long coke bender at a frat house. You have got to be kidding, I thought. This was like Brett Easton Ellis's *Less than Zero*, but without any of the style and without any of the wit. Like Studio 54 without any fabulous people. Come now. Shape up or ship out.

Another reason for avoiding recreational drugs, even after I moved to the more pleasant hippie side of campus after that, was that I simply am not cool enough to pull it off. I would be like Woody Allen in *Annie Hall* sneezing into the highly expensive stash of white powder and scattering it across the room. I wasn't even entirely confident using a lighter. So certainly the operation of a more complex bong or pipe was too daunting, requiring way too much finesse and coolness. I kept expecting someone in the middle of my hesitant inhale to stand up, point at me, and coldly announce to the others assembled there, "Imposter! This is a square honors student who obviously does not belong here! I hear she even had an AP class or two."

But for the rest of my college days, my primary motivation in not doing drugs, in any substantial way, was that I seemingly *always* had a paper due the next day. Between liberal arts and journalism classes and column deadlines for the college paper, I always had to remain lucid to churn out those pages. That made me think that the best antidrug strategy for middle-class college students was just to assign more papers.

And so I was never tempted to abuse heavy-duty pain pills, from the time I started to acquire them via prescription in 1991. In fact, I would typically take only one or two and then throw the vial in a brimming drawer with the others, never to be touched again. I absolutely hated being dazed and confused while on drugs, and then having to recover from the "hangover" the next day. Any relief, which was surprisingly minor, usually wasn't worth the trouble. Although opiates have a reputation as a savior, they mostly failed for me, like other pain patients, to get rid of the pain altogether, at best just blunting it a bit.

I was not being an unusually responsible and upright citizen with my caution. In fact, I was following the behavior patterns of the vast majority of pain patients—who do not abuse painkillers and perhaps underuse them because of their side effects and these patients' own internalized cultural ideals of mind over matter. Besides, as an interesting twist, we chronic pain sufferers are less likely than purely abusing users to get any kind of euphoric response from such drugs. Many have observed that they just target the pain and do nothing else. It's as if these drugs are incapable of multitasking and can take care of only one thing at a time: either physical or mental pain.

In fact, I had never experienced enjoyment in my life from taking drugs—at least before the summer of 1999. That was when I was prescribed Xanax.

At first, I did not worry about any risks involved because it had been prescribed by a holistic physician, who, by definition, I figured would be more restrained with drug pushing.

At our last visit, in early 1998, that doctor at Whole Health Inc. had been optimistic about my recovery, without drugs. I had told him that I was feeling a bit better, and he asked what was going on in my life. I had written a comedy, a play, that I was now producing and was enjoying the experience with the audience and the actors. Compared to writing a book in isolation, this was a great relief. "Ah, the power of laughter," he said, almost surprised that this could actually be true. "There has been a lot of literature about its healing powers. Just like with that guy . . . What is his name?"

"Norman Cousins?" I replied, recalling the first "alternative medicine" book I had read years ago.

"Yeah, Norman Cousins," he said, almost pushing me out the door, relieved not to be seeing me again anytime soon.

But like all gentler pain periods, this one turned out to be short-lived; it ran out when my adrenaline ran out. So when I went to see this doctor again a year later, he seemed a bit confused about how to treat me. He flipped nervously through my chart.

"Let me see here, . . . Have you tried acupuncture?" he asked.

"Yes."

"Homeopathy?"

"Yes."

"A chiropractor?"

"Yes, several."

"Alexander Technique?"

"Yes."

"Massage?"

"Yes."

"Supplements?"

"Yes."

He paused, closed my folder, and looked up, and a new look of confidence spread across his face.

"Well, we're going to try a new type of drug, something that you have never before taken."

"Is it an antidepressant?"

"No."

"Is it an opiate?"

"No."

"Is it a muscle relaxant?"

"No."

"Is it an anticonvul . . . "

"No," he interrupted, just a bit too anxiously.

Then he relaxed and continued, "No, it isn't like anything else you have ever tried. It's in an entirely different class of drugs. Take one three times a day, and then we'll see how you're doing later." He wrote out a prescription, tore it off the pad, and handed it to me.

"This is meant to relax you," he said, "to counter the . . . the cascade of stressful events that has happened to you over the years and is perpetuating this cycle of pain."

When I got home, having filled the prescription, I looked up this drug, Xanax, in some kind of a reference book and saw that it was a benzodiazepine, a tranquilizer. It was in the same family as Valium, and as Klonopin (It's also in the same class as Rohyphol, or "roofies," the date rape drug, which offers sexual predators the convenience of instant sedation of the victim.) Of all the drugs I had taken, Klonopin was the one that had given me the most grief with withdrawal. So I put the Xanax in the overflowing drawer of unwanted and discarded drugs, deciding never to take it.

After all, I knew this drug was risky, but I was not yet well informed about its notoriety. It turns out that tranquilizers are some of the most hated drugs in the women's health movement, which emerged in the 1970s to give women control and knowledge of their health care. At that time, Valium was the first-ever blockbuster drug, the Prozac of its day, about as common in medicine cabinets as aspirin. Between 1969 and 1982, it was the most heavily prescribed drug in America. In fact, the first episode of *The Brady Bunch*, in the late 1960s featured the mother, Carol, taking a Valium to get over her prewedding jitters.

Today, feminists continue to warn that these widely prescribed tranquilizers may actually still be false chemical solutions to justified social unease. Instead of pills, organizing for social change is the way to improve women's lives, they say.

But as with others in constant pain, high-minded feminist social critiques were the last topic on my mind at that time. About four months after deciding not to take the Xanax, I reached a crossroad. I had endured several con-

Tranks and Chronic Pain: A Feminist Nightmare

One of the most classic and enduring complaints about doctors' sexism in treating chronic pain is that they are much more likely to prescribe tranquilizers to women than to men. "Women are the primary gender featured in tranquilizer ads, often as middle-aged chronic complainers of a variety of problems. Relief for both doctor and patient may be found in a mild downer," observed Jim Hogshire in *Pills-A-Go-Go.*

Feminist writers also recall times in the 1960s and 1970s when doctors routinely prescribed tranks to enforce gender roles, as for the dubious ailment of "housewife's syndrome," when housewives were "unnaturally" bored and unhappy.[1] A notorious 1970 ad for Valium, headlined "35 and Single," condescendingly related the sad-sack story of Jan. Nine snapshots chronicled her progressively more pathetic life, starting with her younger and happier days at the beach, moving on to her growing older and uglier, posing with her father. The final photo in the series captured her in the present, alone and expressionless, with her hair newly shaped into a Marian-the-Librarian severe style. "You probably see many Jans in your practice," the ad read. "The unmarrieds with low self esteem. Jan never found a man to measure up to her father. Now she realizes she's in a losing pattern—and that she may never marry. . . . Valium 10-mg tablets help relieve the emotional 'storms' of psychoneurotic tension and the depressive symptoms that can go hand-in-hand with it."[2]

secutive nights of poor, light semisleep, the type that you wake up from not even sure that you have ever lost consciousness in the first place. In the middle of the night, hobbling in pain, I walked back to the drawer. I thought that maybe if I just took one, I could get some sleep and then feel better the next day. Then I wouldn't take it again.

I soon found out that the doctor had been correct on one count: This was unlike any other drug I had ever taken. It actually worked. And immediately. Instant gratification. What a change of pace, I thought. Right after swallowing it down, I felt the strong grip of anxiety, which had been intensified by hours of frustrated sleeplessness, melt seamlessly away. I even rested with a new feeling of well-being, which I had never before had from any drug. I realized that even though it was in the same family as Klonopin, it carried a different grade of high—just as the buzz you get from beer is different from the one you get from champagne. This pleasant effect was also unlike that of sleeping pills—even the modern ones like Ambien. You just

waited and waited for those to knock you out, without enough consideration to relax you first, if they ever kicked in at all.

So this is what all the fuss is about, I thought. This is why all those people
take drugs. No wonder.

But this time, I fell into a nourishing and gentle sleep and woke up eight
hours later, completely refreshed and relaxed. The pain was greatly diminished, as it was on those rare days when my sleep was deep and other conditions were in my favor. I had my whole day before me, which otherwise
would have been lost to pain and fatigue.

Three nights later, I had insomnia. I decided to take Xanax again. The
result was the same positive effect of sleep followed by refreshment.

Xanax was making life so much easier by just erasing problems. Or rather,
helping sleep happen *despite* problems. I found that if I was nervous about
waking up early for a meeting, no problem. If I read a stimulating book and
my mind was too active, no problem. If I'd just had a bitter fight with someone seconds before, no problem. If I'd just heard a loud, strange banging
noise in the kitchen and I didn't want to investigate it, no problem. I just took
the pill, and sleep came. Problems solved.

In these first few weeks, I was elated to have some relief, yet also very cautious and conflicted. I had seen enough after-school specials, not to mention
VH-1 *Behind the Music* programs, to know that I was entering risky territory.
This Xanax was clearly highly addictive. If I continued taking it, I soon would
surely be addicted to it, as would any human alive.

But then again, so what? Why was that necessarily a negative? Did that
fear justify stopping this very rare newfound pain relief? Throughout history,
the culture has determined which headache drugs are considered nefarious,
and opinion changes from decade to decade. At one time, cocaine, cannabis,
heroin, and LSD had each been used for headache relief. And then there is
always a new one, like Xanax, to come along. Which were designated as "evil"
from year to year seemed almost arbitrary.

I had recently talked with an older and very well respected professor, who
also had chronic daily headache. She had told me that she basically had been
largely cured years earlier by a strong drug cocktail from Chicago Headache
Clinic, which she still took nightly. Unlike me, she seemed not to have any
side effects and was able to handle well the large amounts and varieties of
drugs. I asked her if she was addicted, and she replied, "I don't care if I'm
addicted. It works. Now I don't have to worry about the pain. Besides, just
not having to worry every night about if I will be able to fall asleep is worth it.
I feel as if my life has improved immeasurably. We have enough problems

with the pain and the insomnia. Why not get rid of them if we can? I like drugs. They take you off the hook. We are lucky to have them."

I began to think about the difference between addiction and dependence. That professor wasn't really addicted to drugs; she was dependent on them, as official medical guidelines back up. She was not abusing them, which addiction implies. She was not robbing old ladies on the street to get the money for more. In contrast, *dependence* describes a chemical physical reaction, no more. The body may be chemically dependent on the drug. It isn't an emotional and compulsive thing. Unlike with addiction, this dependence is a way to function better and be more productive in life, not withdraw from it. It is in the same category as diabetics being "dependent" on insulin, as depressed people taking Prozac to function. Who would begrudge them such "dependence"?

The professor had a compelling point. But a complication, affecting the social acceptance of taking such a drug, was that I was dealing with physical pain, not a widely recognized disease in and of itself. Also, some people, including chronic pain sufferers, have abused prescription drugs in the past, ruining things for the rest of us. This fear of misuse has led to social norms dictating that taking addictive painkillers is permissible in only the direst of circumstances. In society's view, if I were on my deathbed with cancer pain, a decision to take addictive painkillers would be justified. Then no one, including me, would question my actions as immoral or weak. After all, it's OK to get dependent on a drug, as long as you croak right after and don't have any fun with it. That's a fair trade, just like some people's reasoning that it's OK to have an abortion if you've been raped, but not when you've willingly had sex—and the chances are that you could have derived some enjoyment out of it.

But I could control another factor—by helping to make this drug taking more socially acceptable. I could make it open, not a secret. This nonsneaky approach seemed to define for me at least some of the difference between addiction and the more acceptable dependence. To make sure I was being responsible and undeviant, I would tell all my doctors and my family about taking Xanax, broadcast it to the world.

And I would take Xanax only at night, not three times a day, as originally prescribed. And I would never just start popping them, as I knew addicts did, to cope with varying levels of stress during the day. One family member assured me that millions of people took Xanax regularly and it was one of the most widely prescribed medications in the country. In fact, it was one of the drugs most commonly used by chronic pain patients, as I later read, with at least 40–60 percent of patients admitted to chronic pain programs reported to be on at least one benzodiazepine.[3]

I knew that it would be tough getting myself off the Xanax one day. But I also reasoned that I had been able to navigate that process on my own with Klonopin, from a very high dose to nothing. Now I would be taking only one 0.25-mg Xanax pill, much less than the standard dose of about 3 mg. And now I was older and wiser with drugs, knowing to taper them off very gradually when the time came.

But when I told Dr. Smith about my use of Xanax about a month later and asked him for a refill, he was immediately alarmed. "That is a highly addictive substance!" he said.

I told him that I was feeling generally better, and that I was more productive than I had been in years. I also thought how the six-dollar bottle of generic Xanax lasted a full month and was considerably cheaper than those acupuncture treatments that I'd been having twice a week at sixty dollars a pop, and that had more uncertain effects.

"OK, but don't go past 0.25 mg a day," he said.

"Well, that's the thing," I said. "That dose isn't working anymore. I need to take more."

He was hesitant but said that I could go up to 0.5, still a relatively low dose. It worked, but then, to my disappointment, after a few weeks, I realized that 0.5 was no longer effective. My body was starting to build a tolerance to the drug, needing more of a dose for the same effect. But I made a firm resolution not to raise the dosage any more, not to cross the line.

I e-mailed my consultant friend, Wendy, about what to do. This is her e-mailed reply:

They put you on Xanax? That is a benzodiazepine and they are very addictive. Benzodiazepines calm you down because they bind to some of the same receptor sites in the brain as alcohol. The latest trend is to give Xanax to old people (I guess that's not surprising, since they are a population prone to nerve problems and doctors have a tendency to just drug them up). Other benzodiazepines are Valium, Ativan, and Klonopin (which I know is extremely addictive, I remember you telling me it was the drug of choice for a singer featured on *Behind the Music*. Klonopin is a little different from the rest because it has antiseizure properties.)

Anyway, withdrawal from a benzodiazapine can cause rebound tension from excess nerve firing (because your brain is so used to being calmed down artificially). Withdrawal from very high doses can also cause seizures. I wouldn't worry about withdrawal seizures from a low dose. . . . One more thing: Benzodiazepines and other downers can cause you to become depressed. I really believe that my depression over the past year and a half was caused by medication.

The decision was clear: I had to get off this drug altogether. Since the day I went on it, I'd also had some new stomach problems, diagnosed as reflux. I wondered if there was any connection between the two, although the doctor said that Xanax is often given to relieve stomach problems. Also, the depressed political consultant–pharmaceutical expert I had met had told me something about Xanax being "short-acting," which I did not understand. For some reason, that was undesirable.

Besides, I was having doubts about the difference between addiction and dependence. Did a difference even exist? Was I fooling myself? Was it like the joke about the difference between pornography and erotica: porn is what *you* do, and erotica is what *I* do. Addiction is what you do, and dependence is what I do. Are they really just the same thing?

In the spring of 2000, when work on my sex book was completely done and I had finally come to a period without deadlines during which I did not have to function lucidly, I followed my doctor's directions for stopping the drug in a few days. On the first night, I took half of my regular dose. The next day, I lay on the bed shaking, drifting in and out of sleep. I got up and my vision was off, a bit distorted. I was very anxious and depressed, to a disorienting and odd level, as if some basic chemicals in my brain were now truly missing.

Taking Wendy's advice, I decided to continue the process in my own way, tapering the drug much more slowly. I used a razor blade to cut the small tablets in quarters. But two weeks later, when I was finally totally off the drug, I was unable to sleep—it was as if my body had forgotten how—and the head pain became excruciating. I was also committed to a speaking engagement in the following month, the first of a string to come, for which I had to be alert.

So, I grudgingly decided to go back to the original 0.25-mg dose and try again later to get off it completely. After all, it was a minuscule amount, and I definitely was not abusing it. In that moment, I knew I had made the correct decision.

But I doubted it when I got off the plane in Rochester, Minnesota, and waited for the student from a neighboring school to pick me up near the baggage return. I was doing all I could just to function and didn't know how I would make it through the lecture. It took all my willpower *not* to hop into a very alluring small golf-cart-like transporter that was marked, "Mayo Clinic"—and disappear.

In reality, this vexing yet banal problem of drug dependence is common in chronic pain patients. It was nothing incredibly dramatic or self-destructive, nothing that would ever make it into a good beatnik novel or after-school special. True "drug abuse" doesn't usually happen for pain patients. Their greatest risk is developing an unpleasant state of helplessness, where the drug isn't working anymore—or never did in the first place. But then, without systematic doctor guidance (or even knowledge about how to get off such a drug), a patient has to keep taking it anyway to function, meanwhile suffering its side effects. Doctors are commonly insensitive to the difficulty of getting off an addictive drug for someone in pain, for whom a low dose may have major withdrawal effects. Whereas other patients may just taper off a much larger dose in a day or two with some minor discomfort, the chronic pain patient may be immobilized by pain and anxiety. When tapering, we may be hypersensitive to any fluctuation in brain chemistry, no matter how minute.

About a year later, the time had come to try to get off this drug again. I had suspicions that the Xanax was making me feel worse. For the last few months, I had been made unreasonably anxious and depressed by normal things that never before had made me anxious and depressed. Although I certainly was not a stranger to such emotions, before they had always happened for a definite reason and more-or-less in proportion to the irritant involved. But in those months, I started to feel as if my mind was following the same sad course as my twelve-year-old Mitsubishi Galant, which was now breaking down on a more regular basis, and in more precarious places, such as a busy three-way intersection on my way to a book reading. This anxiety was so extreme that I felt as if I didn't recognize myself. Instead, from a distance, I was observing a different person, some character I was watching in a movie.

One day, I was suddenly afraid to ride my bike about a mile east in traffic to the lakefront, a ride I had taken for years without hesitation. Minor writing deadlines, which would not have overwhelmed me earlier, now unhinged me. With my short-term memory dimming and my attention span decreasing, I made more silly errors than ever, such as not being able to find my credit card, reporting it stolen, and then immediately afterward finding it tucked in an obvious place in my wallet. Another day, I suddenly started checking the stove to be sure that it was off before I left my apartment, more than once. I panicked in packing for a trip, as I never had before.

Another source of anxiety, as is true of so many people in their early thirties, was that the charms of my low-rent "bohemian" lifestyle were wearing thin. I returned late one night to walk up three flights in total darkness, as the lights were all out in the hallways of my building. As I had in the past, I changed the bulbs. But when I was screwing one in, sparks flew out of the socket and I got a strong shock leading from my arm to my left eye. It made me wonder how safe my building was, after all. Later that night, I felt anxiety build when I was awakened by the smell of smoke. The next morning, I learned that a store a block away had burned down.

This seemingly unprecedented level of anxiety escalated, and I stood back again to observe myself. This feeling was actually vaguely familiar, not so strange after all. This was exactly how I had felt the year before when going through withdrawal from the Xanax, even though, this time, I had not reduced the dose at all. It was as if, after two years on the same dose, my body wanted more. As during that brief withdrawal the year before, my vision was a little loopy, my glasses suddenly seeming not strong enough, and then too strong. The withdrawal was the same as that felt by a person who is used to drinking one beer after work and then must have two to feel all right. Just one beer doesn't work anymore, leaving the person feeling more anxious than if she had never had any alcohol at all.

Even after increasing the dosage a bit to try to balance my brain chemistry, I had a new symptom of waking up suddenly after four hours of sleep. Then I remembered the words of that depressed political consultant. Now I realized what he had meant when he had warned me that Xanax was "short-acting." It went in and out of the system in about four hours. The positive result had been, at least in the beginning, that it worked quickly. The bad part was that this sudden start-and-stop effect became increasingly jarring to the body. Its action contrasted to that of long-acting drugs like Prozac—which take awhile to work, leave your system gradually, and do not produce such abrupt highs and lows.

As an added source of stress, I wasn't really sure about this theory, of the body wanting more drug and now going through its own withdrawal period. Was it the Xanax or was it just me? A problem with drug withdrawal is that, like pain, it makes you act a bit, well, crazy, with increased anxiety. Often people like me who have taken tranquilizers have had some anxiety to begin with, so it's hard to know if the increased amount of it is from the drug.

Dr. Smith referred me to a psychiatrist, who agreed with him that the dose was too small to cause such anxiety. She suggested I take Prozac, but I warned her that it gave me insomnia, that I was "different from others and couldn't tolerate such drugs." I thought of returning to the holistic doctor, who had originally prescribed me the stuff, but then I remembered the surgeon's reaction after my operation and worried that the holistic doctor would also react defensively, blaming me for the dependence and difficulty stopping the drug. In desperation, I called the 800 number of Upjohn, the manufacturer of Xanax, asking the operator if mine was a normal reaction. "People call me taking more like 4 mg with this effect," she said.

In any case, I knew that the necessary process of withdrawal would be extremely challenging and time-consuming, perhaps lasting up to a few months. So, that July, now unable to function because of escalating anxiety, I decided to stay temporarily at my parents' home in the suburbs. The plan was to spend no more than two weeks there, where I would have support, moral and otherwise. My parents, now retired, were home and were always reliable in times of need. Meanwhile I would maintain my life in the city, conducting business via cell phone and asking my neighbor to pick up my mail.

At my parents' home—I reasoned—I would finally unravel, because I could. And then move on. Best of all, unlike with a real detox center—which was not even a valid option for me, especially on such a tiny dose of the stuff—it was free. And here I could be in control of the tapering pace of doses and not be the victim of some unreasonable Nurse Ratched. I was also relieved that this sojourn filled the Number One service of a detox center: acting as an excuse not to socialize with other people. While I was feeling shitty, the pressure would be off to be "on" with others.

By coincidence, I arrived at my parents' house the same day that (fellow Aries, as I somehow knew from my regular women's magazine horoscope reading) Mariah Carey checked herself into the hospital suffering from "exhaustion." I cringed as I watched the entertainment news commentators raising their eyebrows over the word *exhaustion*, saying it was an obvious euphemism for just going batty.

Dr. Chung, whom I had just gotten back in touch with, had suggested the move. He reassured me that it wasn't a sign of weakness or regression. He said that in China, seeking the comfort of family in a time of crisis was considered normal—not a sign of mental deformity, as in Western culture.

"While you heal, you need to be where you feel grounded," he said.

Yes, this was more grounding than any hospital ever could be, especially with the gold foil wallpaper in the bathrooms and the hundreds of square feet of shag carpeting, which eased my anxiety on a primal level. The yellow wallpaper in my sister's and my old room—featuring a Gloria Vanderbilt print of giant daisies and tulips that had been chic when hung in the mid-1970s—

was reassuring, not unnerving. Even Charlotte Perkins Gilman would have approved of it.

On my first night back in the suburbs, already braced with strong anxiety and eager to get the tapering started, I took a razor blade and cut off a sliver from one of the two white pills I was taking. Then, about four hours after going to sleep, I darted awake, completely and utterly so. I felt so anxious that I could not lie still. I had to keep moving, pacing, and stretching. I wanted to pound my head against the wall to relieve some of this anxiety. Hmm, I thought, even at this more mild level of withdrawal, I now understand that scene from the film *Ulee's Gold* in which the heroin addict is handcuffed to a bed and is struggling to break free, unable to sit in her own skin. Or that one from *Trainspotting* in which Ewan McGregor hallucinates about the baby crawling on the ceiling.

I waited until 8:30 A.M. and called Dr. Chung, whom I had been consulting for the past few weeks. He advised me to exercise to relieve stress. Later that day, my mom and I went to the park district health club, a great haven, with its spacious facilities and shiny glass-enclosed track. With immense concentration and difficulty, I got dressed and found my way to an elliptical machine. I got on and turned on my headphones, so that I could tune in to one of the TVs ahead of me on the wall. I suddenly had a horrible thought: What if the batteries were dead? I could not use this machine without the medication of television, I thought. And I did not have the wherewithal to figure out how to buy and install new batteries. What would I do if the batteries were out? I asked myself, in a panic. But luckily, the crisis was averted and the headphones worked well. I started moving up and down on the elliptical machine, feeling pacified by its steady rhythm.

After I disembarked from the machine about an hour and a half later, I felt some relief. The worst anxiety was gone. Those endorphins, the ones I had read about for my sixth-grade project, had kicked in. Gleefully, I went out to dinner to a Chinese buffet with my parents, but in the middle of that strip-mall restaurant, I felt great fear. The next day, I noticed that I was becoming agoraphobic, not wanting to leave the house. I needed to go to Osco Drugs to buy some toiletries, but the thought was too daunting. I had never experienced this feeling before in my life. I walked outside and was startled by something behind me. Good lord, I thought, now I'm even literally scared of my own shadow.

But I still decided to force myself through this extreme anxiety, to drive to the gym to continue the endorphin-summoning exercise regimen. I also took walks outside, which were more reflective, for better and for worse.

Even after all this time, I saw that the houses in my parents' neighborhood were still familiar, all resembling different riffs on the Brady Bunch theme, with the aluminum siding and two-car garage as the central focus. They had been built on the site of a former golf course in the early 1960s to accommodate members of the baby boom, and they were still stuck in the era of my childhood. It was the ideal place to grow up—not too rich, where you're sheltered, and not deprived. Safe, nice grounding near a major urban center. Just right.

I passed the cul-de-sac where my sister, my brother, and I had played. That was also the place where all the snow from the nearby blocks was dumped. We would build elaborate networks of tunnels attached to several snow forts. The best part was lying in there after the rigorous digging to rest and enjoy the incredible quiet. As an adult, I identified that sense of enclosure with being inside an MRI machine (even though an MRI is noisy). For that reason, I had never minded MRIs, as they evoked those pleasant snow day memories.

Other sights caught me more off guard. One day, I was cleaning out my car and looked up to see a dazed-looking old man approach me. I waved, but he registered no response. Then I saw that he was being followed by a string of about six others—each walking alone, who were also expressionless. It turned out that a group home was now two houses away, in the same ranch house where I had baby-sat as a teenager. These men were totally drugged up, beyond the ability to make a facial expression. Years earlier, in my darkest moments, I had feared that I would become "one of them," a Charlie from *Flowers for Algernon*, and now the picture was complete.

As I took walks, I also thought of some unsettling memories of varying degrees of seriousness from the past. I passed the house of the boy who had toppled my beloved snow fort complex. There was my old grade school and the playground where we'd played SWAT team, a glorified version of catch, in second grade. And there was the exact spot where I had fallen backward on the Timbertown and gotten a concussion, an incident I had always wondered about as being the root cause of all this suffering. I remembered going back to class and a little later raising my hand to tell the teacher I was seeing double.

I walked most of the way home and then spotted a neighbor's house—and I was carried back about twenty years to the afternoon when we had come home from school to find the household's three teenage children huddled out front with police cars and paramedics. The son broke away and walked by our house. I asked him what was wrong, and he didn't answer. Since then I had learned what had happened: His mother had found a way out of her deep depression.

It was the easy way out. No more trying to keep pace with others. No more pretending everything is OK. No more mind over matter. No more irrational fears. Better yet, no more rational ones.

The weeks passed in the suburbs, and I was experiencing no real improvement. Constant and frightening anxiety still gripped me, making me feel as if I was observing myself from a distance. This was the longest I had been at my parents' house in years, even more than the month I'd needed after surgery. I was now having my mail forwarded here, instead of just having my neighbor pick it up for me. Even more foreboding, Mariah Carey had vanished from the media.

One night, I took out the razor to cut the Xanax on the bathroom counter, just as I remembered my old college roommate doing on that Old Style mirror. I was afraid of cutting the counter, so I took out a strip of flat cardboard that I had with me—ironically, the bookmark from Transitions, a New Age bookstore in Chicago. I looked at the inspirational quote, taken from the 1973 book *Hope for the Flowers*, inscribed on it in poetic script:

"How does one become a butterfly," she asked.
"You must want to fly so much that you are willing to give up being a caterpillar."

But then again, no caterpillar had ever taken on the challenge of getting off a short-acting trank, I thought. I hesitated for a while. Then I realized that I could not bear to slice off even a sliver of the pill. I was not following the month-long tapering schedule I had sketched out on my calendar. At this rate, I wouldn't be off this drug for months and months, if that. Would I lose my apartment? Was I going to move back in here? If I did, how long would it take me to get my act together to leave?

Mountains of white pills loomed ahead of me in the distance. This near-constant anxiety and increased pain were unbearable. It seemed as if it would never end. I could not imagine *not* feeling this way, being normal again. I was stuck in the Valley of the Dolls, or rather the *Doll*, as I had been taking only one paltry 0.5-mg pill a day, my maximum dose.

I needed more information. I took out a still-unread booklet, "Benzodiazepines—How They Work and How to Withdraw," that I had bought months before via the Internet. It was by an English doctor, Professor

C. Heather Ashton, D.M., F.R.C.P, School of Neurosciences, Division of Psychiatry, The Royal Victoria Infirmary. I was riveted to read that Xanax came in more concentrated doses than other benzos, so that 0.5 mg of Xanax really equaled about 10 mg of Valium, a substantial dose, after all. This Dr. Ashton also made a distinction between long-term and short-term use, saying that they were fine to take once in a while for panic attacks or extreme anxiety, but that they lost effectiveness after a few weeks. Then she described a common reaction of patients on typically small "therapeutic" doses after a few years: some kind of breakdown. The symptoms she described from such a Xanax reaction matched mine: the loss of short-term memory, the dizziness, the distorted vision, the shaking, the agoraphobia. Maybe what I was going through wasn't just me.

I knew I needed help getting off the Xanax, no matter what the source of my crazy anxiety was. In any case, this stuff was probably contributing to the turmoil. And my time-tested method of tapering off gradually wasn't working. Perhaps there was some drug I could get on that could help me, like the ones Dr. Ashton described in her booklet. Didn't someone out there make a Xanax patch?

I started to have a new appreciation of alcoholics who had recovered. On a talk show on anxiety disorders, a doctor talked about how a great number of alcoholics were using booze to self-medicate to quell the root problem of anxiety. So, I thought, those who had recovered from alcohol abuse had probably found a way to live with such powerful negative feelings and fears. I thought of my neighbor in Chicago, who had told me she was a former drug addict and alcoholic who had hit the depths of despair, who now seemed the pillar of strength and competence. Her door was like a beacon in the building, with its mezuzah and god's eye made of sticks and yarn. She nursed mountains of flowers and other plants on her porch, which lit up the back of our building.

And so, desiring the type of support she had gotten, I decided I needed an addiction professional, a search that was much more difficult than expected. I took out another book bought years before and not yet read, *The 12 Steps of Chronic Illness,* and looked up the number in the back for the world-famous Hazelden Clinic. The operator referred me to the Chicago office in a posh neighborhood, which told me about an outpatient program, involving hours of group sessions a week in the evenings. "But detox is up to you," the woman said. The cost was more than five thousand dollars, out of the question. Besides, that option sounded like overkill (even for me).

On the Internet, I looked up a list of Chicago addiction specialists. One was in Dr. Chung's building in the Loop. I decided to stop in her office in person the next day, when I would be there anyway for an appointment with Dr. Chung. I would feel out the place and figure out if it was something I wanted to pursue before plunking down the cash for a visit. So, before my appointment with Dr. Chung, I took an elevator up to this doctor's floor and saw a very small psychiatrist's office down a dark and narrow hallway. I walked in and introduced myself to the doctor, who was in the waiting room talking with a patient. "Sorry," she told me, cautiously, "I help people do that, but only when they're hospitalized. And I'm not taking any new patients." On the way down in the elevator, I realized how nutty I must have looked, blurting out my problem to her within a few minutes of meeting her.

A fundamental problem was that this doctor did not know me. I needed to go to someone who had helped me before. So I got my phone book and dialed the direct number of Suzen, the myofacial therapist at Whole Health Inc., who had been a voice of reason a few years earlier with my surgery. Perhaps she could just minimize the pain so I could get through this withdrawal more easily.

I dialed her line, and there was no answer. It just rang, with no voice mail kicking in. I dialed again, thinking I may have gotten the number wrong the first time. The same result.

I looked up the main switchboard number of the clinic and called it.

"Hello, is Suzen there?" I asked.

There was a long pause.

"Suzen passed away last year," the voice said.

I paused for a while. She had only been in her thirties, at the peak of health.

"What?" I said. "What happened?"

"She had an aneurysm. That's all I know."

I walked around for a while in a daze, unable to believe what I had heard. Suzen was so young, with so much left to give to the world, so much dedication to others' welfare. It made utterly no sense.

And to make a more selfish point, I also felt utterly alone, as though there was no one left who could possibly understand what I was going through. I had few options left.

"I think I'm having a nervous breakdown," I told my mother. She had just finished her nightly viewing of *The Nanny* in syndication at 9:30 P.M. Central Standard Time and was now free to talk. I liked watching her watch that show and laughing often. It was somehow a comfortable ritual, adding probably the only structure to my life.

She thought about it a minute, and I could see her going back mentally to her social worker days.

"Hmm. I don't think so. I remember that people who have nervous breakdowns have an inappropriate emotional affect. They laugh at things they aren't supposed to laugh at. They may not make sense. You look perfectly fine to me. You're not walking around blabbering things."

"Still, coherent or not, I think I'm screwed," I told her.

"I don't have to worry about you now? You're not going to do anything drastic?" she asked, now concerned. She seemed to suddenly realize that I was in a different spot than all the other times when I'd stayed with my parents to wean myself off drugs.

"No, I answered. "Don't worry about it. I have too big an ego to do that."

I meant it and was now relieved to be saying it out loud, Eastern philosophy of detachment be damned.

After thinking through all my options for the past few weeks, I had come to the conclusion that I would not take the easy way out. I later identified my feelings at this point with the words of Jeff Tweedy of the band Wilco, who was quoted as saying about how he felt having a terrible breakdown due to recurrent migraines and drug withdrawal, "I didn't want to kill myself, but I wanted to die."[4] Dying sounded fine, just for a little while at least, to get some relief—but suicide was too drastic. After all, the desire for self-destruction and the desire of wanting pain to end can be two different things.

In addition, the sex book was coming out in Japanese in the spring, and I wanted to be around to see that wonder for myself. Also, there were my parents to consider. I was worried in particular about what my death would do to my seventy-two-year-old dad—not the sadness of losing me, but the injuries he would sustain from cleaning out my apartment, which was loaded with boxes of papers, books, and tons of files. Being independent-minded, I knew he would resist getting anyone to help him. I kept imagining him trying to maneuver by himself a giant five-drawer legal-sized file cabinet down three flights of stairs, losing control of it, and then being crushed to death. That was too much to have on my conscience.

20

Urologists in Orlando

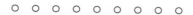

A FEW WEEKS LATER, I pulled myself together and called Elizabeth, my long-time commonsense-heavy physical therapist friend. She told me to think positively, to picture this phase as a storm that I would have to wait out. She agreed that I should see another doctor I trusted and already knew to help get me off this Xanax.

Finally, I got in to see the one psychologist I had seen whom I had liked, who, years earlier, had taught me meditation. After I briefed him, he actually said he had observed this same extreme anxiety in other patients on "small" doses of Xanax, and that the drug was probably at least contributing to this feeling of chaos.

He also surprised me by explaining that Xanax was much more addictive than Klonopin, which had been my baseline for comparison. "But the good news is," he said, "that unlike chronic headaches, depression and anxiety are highly treatable." He reminded me of some herbal aids, such as a potent Alvita valerian-mint tea I had taken years ago for better sleeping. It turned out that valerian was the herbal equivalent of Valium, but not addictive. I needed two bags of tea to get an effect, and it was far less potent than a benzo, but it was still useful to have as a tool.

There is no way to enlightenment. Enlightenment is the way.

But his main suggestion was that I get on a medication to ease the transition from Xanax. A psychopharmacologist would know better what to do than he would. This is basically the ultimate type of drug expert, someone who studies drugs for a living.

I called one I had seen years ago at Rush, who had been highly recommended by the depressed political adviser, and I learned that a new evaluation would cost four hundred dollars. The cost was high, even with the insurance covering a part of it, but I didn't see what choice I had. I was glad that
there was an appointment open in the near future, so near that I didn't have
to write it down. I knew I'd remember it anyway as the same day that yoga
started at the health club, September 11, 2001.

Early that afternoon, my parents and I drove into the city to see the doctor
even though we were obviously badly shaken by the morning's events, which
we had see on TV. We silently listened to the radio in disbelief, as we
observed that ours was one of only a handful of cars on the Dan Ryan
Expressway going north into the city. Everyone else was leaving the city in a
rush, as there was still confusion about whether the attacks would continue
in other cities. "Well, if you didn't have an anxiety disorder before, you have
one now," my mom said, half jokingly. We had called to possibly cancel, but
the receptionist said that she couldn't guarantee that we wouldn't get charged
if we didn't show up. So, we were on our way to Chicago.

We pulled into the parking lot, and I almost walked into an angry and
disheveled patient in a wheelchair who was wildly swearing and waving her
hand at a bus, which had just left her behind in its fumes. We robotically
went up the elevator into the waiting room, which was full of patients.
Apparently, others had also not let that morning's cataclysmic events get in
the way of their shrink appointments.

An older well-dressed woman started talking loudly to my mom about the
day's horrors, and we immediately knew that she was in the right place. She
had just been on the phone with her son, who was a rich trader of some kind
in California. He was excited that he was going to make a killing now in the
gold market, now that the stock market was probably kaput. She added that
she had absolutely no bad feelings about the terrorist attacks, as long as her
son was OK. She then paused and explained that the reason she was there
was that she had an inability to feel empathy. Cutting the silence that followed, a professional and uptight-looking couple returned to the waiting
room, after having apparently seen the doctor. The man made a point of paying in cash, not wanting this visit to be on his insurance.

When I saw the doctor, he was surprisingly amiable and attentive, despite
the chaos of the day. After I gave him a medical history and apprised him of
my current impasse, he gave his assessment. His advice: *Increase* the
dosage. This view, which contrasted to others, reflected the reality of doctors' conflicting views on drugs, even in the case of those like Xanax that

have been around for many years. Dealing with drugs is both an art and a science, indeed.

In this doctor's view, my problem was that I was not taking enough of the drug. In his practice, he had seen others successfully increase their dosage every few years when their bodies became tolerant to the last one. Although he did not use these words, in his opinion I was probably *pseudoaddicted*, an actual medical term meaning "undermedicated with an addictive drug." In these situations, patients often take on traits that make them appear falsely to doctors as if they are abusing drugs, such as being visibly agitated and in search of a higher dose, often actively switching doctors in the process.

I said I didn't think that was a good idea, remembering one day a few months back when I had experimented and taken 0.75 mg and then felt much worse the day after. I just knew in my gut that I wanted off of Xanax. Then, going over my chart from years before, the doctor pointed out my need to take an antidepressant. I explained that I had not been depressed beyond reason before the Xanax, especially for someone with a chronic headache. Besides, that was impossible, as I couldn't tolerate antidepressants. But he pointed out that no matter what the cause of this strange period of anxiety, an antidepressant might be a good idea. He urged me to consider new ones that were just out in liquid form, that could be started more gradually and calibrated at very exact levels. I said I would think about it.

I went to my regular internist downtown the day after, following up on yet another appointment. It had been made at the suggestion of my dad weeks earlier, and I hadn't bothered to cancel it, especially because my deductible from the year had already been made and this visit would basically be free. I had not thought of this general practitioner as an option in this circumstance because she was not a headache specialist. But I had always liked her. Besides her obviously being very bright and knowledgeable, we just clicked. She was only a few years older than I, and I talked to her as I did to Dr. Chung, in the same comfortable tone I used with my friends.

We sat down in her office and she listened to me describe this new phase of high anxiety. At first, I rushed but then slowed down when I realized that she wasn't in a hurry to boot me out. Then, instead of questioning me, a look of recognition registered on her face.

"You know, I could fill up a whole room of people who have told me exactly the same thing about their reaction to Xanax," she said. "Feeling this much anxiety after being on it for about two years, as you have."

"Even on this dose?" I asked.

"Even on that dose."

"But this is something you can't do on your own," she said. "I have had success using Prozac in getting people off it."

I reminded her that I was different, that I couldn't take antidepressants because of the side effect of insomnia. Then I remembered the news from the last doctor about the new liquid form of Prozac and suggested that.

Again, she brightened up. "That's right," she said, reaching for some kind of a reference book on her desk to look up doses. She advised me to get a baby dropper, which I would use to take the liquid in very tiny incremental doses, much smaller (and more tolerable) than those I would be able to get in pill form. We would take about two months to get to the equivalent of 20 mg of Prozac, a standard dose, and it would probably kick in fully about six weeks after that. Then, we would start tapering off the Xanax. As always, patience would be needed.

I asked about the side effects of Prozac, and she took out a piece of paper and a pen and drew a large X on a graph. I was a little more anxious, still worried that she was about to kick me out at any moment, that our time was running out.

"Do you see the top line of the X going downward? That represents the side effects," she said. "They start off strong but then diminish over time. At the same time, that other line of the X going upward represents the effectiveness. As the side effects diminish, the drug itself becomes more effective. Your problem with it has been that you have never been able to give it enough time to kick in, and for the side effects to go away. But with the liquid, I think you'll be able to do it."

There is no way to enlightenment. Enlightenment is the way.

She sketched out an elaborate schedule, increasing the dose every few weeks. Then, she offered to have me call her every few weeks to check in, or more often, if necessary—and she would tell me how to raise or maintain the dose, according to how I was feeling. I was shocked that she had volunteered this contact, which would amount to about a dozen personal calls, for which she would not be paid anything extra. And I would be speaking with her personally, in contrast to headache specialists, to whom I was just able to relay a single message and then wait for a call back. This was clearly a benefit of seeing a non-headache-specialist. She was not as bombarded with calls from patients and was less guarded about taking calls personally.

I also asked her follow-up questions, many that had been in the back of my mind for years. One was whether a large dose of hormones I had taken in June, two weeks before starting the withdrawal, could have made my anxiety worse. (The gynecologist had strongly recommended this course of action for unrelated health reasons, even though I was already showing signs of mounting anxiety.) "Yes, it certainly could have had an effect," she said. I asked her advice about the headaches in general, and she said she was sorry that there were no simple answers. But instead of being disappointed, I was relieved. I was impressed that she was being that honest and direct with me, not delivering promises she couldn't keep. But she still offered some support and validation. She added that she understood what I was going through, as her sister-in-law had that same problem. The daily exercise I was doing, although not a panacea, was a good idea, to combat both pain and fatigue. One of her patients who had chronic fatigue just accepted that every morning she had to do two hours of exercise in order to function that day. "That was the price she realized she had to pay to her disease," the doctor said.

Her words of confidence meant a lot to me, more than I could describe to her. I was surprised to find myself so moved that I was near tears. (But I held myself back from crying, as I didn't want her to think that I was crazy and write me off.) She had listened to me and worked with me to make up a plan. I realized that was the main thing that I, as a chronic pain patient, now sought from a doctor—not an instant cure, just some realistic guidance. Afterward, I was astounded to look at my watch to see that she had spent about forty-five minutes with me.

When I got back to the suburbs, I went to the drugstore and bought the hundred-dollar container of liquid Prozac (no generic was available in the liquid), which was about the same size as a Robitussin bottle. It was a clear liquid but carried an otherworldly glow because of the inorganic orange-pink tint of the plastic bottle. No matter what happened, it was already worth it, just for the validation aspect. For years, doctors had treated me as if I were neurotic in not being able to handle regular antidepressants. I must not have been the only one. I knew that, although Eli Lily was probably a responsible corporate citizen, it wouldn't have gone out of its way to roll out a product just for me personally. Others, besides just children, who require smaller doses, probably needed this type of supergradual introduction to the drug.

That night, I squeezed a few tablespoons, about 1.25 ml, into my mouth. It tasted like Robitussin. Not too bad. And things could improve. If it worked, I thought, I would find more inventive ways to take it, such as in a Prozac cocktail, replete with seltzer, lime, and Cointreau. In that case, to pay it proper homage, I imagined displaying it prominently in my apartment on my mantel, with track lighting spotlighting it from all angles twenty-four hours a day.

Even with this tiny dose, I did feel some side effects, such as lighter sleep and some light-headedness, but they were minor. When I called the internist the next week, she said that those side effects were to be expected and that I should stick to it. I wasn't on my own now to just chuck it at times of turbulence, as I had so many times before. And I was free to ask her follow-up questions: "So one night of insomnia from it a week is fine?"

"Yes," she said.

"And it's OK that the dreams every night are extra vivid?"

"Yes, that may die down."

After we hung up, I still felt supported enough to go on with the plan and not drop it as I usually had done. Knowing that I would talk to her soon was important. I was not alone. I was being listened to. I was being understood. I was being legitimized. This, behold! was a dialogue. This was a partnership.

So, I continued through the weeks, following her directions to gradually increase the Prozac. At this point, I had nothing to lose—except, of course, my sex drive.

Besides, I had loftier concerns. I was following the time-honored process in American society of using one drug to get off another. In the mid-nineteenth century, morphine had been promoted as a tool to help alcoholics get off alcohol. That type of addiction was preferred, as morphine addicts were generally perceived as less violent and more law-abiding. Then, in 1898, the Bayer Corporation introduced its new product, heroin, as an aid to help people get off morphine, to which so many had become addicted. Cocaine (also legal) was also promoted in that era to help wean morphine addicts.

To further ease my transition, I made use of another drug of sorts: television. As strong feelings of anxiety and terror gripped me in the background, I glued myself to the screen. Over the months, I developed a short list of favorites, which followed a delicate balance: They were not too mentally taxing, and yet they were interesting enough to distract me from the pain and anxiety for long periods of time, without commercial interruptions.

Surprisingly, the best network for easing drug withdrawal was PBS. The television in my old childhood room did not have cable but almost magically got three PBS channels: a spiffy one and a low-rent one from Chicago, as well as a modest one from Merrillville, Indiana. Between the three, I always had something to distract me (except in the case of cloying and endlessly repetitive pledge drives, which didn't help the pain).

My first PBS favorite was *Antiques Roadshow*. In watching it, I felt comforted, as if I had never left my gentrified urban neighborhood of gay men and gay-acting straight men galore, spread out as far as the eye could see. It also served as an entertaining lesson in American history. I was tickled when someone showed an old Coke poster from the nineteenth century, in the days when the product contained real cocaine and was used as a headache and nerve tonic. But I discovered the one negative effect of this massive watching of the show only years later. On the rare occasions when I now visit rich people's houses, I can't help but openly appraise their belongings. "Holy smoke," I recently exclaimed to everyone present at the low-key party of a friend's mother. "I saw a guy find a girl's needlepoint sampler like that from the 1800s in his attic, and at a well-publicized auction, he was told he could get like 40 Gs for it!"

A close second was the pleasant *Travels in Europe* by Rick Steves. This featured another apparently gay-acting straight man (with a production company named Back Door Productions) with very discriminating taste. Without any effort or actual headache-triggering travel over time zones, I toured with him some of the best sights of Europe and picked up some handy tips, such as proper etiquette in France. "When you want the waiter's attention for more bread, just hold up the basket," Steves instructed. "Don't snap your fingers and yell, 'Garçon!' That's rude."

Late at night, when most of these stations had signed off and while I was still in a fog of anxiety, I also sometimes zoned out watching an unusually entertaining infomercial. It advertised videotapes of Dean Martin's televised celebrity roasts from the 1970s. I felt in sync with the 1970s décor in my room as I watched insults being traded among Don Rickles (who was actually very funny), Angie Dickinson (from *Police Woman*), Phyllis Diller, Mohammed Ali—and, hey, that's Ronald Reagan before he was president!

When at my lowest points at those late hours, I also made do with an odd program on a PAX affiliate just labeled in the corner as "worship.net." This consisted of banal pictures of tranquil nature scenes, such as waterfalls and sunsets, with bland harp music in the background and garden-variety quotes from the New Testament flashed at the bottom of the screen. I told my brother about this program, and he correctly observed that it was just like the picture show used in the death scene from the 1970s movie *Soylent Green*. In that movie, as a measure against overpopulation, the government systematically kills off old people, doing so in a special soothing ceremony in which such imagery is projected on wide screens all around them in a special room as they lie dying on a hospital gurney. This ceremony makes a horrible situation seem not horrible.

I felt a bit better a month later when I went to speak at a conference in Orlando, to which I had committed myself a year in advance. It was for the American Society for Reproductive Medicine, which seemed largely to comprise urologists. They wanted me to talk about young women's sexual attitudes on a panel about female sexual dysfunction, of which they were finally gaining some awareness (and also using to develop new potentially lucrative lines of Viagra-like pills for women). I wanted to raise awareness of this issue, and besides, they had put their money where their mouth was.

As I walked around light-headed from the Prozac, the atmosphere, especially in the exhibit hall, felt surreal. This was the opposite of the feminist conferences I had attended in the past, which had naturally been woman-centered. Here I passed large freezer tanks sold for storing sperm, with blown-up pictures overhead of the little critters. These tanks were attractively displayed as if they were regular household appliances, like the newest dishwasher, with a pair of rubber gloves draped over the top as an adornment. The urologist who had sponsored my visit wore a little sperm pin on his lapel, opposite his other one, of the American flag.

But that weekend I was more disturbingly confronted with Big Pharma and my remaining fears about it, as pharmaceutical companies were ubiquitous there as advertisers and sponsors of events. I passed a towering and glowing black metal pillar by Pfizer, which had sponsored the elaborate opening banquet. It was the ultimate monument to pharmaceuticals, inspiring the level of awe from onlookers usually reserved for war memorials and Sunday mass. On it were etched the names of fifteen of its most prominent drugs, with the letters lit lovingly from behind. I almost gasped realizing how far my treatments had gone, that I had been on about 20 percent of them over the past decade—such as Zoloft and Neurontin—all in an off-label effort to relieve the headaches. I could at least count my blessings that I had been spared trials of Viagra[1] and Lipitor, also made by Pfizer.

When I wandered into the banquet hall, I found I could sample from an elaborate buffet—there was a array of fish, land mammals, and fowl. In contrast, I had always walked around feeling slightly anemic at feminist conferences, where that food group of protein was often forgotten, in favor of tubs of more politically correct bulgur-wheat salad. Now with a brimming plate, I searched for an empty seat at one of the large round tables. The only one I could see was at a table with about ten undistinctively attractive women in their twenties.

Good Lord, I realized, almost dropping my chicken wings dressed with mango salsa. These women were the drug-rep Sirens, all together now in one place! Over the years, as I had gone to doctors, I had only seen them working alone. And now, I had stumbled upon their hive!

They even ate perkily, I thought, watching them stealthfully across the table through my peripheral vision. Later, looking through the conference programs, I spied pictures in multiple ads of their patron saint (and my nemesis), the ultrafulfilled Ortho Tri-Cyclen girl.

But—and I don't think it was just the Prozac—as I continued to see the Sirens intermingling with the crowd through the weekend, I started to soften a bit. I viewed them as more human, not as the succubi I had imagined. They were always helpful, as when I asked them for free pens or pads of paper at their exhibits in the large hall, even when I said up-front that I was not a doctor. I asked one of them what that new drug she was promoting was for, and she perkily answered, "It's for urinary tract infections!"—as if she were relating to me the great news that I had just made first cut with the Tri Delts at sorority rush. "Oh, lovely!" I responded, pocketing the free refrigerator magnet.

But no one had made me take that magnet, I thought. Gradually, I realized that the problem was not really with them, these salespeople, but with how doctors seemed mindlessly to obey them. Doctors had a choice *not* to take all their knickknacks, giving the appearance that they were willing to be bought and sold for any shiny new object. They also were obligated to look critically at the drug information they are given and not automatically turn to the newest (most expensive) drugs. They had a duty to take the time to learn about the drugs and get patients safely on and off them, meanwhile considering all the reports of side effects, even those that hadn't made it to the medical journals yet. Taking drugs was a skill for the patient, which had to be nurtured and supervised. Just giving a patient a powerful drug and then turning her or him loose was like teaching someone how to drive by just handing over the car keys and a driving manual—and then considering the person high-maintenance who wanted an instructor to ride along.

In the next few months, I had more positive thoughts, for clearly chemical reasons. I felt the Prozac actually kick in and work.

I knew this for a fact because of faultless diagnostic tools: I didn't mind going to baby showers, and I now liked the suburbs. That thing on the fridge that you can put your glass into to get ice and water right there was just too cool.

Best of all, since Prozac worked on me, I knew now that I wasn't bipolar (or at least classically bipolar), as bipolar people tend to go into manic episodes when they are on this drug, as their depressed side diminishes and loses control as a balancing agent.

The best part was that I did feel my old personality gradually return, and I became more like my real old self than I had been in years. That growing sense of hollowness and emotional numbness, which had in the past year developed to define my prevailing mood, had diminished. The internist was right, that most of the side effects would diminish as effectiveness increased. This experience contrasted to my experience with other drugs in the past that had sabotaged my thinking and made me into a drugged-out zombie. Even if I hadn't been on the Xanax, Prozac probably would have helped me deal with anxiety and depression, which had been mounting over the years, either chemically coexisting with headaches or caused by the suffering associated with them.

I was now free to be productive and work on the proposal for this book, which had long been in the back of my mind. Even though I still had pain—and some remaining anxiety and depression, but at a more manageable level—at least I was at a point where I could begin planning ahead again.

When I spoke to the beloved internist next, I thanked her, telling her, "No doctor has ever helped me as much as you helped me." She shrugged, just considering this a basic part of her job.

I had gone through a long journey with drugs, and now it was time to make peace with them, while still maintaining a very critical distance. This conflict had gone on long enough. After more than a decade, I was now more realistically seeing the "big picture" of Big Pharma—its limits and benefits.

The experience with Prozac had been a revelation. These drugs—the same ones that had given me terrible side effects and had just made me feel worse in the past—were not evil. Prozac was clearly useful, when used correctly. Even Xanax had its place, as it is so fast-acting, to be used on a noncontinuous basis for people with panic disorders. That sure beat giving such a person a Prozac and then saying, "Just sit here and wait about six weeks until this kicks in."

This difficulty of correct drug administration is especially in evidence with new drugs, when the full range of side effects has not yet been widely observed and reported. I had the benefit with Prozac that it was more than ten years old. As a result of its longevity and feedback from patients, it had also been improved, now being offered in a liquid form. I also benefited somewhat because Xanax was an old drug, with anecdotal reports available about the wide range of side effects, such as that report from the British doctor I found on the Internet. With the right level of communication and education, I saw that drugs could help.

At that time, I also made some peace with shrinks, likewise the source of painful judgments in the past. In the fall of 2001, I sat in my parents' living room and looked at their bookshelves, filled with their old psychology textbooks from the 1950s and 1960s (intermingled with a few Philip Roth novels and the memoirs of David Ben-Gurion). Perhaps this field, which had been mired in sexism and myth, still had something to offer me.

I then decided to see another professional in her thirties, as the internist had been, a new no-nonsense conventional therapist. She was recommended to me by a corporate friend, as someone who could help me manage my life and my remaining struggles with anxiety. I had gotten a lot out of a more spiritual approach, but now I needed someone less ethereal and more Dr. Phil–like to give me concrete coping tools.

Six months after I had arrived in the suburbs, I finally felt strong and capable enough to return to my apartment, and to begin to learn how to live with the Headache again on my own. Immediately, I made some changes: I made the long-neglected place as welcoming as possible, giving it more of the comforts and grounded feeling of my parents' house (sans shag carpeting, which had nevertheless grown on me over the months). With the help of a friend, I cleaned and organized my apartment thoroughly. Now my plants, which I had taken back from my neighbor and which in past years had been half dead, were thriving under my care. Over the next several months, I tapered off the Xanax, with relative ease, ignoring the occasional resulting blurs in vision and waves of anxiety.

Most essentially, I also started on the road, at last, to acceptance. This involved at least looking into some new educational resources on pain that I never would have considered in the past. At these times of high anxiety with pain and drug withdrawal, I again thought of my energetic older neighbor in Chicago, Carol.

Carol's obvious success in recovery made me curious about why the Program (AA), as they call it, was so powerful for so many people. I had experienced firsthand the incredibly strong grip of an addictive drug, even at a relatively small dose, and knew these spiritual tools had to be incredibly potent to fight primal brain-chemistry-altering compulsions and their accompanying anxieties.

Although the famed twelve steps are something that I had entirely dismissed earlier as anti-intellectual, eye-glazing, and just plain pabulum, I started to think that their core teachings might actually have something fundamental to tell me about the recovery process, about living with terrible pain but not letting it destroy my life. I didn't have to buy the whole thing. I could do what I have done with everything else, like therapy, progressive politics, Judaism, and feminism—just garner some nuggets of wisdom while discarding the nutty parts. So I finally read the book *The 12 Steps of Chronic Illness* and talked to Carol a bit about what I was going through.

That was when she told me the story about the pterodactyls. And then I knew that she would be able to help me.

She recalled a low point in the dark and scary period when she was withdrawing from drugs and alcohol. One night, after returning home from work, she put her key in the door to unlock it and was suddenly braced with fear. She imagined a group of pterodactyls swirling around her apartment, and she was afraid that one would escape through the keyhole when she took her key away. But she took a deep breath, opened the door, and walked inside to face her demons. Meanwhile, she trusted that things would be OK. She did not have any great secret to how she had overcome periods like this. What it took was some intense, difficult, and always ongoing spiritual work and dedication. That was what "letting go" really involved.

In earlier years, I had not seen any value in this concept of acceptance, mainly because I had equated it with just giving up and being defeated. But this book portrayed acceptance as a kind of strength, as a way to "surrender" in order to eventually gain more control. The metaphor used was of someone steering a sailboat, recognizing (and not denying) the winds working against her or him, but then working as hard as possible to steer the boat out of danger.

Soon after this process, working at a slow but steady pace, I began researching this headache book, excited to begin filling in large gaps in my medical knowledge and pursue these concepts of acceptance further. Although I did not expect to find a cure while working on this book, I knew that the most important discovery and conclusion that I could come to was how to live *with* the Headache, which I still had in full force, and even "make friends with it" (as is the lingo in pain circles). The future, although still bound to be difficult, was full of possibilities. For the first time in a while, even though I wasn't exactly trim, my personal life was picking up. While on the elliptical machine at my new city gym, I watched *Entertainment Tonight*, a mainstay of my drug withdrawal period, and saw some good news: Mariah Carey was now on a world tour.

Part Five:

CLOSING REMARKS

21

The Waiting Place (2005)

o o o o o o o o o

ALL THESE YEARS OF INQUIRY AND STRUGGLE basically bring me back to one of the great philosophers of our day: Dr. Seuss.

In December 2001, I read an oddly comforting cover story in the *New York Times Magazine*, which, as I'll soon explain, relates to that children's author. The article, called "Pain: The Disease," by Melanie Thernstrom, reported about emerging widespread research in the field that frames chronic pain in a new way, not just as a symptom of something else, but as a bona fide neurological disease in its own right. (In the months that followed, I started to notice this model articulated in my own specific area of study, with "migraine" more and more referred to as "migraine disease.") Thernstrom described chronic pain as "a pathology of the nervous system that produces abnormal changes in the brain and spinal cord," meanwhile basically sucking up feel-good serotonin and leading to chemically induced depression and anxiety.

This emerging framework was now, at last, giving chronic pain urgency and legitimacy for treatment, pointing out that over time it can damage the body by wearing it down. And that is both good and bad news. On one hand, I don't want to think of myself as having a possibly degenerative illness, but then again, validation is the sweet mother's milk of humanity, whose majestic succor we all eternally crave and seek. So, as a consciousness-raising tool (read: See, this is a real problem and I may not be so crazy, after all), I forwarded the *New York Times* story via e-mail to many of my friends.

One friend, with two small children, responded that in reading the article detailing the miseries of chronic pain, she kept thinking of Seuss's classic book *Oh, The Places You'll Go!* a treatise on the natural cycles of life. In the book, Seuss described an inevitable unpleasant place, "The Waiting Place," where all of us are doomed to spend time when life just is put on hold and you can't do a thing about it.

I agreed with the observation that this is what having chronic pain is like, but then I also thought: To a chronic pain patient, The Waiting Place means more. It does not represent just a temporary stop now and again; it's a way of life. For when all else fails for a pain patient—when neurology becomes destiny, when the potions and powders and pills and positive thinking just don't work—*waiting* is all we have left.

We wait sometimes for an hour to feel better, so we can then finish writing a report. We wait three nights to return a phone call to a friend. We wait a week to get the energy to scour a bathroom tub. We wait an entire summer to withdraw from a powerful drug, meanwhile moving through the edginess and tremors and insomnia and blurred vision that it leaves in its wake. We wait an entire year, pill by pill, to see if a class of drugs will work over time, in higher and higher doses.

This waiting is for more than just the physical pain sensation itself to diminish. At any one time, we also are focused on multiple numbers of overlapping cycles of every possible duration—both internal and external—that help determine our constantly shifting levels of pain. If our pain is worse in the morning, we wait for evening. Many of us wait for a stormy spring season or an extreme hot-weather spell to pass. Women of a certain reproductive age tick off those five days of bleeding, perhaps more dreading those several days leading up to it when estrogen levels dip precariously.

In this process of trying to live in the moment, we face constant tensions and contradictions, many all at once: the struggle between pushing through the pain or ministering to it; the struggle to be dependent on others or stand on our own; the struggle to continue an expensive and time-consuming treatment or move on; the struggle to accept our disability while not overly identifying with it; the struggle to take responsibility for our health, but then not feeling guilty when the pain persists.

And during this time, here is the real challenge: while we wait for pain to release its grip, we try not to put the rest of our lives on hold, and to manage to participate in other parts of life as best we can.

And for a personality like mine—I have always been proactive, have confronted problems head-on, and lack any kind of patience gene—this acceptance of waiting and the reality of the things that simply can't be changed has been a major life lesson of the headache, and of this book. (However, as I continue to maintain, I do *not* consider this pain a "gift," as more dewy-eyed people would call it. I always picture a gift as something you can return.)

But with a considerable level of denial and frustration and self-flagellation, even I have picked up some wisdom through the years, based on my own foibles, in how to get by through all the pain. This knowledge has been, fortunately, deepened over the past few years by the groundwork for this book in reading medical literature and interviewing doctors and other chronic headache patients, mostly other Tired Girls, in my path. I have come across some in my everyday life and lately have more actively sought out others both in person and in an online support group. These fellow travelers have all broadened my knowledge about what can at least help the individual patient move forward and, just as important, what *social and political changes* have to be made in the bigger scheme of things to reduce these lonely struggles.

But in navigating the contradictions of the Waiting Place, I have proven myself an exceptionally slow learner. So slow, that often it's been tough for me to notice that I've made any progress at all. At some point in 2001, I got a clue. I saw Lisa, the psychospiritual therapist, one last time before switching to a more conventional shrink to learn better practical management of my life. I was complaining to her that after all the earnest self-improvement work I had done and all the money I had spent, I was right where I had begun. The pain was still there.

"But there is a difference between getting cured and getting healed," she said. "Spiritually, you are at an entirely different place from where you began."

After thinking about this, I realized that she was right. Time does not necessarily heal physical pain, but it does help with other related wounds.

It is precisely such spiritual wisdom, which I'm still acquiring at a very rudimentary level, that I have found is most vital to coexisting with chronic

pain, to actually living in the present, even during the worst of circumstances. When I think of what has actually helped me get by over the past
(nearly) fifteen years with chronic daily headache, I most appreciate spiritual
teachings, mainly from Chinese medicine, spiritually oriented therapy, and
my own diverse readings in this area.

Around the time of that conversation, I took out my still unread book
about healing, *Chronic Illness and the Twelve Steps*, by Martha Cleveland. It
well articulated the necessity of spiritual growth. "All humans go through life
on a tightrope," it says. "Some of us are forced by circumstance to look down,
and we are not the same as those who don't. We know, deep in our soul, the
potential for vulnerability and catastrophe. For us, that potential has become
real. Our chronic illness or disability has come to us, and we know that it
won't disappear. But we have found another way" (163).

Although definitely not always potent enough to overcome strong pain and
depression, these ideas have provided an important and fundamental framework for *acceptance,* and then moving on as best as I can, within limits. I realize that throughout these always-difficult years, I could have done without
the doctors I have seen and most of the crappy drugs they have administered,
but I cannot imagine life having gone on without this less concrete source of
support and insight.

One key aspect of spirituality in coping with pain, I have found, is that it is
something that you can use for the *long term*. It stands out in a quick-fix
world where medications, if they work at all, typically poop out in effectiveness, create worse "rebound" headaches, or eventually wear down the types
of organs, such as the liver or kidneys, that you might want to have around for
use in the future. A basic reason why spiritual wisdom endures is that it never
runs out of supply (as long as it is continually nourished). "The strength of
the spirit prevents its being used up," goes the quote by Lao-tzu (which also
heads the April 12 entry in the very useful book *Living with It Daily:
Meditations for People with Chronic Pain* by Patricia Nielsen).

Spiritual awareness also endures over time because it goes against, and
often beyond, the sometimes-limited Western concept of treating disease by
waging a "war" with it. Unfortunately, this type of aggressive campaign is not
practical in the long term, over years and years, without also, incidentally,
annihilating the patient. The truth is that *any* doctor can relieve any pain, no
matter how severe, in the short term. Just shovel narcotics down the patient's
throat and don't stop until the pain goes away, or until the patient simply
doesn't care about it anymore.

To achieve this greater understanding of the body and its needs, a useful—and more sustainable—spiritual concept is *mindfulness*, or active consciousness or awareness of the ever-changing body. In an interview by Joan Duncan Oliver in the Buddhist magazine *Tricycle*,[1] meditation guru Jon Kabat-Zinn further explained the difference with the short-term tactic of distraction, and the long-term spiritual mindfulness, which he defined as "bearing witness" to the pain—not denying it, but also separating oneself both mentally and physically from it to reduce any preventable aspects of suffering. Laboratory tests on the mind's role in enduring pain help back up this approach. Kabat-Zinn gave the example of the standard cold-pressor test to measure pain, which perhaps would make a good segment in the reality show *Fear Factor*. It involves a tourniquet being placed around the subject's biceps, to restrict blood flow and cause more sensitivity to pain. Then the subject suspends the hand in icy water and is measured as to the time she or he can stand this very uncomfortable activity.

"What they found was that in the early minutes of having your arm in ice water, distraction works better than mindfulness," he explained. "You're less aware of the discomfort because you're telling yourself a story, or remembering something, or having a fantasy. But after the arm is in cold water for a while, mindfulness becomes much more powerful than distraction for tolerating the pain. [With] distraction alone, once it breaks down and doesn't work, you've got nothing."

Additionally, spirituality serves a unique function to help the often-isolated chronic pain patient to feel more connected to the world. This has been a major focus of conversations through the past several years with my friend Janet Johnson, who also suffers from chronic daily headache (and is now a professor of political science at Brooklyn College). Janet's main spiritual influences have been a past therapist, who has a degree in divinity, and the regular practice of yoga (which she doesn't find as boring as I do). "I mean yoga means yoke" (which means to be joined or linked), she said. "So the focus is on your wholeness and the divinity within yourself and then your connection to the whole rest of the world."

She recently explained to me that spirituality has helped her get through the extreme "self-absorption" of being in pain, which is also a major source of suffering: "I think spirituality's important because it gave me a sense that there are things beyond myself. With headaches, you're alienated from yourself because your pain is so bad, and you don't want to be there. At the same time, you're alienated from everybody else because you have headaches: 'I don't want to go and be with people.' If I'm on meds, then I'm kind of spacey and can't quite communicate my ideas. So there's this kind of way that it becomes very selfish and self-centered. So it's in this way that spirituality recognizes both your wholeness and also your connection."

She also emphasized the basic necessity of using mindfulness to achieve self-awareness. For the chronic pain patient, this is not just a lofty ideal; it's a basic matter of survival. One must learn to observe his or her body to know what types of stressors aggravate the pain, and to know when it is tense so as to be able to take steps, when possible, to relax it. Of course, such awareness has its limits—all the self-knowledge in the world often cannot make severe pain go away—but it's an important tool to have available.

Somewhere along the path to emotional recovery, another major spiritual lesson for the chronic pain patient is that one can be both happy *and* in pain. Just before starting this book, I realized this. I was sorting through pictures I had taken over the past decade before putting them into albums. I noticed immediately a strange aspect of these photos: I was mostly smiling in them, and I was generally not "faking" it. Even during many times when I was in terrible pain, I really was enjoying myself. Despite everything, I still have a substantial number of genuinely fond memories of that period. Of course, there were countless times when pain did ruin my day and, more dramatically, dampen my will to go on living, but there were also times when it did not. I have gone to parties or weddings either putting on an act, feeling that I was there in body only, or being truly engaged with those around me. These two feelings have often been present at the same event in the same few moments.

Yes, of course, as for everyone on the planet, being both happy and in pain is not always possible. We are only human. On days when the pain is especially severe, the struggle to mentally and emotionally detach oneself from the pain in a properly transcending Buddhist fashion may be too great. But even in those most dire cases, sometimes one can limit one's emotional and mental suffering. One quote—also from the pain affirmation book *Living with It Daily*—that best sums up this challenge to me is from Helen Keller: "Everything has its wonders, even darkness and silence, and I learn, whatever state I may be in, to be content" (June 11 entry).

But this state is reachable only through *acceptance,* a vital ingredient in any healing process. As discussed, for years I resisted this process, fearing that it meant the same thing as giving up, as sealing my fate in a lifetime of suffering. But I slowly realized that accepting limits could mean exactly the opposite, that is, being able to go on to the next step of living life in the present moment. One who doesn't recognize the real limits that exist is constantly wasting energy and time butting up against them. As a major point, this step does *not* mean stopping the search for pain relief; acceptance is not the same thing as resignation.

While working on this book, on my worst days, I have personally pondered this challenge of acceptance to minimize suffering. I knew I was at a turning point when I woke up one rainy morning, realized it would be "one of those days" when thinking clearly would not be possible, and did not get upset and frustrated, as in the old days. Instead, I cradled my head and neck in ice packs and watched Turner Classic Movies almost all day, grateful for an all-day showing of Jean Harlow movies (from the brief 1930s period in "pre-Code" Hollywood, when women were allowed to be complicated). This was a very minor and rather "unproductive" way to pass the time, but it was one that was within my reach that day, under present circumstances. Yes, I realize that most people do not have the luxury of my flexible schedule. And again, despite these "enlightened" attitudes, I still suffer more than my share of frustration with the pain. But the main concept here, which any garden-variety AA serenity-prayer sampler will tell you, is that acceptance "of that which we cannot control" often leads to at least some peace.

But taking this first step, of accepting the real disability caused by one's pain, is not as easy as it may seem. Doing so actually goes against the grain of some of our culture's most fundamental beliefs about being able to cure pain through hard work, the right attitude, and/or the right technology. We are denying the ubiquitous messages of those pain-reliever ads that make us feel freakish if we can't cure our pain and in less than five minutes. ("I get headaches, but I don't let the headaches get me" goes a 2004 television commercial for Excedrin.) We have very few, if any, role models to follow in popular culture of people living still-satisfying lives *with* pain, *not* only after having gallantly totally cured themselves completely and, say, winning the Tour de France.

Other cultural influences against acceptance hit some harder than others, based on race, creed, and color. Although chronic pain affects everyone across cultures, educated white people are more likely to be *diagnosed* with it. Besides better access to health care, a major reason is a greater sense of entitlement to recognizing and treating such problems. The statistics show this, as well as common sense. I discussed this point with a friend of a friend, Nichole Wicks, thirty-two, who called me for advice in early 2004 after suffering four months of constant "grinding" head pain that had made working impossible. A few days before we talked, she'd had to quit, and she was feeling guilty about it.

I asked Nichole, who is from a suburban middle-class background, how her race influences her attitudes toward pain. "African-American women, throughout history we've always had to work despite the pain," she explained. "While people are being dragged off or, you know, locked up or disappeared or whatever, we've always had to work through both emotional and physical pain, so that either the family can stay together or the community can stay together.

"And you know, I definitely think that hurts many black communities today because now they can address things like, for example, clinical depression. I don't think many people in the black community would even comprehend what that means. You know, it's kind of like the old motto of 'Brush yourself off; life sucks, but you have to plow through. You can't let this get you down.' I definitely have some of that in me."

Also in 2004, I witnessed this attitude in fifty-eight-year-old Hazel Reese, an African-American former phone company employee in Chicago who retired early because of her pain. Reese's story makes mine look like a picnic, with enough challenges to make anyone very depressed. Besides having constant head pain similar to or greater than mine since the age of thirteen, she also has suffered serious immune disorders, severe domestic violence, and a total of about forty hospitalizations. She has lived in one of Chicago's most notorious housing projects, Cabrini Green, and supported three sons as a single mother. In her twenty-four years of work at the phone company, she never missed a day of work because of her headache.

But revealing her overall optimistic "nonvictim" outlook, the title of her new self-published autobiography chronicling her struggles is *I Will Not Complain!* In the book, she explains that this title is taken from the title of a verse by the Reverend Paul Jones, who talks about the virtue of trusting the Lord to get by, through pain after pain. (I told her that to reflect my contrasting middle-class background and lower tolerance of protracted struggle, my book should be called *I Will Complain!*)

Another great personal challenge for all is that acceptance is actually ongoing, a process that one undergoes over time. A few years ago, one doctor told me to "get some acceptance," but I had no idea what that meant. Instead, I interpreted it as his saying, "I am giving up on you. You annoy me. Please go away now." This bumper-sticker-level advice to "just accept it" is as limited as Nancy Reagan's 1980s slogan to prevent drug abuse: "Just say no." One has to go beyond the surface to address the underlying concepts necessary to achieve the desired state of mind, which may involve redefining one's core values, sense of identity, career goals, and relationships.

After all, accepting that you may have a disability—whether you use that term or not—involves a process of grieving for a lost self. You are mourning for a death: your own, as you had once imagined yourself to be. This process is actually much like that popularized by psychologist Elisabeth Kübler-Ross in her famous theory of the stages of accepting death, which include isolation, anger, depression, and hope for the future. Meanwhile, because of the ongoing nature of chronic pain and other chronic illnesses, as I've found, these stages often repeat themselves endlessly, even in the same rainy afternoon.

For me, this acceptance has been an exceptionally slow process. About five years after that lunch in Chicago in 2000 when Janet Johnson asked me if I considered myself disabled, I finally was able to answer her with a yes. Of course, this was a difficult realization. The notion that someone with chronic headaches could be disabled defied my own concepts of disability, along with those prevailing in society. Like everyone else, I pictured a disabled person as visibly handicapped, like Dickens's Tiny Tim.

Although I certainly would not want to trade places, I started to more realistically examine my actual level of impairment, which is often considerable, at least compared to the state of the "able-bodied." This impairment was made clear to me, for example, when I met a conventionally disabled woman at a Michigan "summer share" (or group weekend retreat) that a friend who had moved here from New York City (where these arrangements are common) organized. This woman's disability is the opposite of invisible. In fact it's tough *not* to notice. She has one arm, which is how she "came out" at birth. But through the weekend, I observed how actually *undisabled* she was: able to drive, able to cook, and able to keep up with what everyone else was doing without help. And I knew that she had attended a prestigious women's college and worked an office job during the week—with hours I would never be able to keep. I asked her what she is *not* able to do because of her handicap. Her only answer, after a few minutes of thinking, delivered in a joking tone, was "Play the guitar and cut vegetables neatly."

Still, of course, her life is no cakewalk, as she also revealed to me, in terms of how the disability has affected her self-image and creates the constant annoyance of other people (like me) constantly defining her by it. She joked that she had been mildly insulted during her cashier job in college when customers routinely cheered her on for daring to work.

But in contrast to her that weekend, I was able to participate in a fraction of group activities. And when I did take part, I was embroiled in a constant silent struggle to keep up with people and do "my share" of cooking and other communal tasks. Ironically, a major problem with her is people overidentifying her with her missing arm, and a problem for people with inherently invisible chronic pain is the opposite, not being validated or acknowledged in any way by society.

Other sources of insight into what makes disability have been less personal. Some of the facts and figures I found in routine research for this book also were eye-opening to me. In the 2004 book *Migraine and Other Headaches*, the authors compared those with severe chronic head pain to others one would more commonly accept as disabled. "In general, headache sufferers are worse off than people who have arthritis, roughly similar to those who have congestive heart failure severe enough to interfere with walking up and down stairs and only slightly better than people with AIDS," wrote neurologists William B. Young and Stephen D. Silberstein, summing up medical research in the field for a popular audience (6).

Making matters worse with issues of accepting disability, many doctors don't even know about the existence of chronic daily headache, or headaches that last more than two hours. The result is a general portrayal by them and in the media of the disorder as a marginal complaint, limited to only the most neurotic of patients.

But part of my own acceptance has also been made possible through homework on the basic neurology behind chronic daily headache (at least as it is currently conceived). Again, being an educated patient isn't just a nice-sounding ideal for those with chronic pain. When you are without a doctor, which accounts for the great majority of the time, you are all you've got to shepherd yourself through.

Needless to say, I was more fortunate than most chronic headache patients in having the opportunity to attend medical conferences and request obscure journal articles from Italy through interlibrary loans. But I also benefited from easily accessible educational web sites and newsletters from the major associations, which often boiled down the latest research, including that of the National Headache Foundation and the American Council on Headache Education (yes, that's ACHE, on purpose).

But reading articles meant only for the eyes of doctors has been most startling. The truth is that doctors are much more direct with each other than with patients (or the media) about the real obstacles that exist for chronic pain patients, specifically those with chronic daily headache. The real story of doctors' current overall limits is like highly classified information. The result is large populations of patients who blame themselves, feeling as if

Ye Olde "Chronic Daily Headache"

Although, considering recent historical classifications, "chronic daily headache" may seem like a new concept, it is actually a new label for a long-recognized illness. In fact, such disabling chronic headaches have been recognized in medical literature for centuries. In his classic 1888 treatise on neurology, *A Manual of Disease of the Nervous System*, W. R. Gowers recognized frequent migrainous headaches.[2]

This syndrome was even addressed by the well-known physician Thomas Willis, who coined the term *neurology*. His 1672 classic Latin text, *De Anima Brutorum,* describes three types of headaches, a "continuous headache" being listed first, and two types of "intermittent" ones listed next.[3] In his also well-known 1685 treatise, *The London Practice of Physick*, Willis described how he had been called to "see a Lady of Quality, troubled for above twenty years with a Head-ach, which at first was intermittent, but of late is almost continual." (But I assume that many neurologists today would disagree with his explanation that such pain is caused by animal spirits being discharged from the nerves. They also probably wouldn't like his bleeding remedies.)

At the national 2003 meeting of the American Headache Society, I asked the high-profile Dr. Stephen Silberstein, also a coauthor of the new 2004 official International Headache Society medical guidelines, if the general population is aware of this problem. "I don't even think doctors are aware," he said.

"Really?" I said. "You don't even think that doctors are aware of it? What about therapists?"

"Nobody is aware of it," he said.

they are the only ones not "cured" by doctors, and refusing to accept the reality of their problems.

In the past few years, as a result of my own years of guilt and self-blame in viewing myself as the one "unresponsive" headache patient on earth, such revelations have often caught me off guard, although they are common knowledge among pain specialists. I did a double take when interviewing neurologists, such as one who casually remarked that the medications she has available for chronic daily headache "are minimally effective."

I had the same startled yet validating reaction, again in the summer of 2003, with an interview with a young neurologist who was explaining to me her initial attraction to neurology. She said that since most neurological problems like chronic daily headache are currently incurable, she feels she can

The Pert Plus Syndrome:
Crappy "Preventive" Drugs Exposed at Last

A major source of confusion to the chronic headache sufferer is that drugs often do not work. But instead of blaming the drugs, a common reaction of the doctor and other therapists is to blame the patient for being "unresponsive."

But a major discovery I made while researching this book, which surprised me as both a patient and a writer, is that these drugs actually have been at least partly studied and found inadequate for headache relief. In fact, recent, and very unpublicized, studies show that the drugs available for CDH prevention only really work in about 50 percent of patients (and even they should expect, at most, a 50 percent reduction in pain).[4]

The crappy nature of these drugs seems to be a very well-kept secret, with self-help books and doctors in person virtually never disclosing this fact. In all these years, I personally have found only one instance of doctors talking openly about how inadequate current "preventive" drugs for headaches are, and actually providing scientific data as support. But this was only when they were arguing with each other for the effectiveness of *new* drugs (which they personally were being paid to promote and study).

I call this the Pert Plus syndrome. Here's the reason: I remember using Pert Plus shampoo years ago and noticing that it made my hair limp, although the commercial was telling me that it should be fabulously full of body. But then, the maker introduced "NEW Pert Plus." Only then, when trying to sell something to replace it, did the company admit to the inadequacy of the previous product, promising that this one would not make your hair go limp, as I remember it.

Nowhere was this Pert Plus phenomenon more evident to me than in the ample sales materials distributed at the 2003 annual meeting of the American Headache Society in Chicago. This was particularly the case at its numerous "satellite" sessions—which are basically panels sponsored by pharmaceutical companies, often to highlight flattering research on their new products (which they also typically had sponsored in the first place).

The most sophisticated satellite session of this type was held in an upper-level deluxe suite of the Fairmont Hotel, overlooking the Chicago skyline. This unofficial conference event, about the positive uses of Botox for headache pain, was sponsored by the mysterious and addressless "Neurotoxin Institute." (It is described in fine print on its materials and web site as being supported by "an unrestricted educational grant from Allergan," which, to no one's surprise, is the company that makes Botox.) Treating headaches is an off-label use for Botox, so Allergan is not allowed to directly advertise it for this purpose. But nothing was stopping the company from sponsoring sessions by doctors that directly promote this use. As at other medical meetings in other pharmaceutical-heavy fields, sales Sirens were available to serve up plenty of data, along with the open bar, to the fifty doctors present.

In the provided "continuing-education" video, "Focus on Headache," neurologist (and the evening's presenter) Dr. Stephen Silberstein, who is widely noted as the world's leading expert on chronic daily headache, discusses the faults of current drugs in a much more direct way than I had previously heard, especially in any self-help book. He talks about the "pressing need to address patient dissatisfaction" and discusses how the current medications "are not optimal . . . with low efficacy rates." Hmm, I thought for the first time, munching on the rack of lamb provided by the ample neurotoxin-funded buffet, maybe it wasn't just me, after all.

In another satellite panel that weekend promoting the new off-label headache drug Topamax (nonsurprisingly sponsored by manufacturer Ortho-McNeil), I heard a variety of doctors clearly make an assertion again about the inadequacy of the currently available preventives. "Interestingly, a majority of commonly used drugs have little evidence of efficacy. In contrast, almost all options have well documented adverse events, often leading to a discontinuation of preventive therapy," read a summary in the program book leading to the presentation of Dr. David W. Dodick, the well-respected director of the Headache Program at the Mayo Clinic branch in Scottsdale, Arizona. This time the assertion was backed up by the citation of many studies, including a major federally sponsored one from 1999 done at Duke University. (If not for that panel, I would never have found it.)[5]

That weekend, it seemed as if everyone but me (a patient) had known about the inadequacy of the treatments available to treat chronic daily headache. I even discovered this during one of the most odd events of the weekend, taking a group field trip to the Chicago Headache Clinic's new outpatient and inpatient facilities in the upscale Lincoln Park neighborhood. The clinic chartered a trolley on wheels to take doctors from the hotel downtown to the North Side.

On the way there, I was sitting next to a very educated and sharp pharmaceutical researcher from Ann Arbor. I told him about my book on chronic daily headache, and he shrugged casually, "Oh yeah, we really can't do much for that." I asked him about other classes of drugs that I had taken, and he shook his head at the poor quality of each one. (I think I went on too long with my questions, as I saw him make a point of sitting next to someone else on the way back to the hotel.) While touring the new Chicago Headache Clinic inpatient clinic, I also got the message driven home to me of the limited types of preventives still being used. Most of the (zombified) patients there seemed to be on the same nasty MAO inhibitors I had taken a decade earlier (at least according to a medication sheet handed out on request). Even at this internationally recognized center, no new breakthroughs seem to have been made, this off-label side-effect-heavy set of drugs from another era still being a staple of treatment.

make a difference in patients' lives through helping them to manage their illnesses. *Incurable*, I thought, zoning out of the next minute of what she was saying. I had never before read or heard this said so directly and nakedly, that what I have is not curable, like other neurological problems, such as MS, epilepsy, Parkinson's, Alzheimer's, autism, and so on. Well, yes, I thought, I guess that in looking at neurology as a whole, this analysis makes a lot of sense. After all, what in neurology *is* curable?

Education has definitely been a healing balm. In my reading of medical texts, I have been greatly relieved, instead of insulted, by the realization: It really is all in my head. Basically, chronic headaches are rooted in neurobiology in the brain. Although I'd previously dismissed the neurological model as just one more competing theory that explains headaches (no more compelling than the possibility of a deviated septum or a deviated mind), now I perceived it as primary and making the most sense of all.

One of the best and simplest descriptions of migraine that I have heard (and actually got from an educational video on Botox and headaches) is of migraine as "a genetic disease with environmental triggers." This helps to distinguish cause from effect. As with other diseases, this model explains that stress (an environmental trigger) can make a difference in a headache, but without the genetic predisposition, no amount of stress will lead to head pain. In fact, scientists have found that some people's brains are, because of their wiring, physiologically incapable of experiencing headaches.

The brain's overreaction to change can cause a variety of problems, which can be easily mistaken for root causes. Migraine takes more forms than the Cheshire cat. As I have explained, the migraine response sets off a cascade of neurological activity, which can create a wide variety of disturbances in the entire body. These include sinus inflammation and neck and shoulder pain, often mistakenly pegged as the root cause of headaches. Such hypersensitive brain chemistry also helps me at last understand why I often need small doses of medications, often increased very gradually, like most of the other chronic pain patients I have met.

This knowledge also provides a reasonable (yet admittedly vague) theoretical framework for explaining my most seemingly bizarre and unique experiences with pain. Specifically, the concept of *central sensitization*, of pain processors in the brain becoming increasingly sensitive over time and carving out more and more new (and painful) neural pathways, has been very enlightening. Although my problem seems to have started in 1991, when contact lenses first set off severe pain, I now think that the sensitization of the nerves had probably been building over time. From the time I first got the lenses, at the age of fourteen, I felt that sensitization grow through the years; I started to wear the lenses for shorter times.

And as central sensitization is thought to happen mainly in the brains of women, it also demonstrates at least part of the reason why we account for most chronic headache sufferers. This model also connects migraines to other female-dominated disorders, such as irritable bowel syndrome, fibromyalgia, and chronic fatigue syndrome, which are also theorized to be rooted in hyperactivity of the brain.

The concept that external triggers lower resistance also sheds some light on the previously perplexing question of headache onset. Triggers spur not only individual episodes, but also the onset of the entire problem itself, which in my case had very likely been developing behind the scenes for years. My resistance, already possibly set in genetics, may have been weakened by a concussion in grade school and then, later on, stress. So I no longer blame that one concentrated period of stress in 1991, preceding the onset, as the total culprit.

All this knowledge has been reinforced in the past several years by advanced types of brain imaging, which make the old ones, such as regular MRIs and CT scans, look as primitive as an Etch-A-Sketch. The new scans have revealed that the brains of migraine sufferers are hypersensitive to stimuli, generally reacting more strongly to exposure to light and sound (even when a migraine is not happening). As others get used to such stimuli over time, the brains of migraine patients become more and more stimulated by repeated exposure. These scans also reveal shifts in activity through the entire brain during an episodic migraine, which seems to begin with a traceable dysfunction in the brain stem. As discussed, in those with constant pain (without a baseline to measure from), scans specifically have revealed structural differences; the brains of those with chronic daily headache exhibit increased iron deposits, for example.

I also gained insight into why so many alternative medicine methods I tried had worked only briefly. I got this knowledge only while reading further about the gate theory, which reveals why these therapies may have worked in the first place. For example, the gentle motions of massage help to interrupt pain signals at the spinal cord, forming a "gate" against them. But now following these same principles, I can understand why the gate stops working. Eventually, the brain gets bored by these new signals from the massage and starts to tune them out, kind of like "white noise." They are no longer "new" and worthy of attention.

Another useful, if also depressing, neurological concept is *comorbidities*, which is a part of standard dialogue in medicine but not yet well known to the general population. (But in the last year, I have noticed pharmaceutical ads discussing depression that list pain as a key symptom.) Evidently, to our misfortune, chronic headaches often come bundled with other ailments, just like the discounted cable-telephone-DSL line service offered by your local phone company. After studying these problems as rooted in brain chemistry, I understand that some of the most common chronic headache comorbidities—including anxiety, depression, and fatigue—are not moral failings. This discovery has led to more acceptance of my own comorbidities, and then to treatment of them, which, when possible (as with Prozac for anxiety and depression, which has had almost no continuing side effects for me), has improved my quality of life overall.

This knowledge also helps to explain, at last, a more nuanced concept of the "headache personality," which for decades has been used to blame the victims as bringing it on themselves with their supposed rigidity and perfectionism. After years of wondering about it, I finally understood this concept when interviewing brain researcher Dr. Nabih Ramadan, the medical coeditor of the newsletter of the American Council on Headache Education. I commented to him about how doctors often just commonly dismiss chronic-daily headache patients as neurotic, and he responded, "The problem with this kind of argument is the fact that you don't have to necessarily have a neurotic personality to have chronic daily headache. And there is some evidence that you have children with daily headaches. And generally those children don't express any personality disorder or personality trait that is of a neurotic character. In essence, they are not exhibiting a neurotic behavior by complaining of pain."

Then he explained where comorbidities, based on shared brain chemistry, come in, as sometimes influencing personality: "The confounding problem is the fact that a lot of these conditions do tend to overlap. So, for example, a lot of the painful conditions—whether it's migraine or chronic daily headache—are coexisting with things like fibromyalgia, with irritable bowel syndrome, with chronic fatigue syndrome. So there is a lot of overlap. And then, in addition to the overlapping with psychiatric disorders such as anxiety, depression, and some personality traits, people tend to focus more on trying to find cause and effect, when, in fact, it's [the dynamic between personality and headache] much greater than that."

I asked him if doctors and therapists are generally aware of this relationship, are aware that these comorbidities do not actually cause the headaches but coexist with them. He answered, "Well, there is some awareness of it, but I don't think it is widely accepted yet. I mean, in order to be effective in medicine, in general, you tend to use this cause-and-effect or black-and-white relationship. But the reality of the matter is that brain physiology is not just an all-or-none phenomenon, and there are a lot of nuances that we have to recognize when we are managing our patients."

Other more concrete knowledge of mine about "living with the pain" has also been recent. An essential practical step toward coping with pain is learning some basic management concepts that can help, at least at times. Particularly useful are the "ten steps" from the American Chronic Pain Association, related in a book and in a video, that many intellectuals will be happy to know have nothing to do with a "higher power." They include principles that may be considered trite by an outsider but are a revelation to a panicked pain sufferer. They include setting priorities and goals, recognizing negative emotions, relaxing, and exercising. I was most intrigued by the fifth step, in my opinion the most original, of recognizing "your basic rights." This sense of entitlement to having one's needs recognized could greatly counter common feelings of anxiety that pain patients have, of trying to always bend to others' schedules and paces. These "rights" follow principles of the disability rights movement—and come to think of it, of the gay rights movement—that it isn't us who has the problem; it's society that has trouble in accepting and accommodating natural human diversity.

Of the fifteen rights, a few that most made me think were the "right to change your mind" and the "right to make mistakes." As I read them, I did feel a wave of antianxiety roll over me (not as good as that from Xanax, but I'll take what I can get). Indeed, for a person in chronic pain, part of the anxiety of participating in life and making plans with others is the uncertainty about being able to come through, to keep appointments. Although I still rarely cancel on people, I am now newly comforted by the fact that I have the *right* to do it. (But a friend just gave me a less lofty reason for having less guilt when I cancel on people: "Don't worry. No one wants to see you that much anyway.")

Another one of these rights, the "right to do less than you are humanly capable of doing," was also liberating. This gives one permission to actually keep some reserves of energy, and not to consider every theoretically "achievable" task compulsory. This concept relates to another basic management tool that I have only studied as an option while researching this book. This is the vital concept of *pace*. It reveals how *external social conditions,* of just being allowed to take things slower, can very strongly define our experience of disability. We already have a basic concept of how this works with people with visible disabilities: A person in a wheelchair, now with ramps and elevators installed to get to class at the university, is less disabled. A person who is deaf, now with an interpreter at the theater, is now less disabled. And for someone with an invisible chronic illness, living life at a slower pace can also greatly reduce the level of "disability" experienced. This has been my main management strategy in working on this book, to do so slowly but steadily. Amazingly, after a while, the pages pile up.

I brought up this concept of pace with my realist physical-therapist friend Elizabeth Hart. She agreed that when her patients are able to get more flexible work schedules, they do much better. She also pointed out that in other cultures, some people might not be as "disabled" as they are in the United States, where that option is not often recognized. "I've had people say, 'Well, you know, I can work for eight hours, but after I have worked for ten hours, my pain is really bad, and by the twelfth hour, I want to die.' And I'll say, 'Then work for eight hours.'"

As I have mentioned earlier, another key management strategy for getting by in the long term is to take advantage of simple low-tech remedies, such as massage, heating pads, essential oils, premium cable channels, and a healthy sense of humor and absurdity. Although definitely not cure-alls, such remedies can make a difference, as I know from experience.

Despite their limits, these spiritual concepts and management techniques can all have one desirable effect in the end to relieve anxiety. They may help free you from worrying as much about the pain. The chronic-pain meditations book *Living with It Daily* cites the following twelve-step-friendly quote from Louisa May Alcott (in the July 18 entry), which sums up the desired state of mind: "I am not afraid of storms, for I am learning to sail my ships."

Neurologist and headache specialist Dr. Paula Mendes explained it in a different way in an interview. Mendes talked about telling her patients to take their coping tools and, literally and metaphorically, put them in a drawer. "Have a drawer in your room with information about what to do, whom to call, and what meds to take, and forget about it. Close the drawer and forget it. Have your life. Don't worry about having a headache."

Of course, like all advice related to pop spirituality, this is easier said than done. People with more-or-less constant pain (about half of chronic-pain patients, according to a May 2004 American Chronic Pain Association survey) do not have the employment option of periods of reprieve when they can just "forget about it." But Mendes expressed some important wisdom about recognizing the problem but not defining yourself by it.

She was influenced by the Buddhist principles of not "getting attached to suffering and living in the moment. If your life is revolving around headache, you get attached to the fact that you are a chronic daily headache patient and something can happen because you have a headache. Just live for right now. Not to say that you shouldn't know exactly what to do when you have a headache; you should be prepared and feel confident that you know exactly what you're going to do."

Besides learning how to manage one's own life, denizens of the Waiting Place also have to learn how to manage others. Namely, therapists and doctors. If not handled correctly, these professionals can actually make one's life worse and create even more feelings of isolation and self-recrimination. With chronic pain syndromes, the risks of misdiagnosis and belittling are especially great because of medical professionals' lack of education, especially in determining cause and effect, such as blaming depression for causing the pain of a depressed headache patient.

As a result, the temptation for chronic-pain patients like me has been to steer clear of therapists and doctors. But our fear of them often deprives us of important support. In fact, a combination of drugs and therapy may be optimal in chronic pain treatments, as specialists in the field of depression have long recognized.

Perhaps a more affordable, and even preferable, way to go with therapy is a free support group—either online or in person. As I found from attending one in Chicago, sponsored by the National Headache Foundation, this is one unique place in life where people do really feel your pain, in deep contrast to regular contact with friends, family, and coworkers, who even at their most empathetic really have no clue whatsoever to what you are going through.

One patient I met in an online headache forum, Melanie Watkins, a thirty-year-old nurse from Alabama, told me about why such a service has been "such a blessing in my life." She is now a moderator of the forum, at www.headaches.about.com. "Until I found that forum," she said, "I didn't know that there were people like me. I did not know that there were people who hurt all the time. In nursing school, when we studied chronic pain I can remember sitting there thinking, 'Oh, nobody can hurt all the time. That's not possible.' And it is possible to hurt from the minute you wake up till the minute you go to bed. And it's very lonely to feel like that."

Another person from the online forum went further to describe the impact of the support group she attends near her home in Vancouver, Washington. "I frankly don't think I would be alive today if I hadn't gotten involved with the support group," said Jean (not her real name), forty-seven, a former buyer in the wholesale food industry. The group helped her several years ago when her health began to deteriorate with migraines that became almost daily after a hysterectomy. At that time, her husband of twenty-five years, who was in the military, left her, insisting that her illnesses were just "mind over matter."

When she went on to explain the group's meaning, her words sounded formulaic, as if they were from a self-help book, but they were very sincere: "With (the group's) support and encouragement, I have found a way to somehow keep going when things were really, really bad. And I've grown and grown, and now I have a life, or the start of a life, that is going somewhere. And I am beginning to like the person that I am turning out to be."

A reasonable goal would be to find a therapist who is trained in this area. I saw the benefit of this kind of knowledge in a few sessions with a psychologist at a well-known headache clinic in Michigan, which I visited a few times in 2003 (after I had met my gargantuan deductible for that year and realized such lavish excursions would be mostly covered). This therapy with someone educated in chronic daily headache, although brief, was entirely different from anything I had experienced. In conversation about sources of stress, I brought up my ongoing guilt about having caused the headaches myself, through pushing myself too hard with my work in my twenties. He had four responses: "First, the thought that you caused this yourself is untenable." Hmm, I thought. Good word, *untenable*. I have to remember that one.

"Second, a lot of people write books under pressure, and don't end up with chronic headaches." Good point.

"Third, you were twenty-four when it happened. That's a very typical age of onset for chronic daily headache." OK, I'll buy that.

"Fourth," he said, with his most helpful and informed point, "studies show that in at least 40 percent of people who have chronic daily headache, the onset followed a stressful event." Then he was able, by memory, to cite the study for me to go and look up. I realized that if it hadn't been writing deadlines, something else would have come along to eventually trigger the Headache.

But seeking a headache specialist in any area, including in neurology, may have some trade-offs. A negative aspect, already discussed, is that a specialist has a lot of other innately irksome, frustrating, and time-consuming headache patients such as me. Headache and chronic pain patients, by nature, need much attention, with longer visits and large numbers of follow-up calls about medications. As a result, picking up the phone and talking to a headache specialist personally when you have a question is not likely to happen.

As a result, a key to the best possible treatment may be a doctor who is willing to basically spend a lot of time with you and learn your particular patterns, of both pain and responses to medication. Since specialists are often less reachable, more commonsense, regular, and detailed treatment may be found from a family doctor or general neurologist (who may not specialize in headaches as a main focus), as any of those I interviewed with chronic daily headache have found. One chronic headache patient I just met, the coworker of a friend in Chicago, found that the doctor who treated her pain most effectively ended up being her cardiologist, who happened to take a strong personal interest in her and to have a wide scope of knowledge. His treatment was more effective than the treatment she had received at a much more costly and heavy-handed headache clinic.

Seeking such personalized treatment is often not easy, the result of an active process on the part of the patient. Neurologist (and headache specialist) Paula Mendes observed the payoffs, telling me that the "pushiest" patients are those who more likely get better: "They know what their options are and they pick what's best for them. They know what's best for them. We (doctors) may think we know, but we [patient and doctor] are a team. I tell you what's available, and I suggest what I think will be best for you, but you have to tell me."

Indeed, as patients will also tell you, the price of good care, like the price of democracy itself, is constant vigilance. As a tool to protect oneself against victim-blaming doctors, in an interview, Janet Johnson brought up the concept of a *healthy witness*, which she learned in yoga practice. As concepts of mindfulness can help one deal with pain, as Dr. Mendes discussed with me, they can also assist with drawing boundaries with others. Johnson explained a healthy witness as basically learning to listen to oneself, to cultivate "a part of you psyche that witnesses what's going on and observes. It's sort of detached from yourself. It sort of observes you in relationship to the world and says, 'That person is not working for you. You need to do something different.' It gives me pause when I feel myself roped into things that are beyond my control, and it's not safe."

In other words, it is all about "intuition," that same protective impulse that any course in self-defense will teach you to respect.

As a result of this new consciousness, Johnson took an especially strong stand against headache specialists (one that I would not recommend to others) in actually throwing away a shopping bag of past MRIs after a negative experience with her first doctor at the Chicago Headache Clinic, where she felt she wasn't being listened to as an individual and was being automatically prescribed a one-size-fits-all regimen. I asked her about why she had taken that step, and she explained, "It's my new theory about only keeping things in my life that keep me healthy and excluding everything else. So throwing them out was my way of getting rid of all the crap that I went through."

Less expectedly, I have found, one's healthy witness also has to be mobilized in the case of "alternative" practitioners. Often mistreatment is more difficult to gauge in these cases because it is done in more progressive and spiritual language, such as with talk of "healing" and "learning to love yourself." A typical problem is being pushed into having multiple appointments for a treatment that does not seem to be working, even after a few tries.

In all these cases, to possibly avoid problems it is also important to focus on the less inspiring matter of finances. Not yours, the doctor's. Before accepting treatment, patients have to follow the money trail, asking themselves how that doctor makes his or her greatest profits, such as from expensive tests and procedures, and how that may bias care. Doctors mainly make money not from listening to a patient, which is time-consuming, but from performing costly and unproven procedures. Often the best treatments are not necessarily the most expensive ones, which are likely to be pitched to you with inflated (however vague) promises.

22

From a New Generation

○ ○ ○ ○ ○ ○ ○ ○ ○

Convenient Bulleted Advice to Nonpatients, and Hope

THERE IS ONLY SO MUCH THAT the lone chronic pain patient can do on her or his own, with energy and resources typically limited, to make life more tolerable in the Waiting Place. The best-laid patient management strategies and philosophies only go so far. They help patients choose among the options currently available but do nothing to expand the quality and number of options *as a whole*.

And that is where others, like those who treat patients and form public opinion about them, come in. They can take steps to improve the quality of life of patients with chronic pain—those who account for the leading cause of adult disability in the United States. Meanwhile they can make them a mainstream part of health care, no longer doomed to peering in from the sidelines, like "old maiden aunts" at that one table of "odd" adults at the wedding. As a great deal of chronic pain is actually not under control, contrary to most popular opinion, this is an urgent matter. According to a May 2004 study by the American Chronic Pain Association, 47 percent of people with chronic pain say that their pain is not under control. And the number is larger, at 59 percent, for those whose pain is ever-present.

Some of my advice to professionals actually overlaps with that I have given to patients. They also need to learn *acceptance* of the disabling realities of chronic pain to reduce double standards and victim blaming. This will all lead to more efficient and effective treatment—which can endure over the *long term*. But I can't list everything that needs to be done, as that could be another book (and this conclusion is already too long as it is).

So, to sum it all up neatly, I thought I'd take a cue from popular self-help books and list the changes that need to be made in convenient, media-friendly, simple-as-pie, and only slightly condescending sound-byte bulleted form:

To shrinks: Although many of Freud's conceptions about the subconscious are still useful, his overly broad theories of chronic pain as essentially a psychiatric phenomenon have been widely debunked. Like thirty years ago. So, keep in mind:

- Yes, psychology and stress can certainly play a role in exacerbating chronic pain, but it is basically a physical disease. One has to have a genetic predisposition to have chronic headaches. And in reality, you could always find a supposed subconscious motivation in *anyone* for having chronic pain. All people have stresses in their lives and things they want to avoid that can be blamed for "causing" the pain. And even if the mind has an influence in exacerbating the pain, that doesn't mean that "mind over matter" can cure it.

- With this in mind, you can even encourage a patient to accept pain, seeing it as a positive part of emotional recovery. For the acceptance of pain does not mean that a person is "self-perpetuating" it by becoming "attached" to it. In this same vein, please don't limit your work to the "behavioral psychology" of "reducing pain behaviors"—as in cracking down on patients' sleeping late, moaning, or cutting down on work. These steps are not enough to get rid of a real physical disease, just as you would not limit your treatment of a diabetic to encouraging the reduction of the "diabetic behaviors" of avoiding sugar and taking insulin, and telling the patient, "Just learn to relax." That would be malpractice.

To neurologists: All of the above, plus this:

- Admit that you don't like the headache patient, the person who most commonly visits you during your day, and there are good reasons why. A pain patient requires time and communication, and at best, you may only be able to reduce part of the symptoms.

- This reality has implications for how you should try to treat this patient. First, please do not be afraid to admit that you do not know something, which is only to be expected. If the patient does not get better, you should not take it as a personal affront.

- Second, although a patient's chronic pain is probably not psychosomatic in origin, she or he does need your emotional support, not as a therapist, but in sticking with her or him through difficult periods and giving personal support in getting on and off drugs.

- Third is a related matter: Even a patient whose pain is exacerbated by stress or emotional influences deserves medical pain treatment. In fact, even a patient who is stark raving mad, coming into your office on all fours and barking and foaming at the mouth, may have real chronic pain that deserves treatment. Using someone's mental history as an excuse to deny treatment is tantamount to a jury's not convicting a rapist because the rape victim was not an "innocent" virgin. (For younger readers, the reasoning goes that if she has a sexual history, she is "bad" and not deserving of legal protection.) As we have rape shield laws, preventing courts from going into a rape victim's sexual history, we should consider "mental health" shield laws for pain sufferers.[1]

- Fourth, speaking of what you don't know, you cannot possibly know every side effect, especially of new drugs, so you should not dismiss new side effects reported to you by patients. In fact, patient feedback about seemingly "obscure" side effects has been invaluable to science in reevaluating drugs and making new ones.

- Fifth, we want to be warned about side effects, which have the danger of interrupting our daily responsibilities, which may be numerous. After all, women today work. We go to school. We read. We have responsibilities. Don't assume that we just stay home all day rearranging our glass menageries and Precious Moments figurines.

- Sixth, please communicate clearly why you are giving an antidepressant to a pain patient: that you aren't accusing the patient of "just being depressed," and that the neurology of depression and that of chronic pain are very similar.

- And when being paid by pharmaceutical companies to do studies on their drugs, please recognize that you, like everyone else, are human and prone to bias. Studies show that doctors think that they can be objective in being consultants to Big Pharma, that they are the *one* exception to the proven phenomenon of gifts influencing behavior. These companies are not paying you for nothing; they know what they are doing and expect to get a return on investment. On a smaller level, please stop accepting every single tchotchke that they offer you for your office (as doctors are regulated to do in every other country except the United States and New Zealand). You give the message, "Yes, I can be bought for an Amerge clipboard and Lexapro Post-It Notes. That's all it takes." Just budget an extra hundred dollars a year to go to Office Depot and buy all that crap in one trip.

- Finally, don't forget that patients who come to you about pain might want some actual *pain relief*. Neurologists are often fixed on daily preventives (which do not often work) for fear of causing a rebound headache. They may also get carried away with identifying and treating the endless numbers of comorbidities discovered on a regular basis. This focus can help matters overall but often also serves as a distraction from treating the original problem: the pain.

- In sum, a problem with how your field is set up is that it is geared to the convenience of the doctor, not the patient. For example, headache specialists don't typically personally take calls from patients. Although this practice makes sense from your perspective (taking more calls in person would indeed be time-consuming), the patient loses out. Meanwhile, without this personalized support, very chronic patients like me go on struggling through life in a state of disability. (An example from my life of this attention's making a difference was when my internist talked to me weekly over the period of a few months to get me on a drug that greatly enhanced my level of functioning. I couldn't have done it without this type of support.) This focus on the doctor's convenience in neurology was typical of the field of obstetrics and gynecology fifty years ago, when women giving birth had no choice but to do what was most convenient for the doctor, such as being put to sleep during the process or being induced to fit into a doctor's vacation schedule.

To all other types of doctors, including shrinks:

- Please learn at least some basic neurology about chronic pain and chronic daily headache. Know that chronic headaches based in neurological imbalances can imitate other problems that you may face daily in your practice: A migraine can misleadingly resemble a sinus problem (as nine out of ten so-called diagnosed sinus headaches are really migraine), an unrelated spinal stenosis, or a muscle contraction disorder of the neck. The danger is in using costly and dangerous procedures to treat those false causes and make the patient's pain worse in the end, an outcome that is, by all accounts, very common.

To "alternative" healers:

- If you don't know something, please don't use your common default diagnosis of blaming all ills on "lack of balance." Even if we lose weight, avoid gluten, and move to an ashram, chronic pain can still continue. Don't insult and belittle us with the argument that the pain is *all* a result of the body trying to communicate a message, like we're too angry. If you told someone with cancer or diabetes that, you would be considered cruel and even stupid. This is a double standard for people in pain, another version of dismissing the pain as purely "psychosomatic," that can discourage real medical research and treatment. In the meantime, don't assume that the mind always has "control" over the body, that it's all a matter of just changing thought patterns.

To the government:

- First, please fund some research on chronic pain, on its causes, treatment, and prevention. Whereas pain accounts for 20 percent of medical visits and 10 percent of prescription drug sales, it represents only 0.6 percent of the National Institutes of Health research funds.[2] Please don't make this so-called Decade of Pain Control and Research of 2000–2010, as declared by Congress, a sham. This means you can't leave all research up to pharmaceutical companies, which have very tailored agendas to push a specific drug. You also have more muscle to conduct basic research that a pharmaceutical company would not fund, with a perspective on more long-term knowledge (such as the long-term effects of opiates in the treatment of chronic pain, which are still not known), and on diseases that are considered "too obscure" one year (but then suddenly common the next, when a famous person gets one). The government also has a duty to test commonly used old off-label drugs, which are now in generic forms and no longer profitable. If there is no apparent direct link to a marketable (new) product, then Big Pharma isn't going to want to go there.

- Second, please make disability payments easier to get for chronic pain patients. Although neurology is invisible, you can still get "proof" of real disability from the paper trail left with doctors and from patient "headache diaries," which tell a lot (and are used commonly to get disability payments for patients with depression). And please make payments more realistic. This is not 1929, when $585 a month was considered a bonanza. The low rate of payments assumes that disability happens on an incentive system; the reasoning goes "If we don't 'reward' disability, then it is less likely to happen." But disability is a part of life, and why should disabled people be further punished by living a life of abject poverty?

- Third, please allow the patients in need access to opioids, such as methadone and Oxycontin. These are not inherently nefarious demon drugs. Any abuse of these drugs is a law enforcement problem, not a medical problem. The responsibility goes to the doctors to strictly monitor and support patients who are on these drugs, not just write out a prescription and abandon them.

- And while you're at it, please get a national health care plan. The problems of people in pain getting health care are part of this larger lack of care. Almost three in ten chronic pain patients have been unable to get a prescription filled because of cost or lack of insurance, according to the 2004 American Chronic Pain Association study. No one should have to cut pain pills in half to get by, as is a common practice.

To insurance companies:

- To adequately treat chronic pain, and ultimately save money, you should reimburse patients for things that actually *work* for them, to make life manageable, such as massage therapy, regular therapy, acupuncture, and an unlimited amount of a certain medication. A perennial example of insurance company myopia is episodic migraine sufferers' only being allotted a certain number of triptans per month. (I saw this with Melanie Watkins, a patient I interviewed, who cannot afford to pay the forty dollars for two very effective Relpax pills every time she has a migraine. As a result, the weekend before our interview, she was confined to bed.) In the end, as these people don't just curl up and die, you end up losing money by instead funding costly, useless tests and possibly harmful procedures, which they *can* get approved. To today's disabled population, who are mostly chronically ill, ongoing health care is a necessity.

To journalists:

- Here's the neat thing about a press release: You don't have to reprint it *exactly* as it is given to you. It's only what the pharmaceutical company *wants* you to write, about how good its new drug is. It is a suggestion, not at all mandatory. You can even go out and get your own sources, such as patients and doctors, whom the company did not preapprove and supply to you. And you're even allowed to write about health issues like pain on your own initiative, without the permission of a drug maker.

- Also recognize that if you interview an "expert" at a pain or headache clinic, he or she has a motivation to talk about how totally *treatable* pain is, as the person is involved in promoting a business. These people don't have much of a reason to talk about how much they do *not* know. And then, after the story runs, you don't have to totally forget about the issue. Later, you can even follow up on your own with any patients you've talked to. It's all very permissible.

- But this doesn't mean that, after lauding a drug as a savior, you should turn around and demonize it two years later, as you usually do, after the reality of the side effects becomes known through widespread patient use. Leave the "virgin/whore" coverage to other parts of the media like *Entertainment Tonight*.

This discussion of complexity in the world brings me to my next point:

To feminist academics and cultural critics:

- Your work has been very valuable in pointing out cultural and social factors that indeed contribute to chronic pain and depression. Yes, injustices that women face can certainly make these problems worse. And problems of poverty and racism can certainly also exacerbate pain, by denying valuable care and legitimacy to these patients. And yes, toxins in the environment probably don't make matters any better. The women's health movement has further taught valuable lessons in being vigilant about the invasive, harmful, and expensive medical interventions that capitalism often promotes over others. (An example is some doctors' extreme step in taking out women's ovaries as a migraine treatment, a procedure that has mostly made the pain worse in the end.)

- But that is only part of the picture. Today, after much success in prov-
ing women's strengths over the past forty years, it is finally time for you
to also recognize the natural "negative" or "weak" parts of women's bodies. We should talk about biology, as well as the environment, as shaping our neurology. After all, although we still have a way to go to prove
ourselves as equals, the coast is clearer. We are now in a relatively
stronger social and political position, not as much risking the loss of
ground if we admit weaknesses, like pain and fatigue, which do happen
more in women. This is a basic step toward being able to organize to
address physical impairments and then moving on. After all, women
with chronic headaches, as well as other types of invisible illnesses, are
crying out for recognition. I would *love* for chronic migraines and other
types of headaches to become more "medicalized" for some new-and-
improved pharmaceuticals to be made available for treatment.

  We reduce the risk of, once again, being condemned as "inferior" if
we emphasize the point that pain and weakness vary greatly among all
individuals, and gender by no means determines if a woman will have
pain and fatigue.

  After all, being able to realistically discuss women's complexities is a
sign of strength, not weakness. The principle that even though a woman
may have weaknesses she still deserves equal rights is not so radical now.

To society:

- Disabilities come in many shapes and forms, including those that are
invisible. As we now generally (with notable exceptions) accept that providing ramps and sign language interpreters for those with other disabilities is reasonable, we must also make accommodations for those with
pain and fatigue. Allowing for varying human paces in education and the
workplace is key. Some innovative programs now lead the way. One
teenage girl I interviewed, Allison, fourteen, with chronic daily headache
and comorbid anxiety, was very excited about starting at a new "therapeutic day school" in the Chicago suburb of Niles in the summer of
2003. (I had met her dad at a Chicago support group.) Before the
headaches had started the year before, when she was in eighth grade,
she was a straight-A student and basketball player. Now, after trying
about fifteen drugs that did not work, she has a chance to continue her
education, after having to drop out of high school in November of her
freshman year. This new school, which also admits teens with depression, gives more specialized attention to these students. It has a total of

about twenty-five students, with shorter hours (starting later in the morning), counselors on hand, and classes with a three-to-one student-teacher ratio. (Her old high school covers the tab for her attendance at this school, and it does not cost her family anything extra.)[3] Such a program innovatively recognizes that most people who are disabled are not *totally* disabled and can still participate and make valuable contributions to society. With accommodations for pace, most disabled people with chronic pain don't have to choose between the usually available extremes: totally dropping out of society, or having to constantly push themselves with extreme punishing pain to fit in at a "normal" pace.

- Also, although terms like *chronic daily headache* may sound silly and generic when you first hear them—like a marketing gimmick to sell more drugs—they are important. What they describe is real. Remember, not so long ago, words like *Ms.*, *sexual harassment*, and *depression* also sounded absurd.

To A-list celebrities:

- Step up to the plate. Face it. A disease is only real to society when a famous person gets it. But I'm talking top names, star power, here. Too bad that in the one organized PR campaign that I know of to folks like you to raise public awareness of chronic pain, the stars involved—while certainly notable—had all reached the height of their popularity decades ago. They are part of a traveling exhibit of inscribed black-and-white photos, "The Faces of Pain" (sponsored by Purdue Pharma), which I saw in the exhibit hall of the 2003 American Pain Society meeting. (By coincidence, the APS conference was held at the Hyatt Hotel in Chicago, right near my first notable episode with my pain, in a nearby bathroom.) The celebrity subjects included Corbin Bernsen from *LA Law* (knee pain), Bo Derek (back pain), and most interestingly, Lynda Carter, who played *Wonder Woman*. The copy near her photo recognized the irony: "If you're Wonder Woman, it's easy to battle the world's villains with a pair of solid gold bracelets and a few well placed kicks. But what do you do to fight pain? In 1999, America's favorite female superhero found herself suffering from chronic back pain. Even a golden lasso couldn't help her get an accurate and speedy diagnosis."
- Other celebrity spokesperson options, although seemingly more promising, have come up short. One of the most popular film characters of our day, Harry Potter, has migraines (as I am told, when his enemy

comes near); it's too bad that he is fictional. Some human sports stars have been widely reported to be bushwhacked by migraines, such as Kendall Gill of the Chicago Bulls and Terrell Davis formerly of the Denver Broncos. But they probably won't appeal to our mostly female demographic of headache sufferers. I did notice in the news in spring 2004 that fellow Chicagoan Jeff Tweedy, from the band Wilco, checked himself into rehab after a breakdown because of drug addiction that happened from treating recurrent migraines and anxiety.[4] But he may be limited to the hipster cohort, and most people wouldn't recognize him on the street. At about the same time, a better-known celebrity emerged specifically with chronic head pain, but that did little to generate sympathy for our cause. That was the widely satirized David Gest, who sued ex-wife Liza Minnelli for repeatedly hitting him on the head and triggering constant head pain. This is not to say that I don't sympathize with him. "Plaintiff currently takes 11 prescription medications per day, some more than once, to treat the pain and injury," reads his law brief, which sounds comical to others and yet is entirely plausible to me, especially if his neurology is predisposed to this condition.

To pharmaceutical companies:

- Please test your drugs adequately before giving them to us, and be upfront about the results, even negative ones.

- Also, please test the drugs for our actual specific problem, so that every drug we take is not "off-label," or originally approved for something entirely different. I'm counting on you to make a new antidepressant or anticonvulsant that will tame the hyperactive nerves now having a party in my brain (without making me into a blithering, obese, drug-addicted idiot in the process). Even if a drug gets rid of pain, I consider the treatment unsuccessful if I am not able to tie my own shoes while on it.

On the face of it, it might seem as if I'm asking for a lot. Why should all these factions of society mobilize all these resources and support for chronic pain patients?

Four reasons, again in bulleted form:

- The Right Thing: "This is a moral issue," said neurosurgeon Dr. John Loeser in his keynote speech to the American Pain Society in 2003, "for only a corrupt society ignores pain and suffering." In other words, basically, not doing so is . . . well, untenable.

- Suicide Prevention: This is the justification that advocates of depressed and bipolar people use to get their problem treated, so I might as well follow their lead. Like depressives, chronic pain patients are at a markedly higher risk of committing suicide. In a study of patients who attempted suicide, a majority (52 percent) had some kind of "somatic disease" or chronic pain problem. Other studies show that people with chronic pain syndromes, including migraine, chronic abdominal pain (some of my age cohort will think of rock singer Kurt Cobain, who killed himself in 1994), and orthopedic pain syndromes (rheumatoid arthritis, in which the immune system attacks the body) are more likely to think about suicide, attempt it, and go through with it. The depression and anxiety that typically come with chronic pain aren't only added annoyances; they interact with chronic pain to create suicide risks.[5]

- Money Saved: To be specific, the total cost in lost productivity from workers with chronic pain is estimated to be at least $61.2 billion a year.[6] And the cost to U.S. society alone for headaches is estimated at $13 billion a year in lost work.

- Pain Nipped in Bud: I'm really not sure if this is possible, that if you treat chronic pain early, in its beginning stages, you can halt its progression over time. But this is what some experts are saying now. This rationale uses the "disease" model of chronic pain, comparing it to something somewhat preventable, such as heart disease (which is genetic but can sometimes be managed, if not altogether avoided, through a healthier lifestyle).

The good news is that these are not just abstract motivations. In the past year, as an encouraging sign, I have been relieved to learn that medical science has just started to respond in the recognition and treatment of chronic daily headache. In the course of writing this book, I have seen medical knowledge of chronic daily headache, as well as chronic pain in general, grow (although it is still at its very beginning stages). (See sidebar.)

But doctors don't act alone, in a vacuum. Pushing medical science to get on the ball and better treat this disease is the tidal force: the market economy. In other words, the consumer. And boy, is she (and also very often, he) pissed.

In this area, I am specifically referring to a new generation of women, who account for a great number of chronic pain patients. Although the stereotype is that pain is limited to senior citizens, many pain syndromes, such as chronic headache and fibromyalgia, typically first appear in one's twenties. And at

Some Beginning Awareness of Chronic Daily Headache

More than a decade after the onset of my headache, I found that some very important (and legitimizing) epidemiological studies had recently been done in the late 1990s and beyond on chronic daily headache, which surprised doctors with their significant numbers.[7] As an official medical system response, in 2004 the International Headache Society published revised official classifications that defined the types of chronic daily headache in more detail than ever before. For example, it classified them according to duration (long or short) and known cause (such as medication rebound or injury).

The most common type of "long-duration" chronic daily headache (lasting more than four hours) was newly named, *chronic migraine* (formerly known by some as *transformed migraine*). This reference to "migraine" reveals some overlapping in categories, with types of CDH being classified as subtypes of other problems. In fact, the term *transformed migraine* also indicates the widespread theory that CDH is really a form of migraine, evolved (or devolved) into a worse state.

In 2004, the IHS guidelines also added two other primary long-duration forms of CDH, including *new persistent daily headache* (one that becomes constant very quickly, over three days at most, and either goes away immediately or persists) and the more-common-than-had-been-believed *hemicrania continua* (characterized by one-sided pain, which I sadly did not have, as it is diagnosable and fully treatable with the anti-inflammatory indomethacin).

an increasing level, these patients will demand validation and better treatment. They stand out as rejecting guilt-laden baggage—both from 1970s feminism, which denies women's "weaknesses," and from age-old sexist theories that women are *only* weak. As they have in other areas of life (such as jobs, sexuality, and relationships), these women are going to demand that some of the most basic ideals of the women's movement be realized, and that women be treated like *complex* humans, like everyone else.

As we are neither virgins nor whores, we are neither hysterics nor superwomen. After all, Wonder Woman was played by an actor, and even she has chronic pain.

Through the natural evolution of ideas over time, even the most politically minded feminist activists are articulating this basic principle. One young woman I interviewed, Nichole Wicks, a chronic daily headache sufferer, ironically had to leave her job as a women's health activist in New York City partly because of what she called a lack of tolerance at her organization for her ailment. She credits her college background in psychology with helping her understand that she has to take care of herself before she can capably serve others. "Trying to save the world, in your own particular way, is very important. But the world will not save you," she explained.

In my last two books, both on "younger women," I have learned much about them that gives me hope. Ironically, as I have studied them through the years as a general topic, they have emerged as a source of possible political change in my own life. A common theme in all this research has been that I am a part of a generation that has been raised with a greater-than-ever sense of entitlement to equal treatment and respect. We feel more open, and less ashamed, in discussing the traditionally "tough" and "embarrassing" issues related to chronic headaches, such as hormones, sexual side effects of drugs, depression, and anxiety. And this is not just attitude; it is supported by real power and status in society, as a result of more than thirty years of the women's health movement, increased access to jobs and education, and the information age. An emerging "pain rights" movement is also starting to exert an influence; for example, pain was declared "the fifth vital sign" in 2000, and relief is now being presented as a given "right" of patients.[8]

Neurologist Paula Mendes, who is my age exactly, told me in an interview that she has noticed a difference in patient demand for information, younger people seeing that as natural (and not being uppity). "I haven't been practicing very long, but from what I see, older patients don't ask a lot of questions," said Dr. Mendes. "I feel as if I'm trying to teach them things. But they're not really that interested. And they're kind of surprised sometimes when I start to tell them what this medication is for and what this is for, and their reaction is 'Just give me the prescription.' Younger patients, they are out there on the Internet. They want to understand what's going on."

This expectation is true across American society, not just in high-powered and high-maintenance urban professionals. Of the six women with chronic daily headache whom I met online and interviewed, all (at that point) were highly educated on the topic. In most cases, they knew more than their primary-care doctors and regular neurologists. They were educating themselves about treatments and neurology on a near-daily basis by participating in discussion groups and reading educational materials on web sites. Most came from working-class backgrounds, had a high school education, and were either on disability or currently applying for it.

But there is a catch. A fault, in my opinion, is that this generational sense of entitlement often does not come hand in hand with a greater political awareness, of a consciousness of the world beyond oneself and the possibilities of organized social change—such as in young women supporting feminism but not wanting to take an active stand for it.

Yet, sometimes, even when people are self-absorbed, this greater sense of entitlement—and naïveté about limits—can work wonders. I am indeed encouraged by the beginning trickle of young women "coming out" in the media for all sorts of invisible illnesses, as no one would have possibly dared in the past. Again, this reflects the sense of entitlement of gays and lesbians of our same generation coming out, not realizing that they are supposed to be deterred by the possibility of others not liking them and limiting their rights.

Some writers on "Third-Wave" feminism (following the baby boomers in the 1960s and 1970s) have noticed this trend, of young women going even further in many cases to challenge past confining roles. Writing in *In These Times*, thirty-something Silja Talvi observed that a purpose of this generation is to question past boundaries—those of traditional society *and* of feminism itself. "These are the women 'on the edge,'" she wrote, "pushing and pulling at the inner and outermost definitions of femininity, feminism, and womanhood. In doing so, they are rebelling not just against the dominant culture, but against a feminist culture that can be just as proscriptive in defining what is 'normal.' . . . Women grappling with their internal edges . . . including those women who are coping creatively with mental illnesses ranging from depression to bipolar disorders."

The most prominent example of a younger woman "coming out" with stigmatized illness, as of this writing, is of thirty-something author Laura Hillenbrand, who wrote the best-selling book *Seabiscuit*. In an award-winning 2003 *New Yorker* essay, she wrote about her struggle to be taken seriously by doctors who were treating her chronic fatigue syndrome. This essay had an immense impact on many people. After the essay was published, my friend Rivka, with chronic fatigue syndrome, told me how her life had changed as a direct result of it, with many people now apologizing to her for not taking her seriously earlier. The power of a broad public forum is boundless.

Such a "coming-out" story would not have been published in another generation. Until 1988, identifying oneself with chronic fatigue syndrome, before it was classified as a real illness, was like announcing you were crazy. Hillenbrand's success and obvious drive have dispelled stereotypes of chronic fatigue patients as being just lazy. She followed other significant writers of this generation in talking about other problems previously denigrated as moral weaknesses, in a genre I would call "sick lit," such as Elizabeth

Wurtzel's *Prozac Nation* (on depression), and Lizzie Simon's *Detour: My Bipolar Road Trip in 4-D.* Perhaps one of the most notable has been Susanna Kaysen's *The Camera My Mother Gave Me,* on vaginal pain, which certainly would not have been written about twenty years ago—without personal shame and without heavy metaphors about patriarchal sexual oppression.

While I was working on this book, I also saw the first spate of articles in the popular media devoted to chronic daily headache. They also raise my hope for further awareness. They also involved young women speaking out. In 2003, such articles appeared in two of the most legitimizing media: Oprah's *O Magazine* and the *New York Times.* Although neither included criticism of doctors and the lack of federal research into these problems, they represented a start. The *O* article was by a woman who has had a constant headache for twenty-four years. The *Times* story was mainly about chronic daily headache caused by medication overuse. Soon after its publication, the Associated Press sent out a widely published story on teenagers with CDH, who also did not feel ashamed of being quoted about this disease in public.[9]

The bottom line—at least as I see it through my own particular lens—is that this new generation of patients, along with those that follow, will more and more demand to be taken seriously. They will insist upon more funding for research, more media coverage, and more general respect. And I'm hoping that in the future they will see the connections between their invisible and socially belittled or misunderstood illnesses (whether they have chronic daily headache, bipolar disorder, chronic fatigue syndrome, or irritable bowel syndrome), and the illnesses of others, all a part of the same basic struggle. And that is the struggle to take women's health problems seriously, even those that may publicly portray us as less than superwomen.

Recently, I have read about one helpful new term that makes these political and medical connections among us, among the Tired Girls. One doctor I have read, Jay A. Goldstein, helpfully described these illnesses being "neurosomatic," a contrast with past descriptions of these primarily female disorders as "psychosomatic," or as being *caused* or propagated by mental or emotional problems. *Neurosomatic* means that all "somatic" (bodily) reactions can be rooted in similar neurology. Specifically, Goldstein, author of the 2004 book *Tuning the Brain,* defined them as "inappropriate handling of sensory and cognitive input of the brain," specifically of the emotion-driven limbic system of the brain. This emphasis on regular "input" validates these illnesses as not just caused by emotion or "stress," something one could avoid with proper attitude or effort.

But to be sure, younger generations of women will continue to demand more and more of a partnership with their doctors. This attitude contrasts with accepting, and even preferring, the paternalistic styles of the past, according to which a doctor just tells you what to do, and you like it. In the 1970s, women started to voice this principle in other, more obviously female, health areas, such as obstetrics and gynecology. And now, at last, neurology, which has been overwhelmingly dominated by male doctors practicing an "invisible" science, is facing such challenges.

Those women patients, aged fourteen to fifty-three, whom I interviewed for this book in the final stages of research would agree. These fourteen people considered having a partnership with their doctor not an ideal but a basic right. This attitude often contrasted with that of their mothers, some of whom shared the same condition. Lynne Schultz, a former veterinary technician from Nebraska, told me that her mother, who also suffered from depression, "didn't believe that there really was such a thing" as depression and migraine. "She kind of believes this is all kind of in your head, and you can just get up and make yourself feel better," she said.

In a similar vein, Melanie Watkins, a nurse from Tuscaloosa, Alabama, said that her attitude of accepting her disorder goes against the experience of her mother, the daughter of farmers. Like her, her mother has "ocular migraine," which involves severe vision impairment during an attack. Watkins said, "She can't deal with it because she doesn't acknowledge that she's ever sick. She doesn't 'give in' to stuff. And I can." Watkins explained that because of her medical education as a nurse and a strong "support system," including her husband, she doesn't see her ailment as a form of moral weakness.

As a result of what I view as their greater generational sense of entitlement, the great majority of the female chronic daily headache sufferers I interviewed reported dramatic clashes with doctors. They typically complained of those who did not recognize the medical realities of their pain, and/or took a paternalistic approach. But instead of just bearing with poor treatment and ultimately blaming themselves for their pain, they took some action. They were very likely to switch doctors or assert their needs, often with a positive result for better care. Here is a representative sample of such recent experiences of women I met online at the about.com online headache forum:

Lynne Schultz, forty, who now lives on disability payments, told me that she now sees an internist for her constant head pain, after giving up on many neurologists who did not listen to her. "I had one that put me on a medication, and the medication did work for my headaches," she recalled, referring to the new highly touted anticonvulsant Topamax (which I was too afraid to try while trying to be coherent in writing this book). "But I was having such terrible side effects with it that I had absolutely no quality of life. I couldn't speak. I couldn't get my words out. I couldn't function. And it was even to the point where I couldn't sweat. This was summer, and I mean I couldn't even go outside because I would just get really, really overheated. And I went to the doctor and I said, 'I'm having all these problems,' and his response was, 'Well, I got rid of your headaches, didn't I?'"

Tamara Davis, a forty-year-old former grocery store manager in Upstate New York, explained why she has learned to be assertive to get narcotics to treat her constant severe migraines, which became daily after a stroke at the age of thirty-three, from which she suffered traceable brain damage. In the years after that, she blindly accepted the poor treatments that her neurologist prescribed for several years, including a high dose of Depakote that did not work (and made her gain a hundred pounds and lose hair) and constant doses of anti-inflammatories (like Advil) that harmed her stomach. "He thought that the prophylactic medicine should take care of it, but it did not," she explained. "And he was more worried about rebound headaches, yet I had headaches every day anyway, so what's a rebound headache?" Finally, after joining the online support group, she saw another doctor, who prescribed her Oxycontin, which she takes every eight hours to keep it in her bloodstream. It has decreased her pain from a 7 (on a scale of 1 to 10) to a 4, making life more bearable. "It has literally saved my life," she said, adding that she has few, if any, side effects, and certainly no high from this "long-acting" medication (which enters the system gradually and creates no sense of euphoria, which the Puritans reading this may fear).

Davis said, "What I have learned is that I should not feel guilty about controlling my pain. If it means taking narcotics, I will take narcotics. Whatever I have to do to take care of my pain, I will do. And I will not let myself feel guilty about it, I will not let people make me feel guilty about it, and I will not allow people to treat me like a drug addict. I have a very real, valid reason to take narcotics, and I am not an abuser. I am a person who is in chronic and intractable pain. And anyone who chooses to criticize me—let them have a migraine. Let them have a migraine every single day of their lives. And I will no longer accept substandard treatment from doctors. I've learned through personal experience that you'll get what you'll tolerate, and if you'll tolerate substandard treatment, you'll get it."

Rachel Benedict, thirty-one, a Dallas mother, stopped seeing a pain specialist after doubting his treatment: "So finally, last time I went in to him and said, 'We need to try something else.' And he said, 'No, what we're trying is fine.' And I said, 'Well, why are my headaches not any better then?' And he said, 'Well, because you don't have enough faith in God.'"

But even the fundamentalist Christians interviewed (who were numerous on this site) did not fare any better with doctors. Relating a similar story was Amber, twenty-one, of Dayton, Ohio, who formerly worked for the National Right to Life Committee in Washington, D.C., as an administrative assistant. She suffers with moderate chronic daily headache, which came on gradually after a few concussions she had as a teen (one in a car accident and another at a church-group field trip to a carnival). Like many CDH patients, she also has almost daily episodes of migraines, which became a fixture in her life after another recent head injury (a slip on the ice). After seeing five local neurologists, she recently made an expensive trek to a prestigious clinic, where a neurologist prescribed her a triptan, despite her telling him of a blood disorder. "Since the triptans work by constricting the blood vessels, I can't take them. But he really didn't listen to me when I told him that." The result: "I took one, and it was giving me horrible, horrible heart pain and making me feel really sick, so I ended up making myself throw up. I was afraid to keep the drug in my stomach." She does plan to go back and see a different neurologist at that clinic eventually, but for now she is sticking to her family doctor, "the only one I feel that I've gotten any respect from. Every time I go to a neurologist, it's like they don't want to entertain the thought that I know anything about my condition."

Another religious woman, already quoted, Melanie Watkins, has learned to be very proactive with her current headache specialist. She decided to leave her last one, who was "older than dirt" and from the generation believing "I'm the doctor, and that's good enough. I say you don't need another explanation." Watkins, who has a bachelor's degree in nursing along with a new law degree, explained, "I'm not used to doctors just saying flat out that's how it's going to be. I'm used to doctors asking my opinions on stuff, and I just couldn't deal with his attitude anymore. I mean I can't stand being talked down to and condescended to. Then I found a doctor who would talk to me, and here is what he told me on the first day: 'I don't tell you what to do. I don't dictate what we do. We're partners in this because it's your body.'"

But probably the most dramatic case of a clash in values was that of Mary, twenty-six (who does not want her real name used), whom I met at the waiting room at a Michigan headache clinic (where I was a patient) in the fall of 2003. She told me in detail how she had finally become tired of blindly doing what doctors told her after three years of constant severe head pain. Two years before, she had dropped out of college to be hospitalized for eight months at the Chicago Headache Clinic, where she had (unsuccessfully) tried seventy-five different medications. Later, like Tamara Davis, she resorted to taking narcotics from her family doctor to get by. Then she went to a second headache clinic, in Michigan, where she was hospitalized again.

There, she learned to take a stand to defend her mother. Her new doctor had become angry with the mother when Mary refused to get a lumbar puncture (spinal tap). He had wrongly assumed that Mary was blindly following her mother's advice and so ordered Mary's mother to leave the hospital, where she was staying. Afterward, Mary felt unfairly judged at a therapy session. "This counselor said to me, 'Why are you so close to your mother?' I said, 'Ma'am, my mother has been my caregiver for the past year.' And she said, 'I don't understand why your mother is your caregiver.' I said, 'Ma'am, I am on five different narcotics. I cannot drive half the time, I don't know where I'm at half the time, and I need somebody to take care of me.' The therapist literally said that it was crazy that my mother had to take care of me. She said, 'You're twenty-five years old.' I said, 'I don't care if I'm twenty-five years old. I'm on five different narcotics.'" Later, another counselor intervened and asked Mary how she wanted to proceed. "And I said, 'I want every doctor and every nurse, every counselor and every physician assistant to respect my mother—is what I want.' And I tell you what, Paula, it was a 180, and it changed, because I was ready to walk out the door."[10]

I hope that change can also be possible not only because of a new generation of demanding women patients, but because of a new generation of female (and male) doctors. I only now realize that, during the almost fifteen years of my life that I have had this problem, women my age have entered the field of neurology in new numbers and have begun practicing. Although I do not want to be simplistic and say that a young woman will always have a less paternalistic point of view than an older man (or a younger man), anecdotal evidence has shown that gender and age variables may be at least two important factors. Also, it may contribute to empathy that women neurologists are much more likely to be migraine sufferers themselves (migraine is reported by a whopping 74 percent of female neurologists, compared to 44 percent of male neurologists).[11]

In 2003, I had the pleasure of meeting two female neurologists in their mid-thirties, both practicing nearby in the Chicago suburbs, who had made this journey to practice medicine. Both were friends of a friend. Talking to them was startling at times, as I have associated neurology with much older males, not with people who look and sound like peers. Each of these women,

Dr. Megan Shanks and Dr. Paula Mendes, independently told me about their philosophies of making the patient "a partner" and educating her or him. They agreed that this partnership is especially vital in the treatment of chronic pain, because everyone responds differently to the same treatments, and because diagnoses are made almost purely as a result of personal communication, not laboratory tests.

"Some patients want a more parental, you know, 'take-care-of-me' type of approach. And I'm willing to do that," said Dr. Shanks, who is from Australia and attended Rush Medical College. "But I'm happiest in a partnership with a patient. I educate patients up to as much as they want to know, sometimes more, about their illness so that they understand it. And that's particularly important in headache because there are so many things you do in your day that can affect your headache, that can have an impact."

Sometimes this figuring out of pain patterns for episodic migraine patients can take several conversations. Dr. Shanks mentioned a patient who told her, "When I don't eat a bagel, I get a headache." Finally, through ongoing dialogue, Dr. Shanks realized that when the patient does not eat a bagel, she eats French toast with cinnamon. "And when that patient eats Altoids with cinnamon, she also gets a migraine," the doctor said. "And she said, 'But that can't be it. Because I looked it up, and cinnamon isn't something that causes migraines.' I said, 'Well that's because you're not on the list. But it does trigger migraines in you.' So sometimes it's just basic stuff, you know, that can do it. And just that kind of pointing out to people, 'This isn't in your head; this really is something that happens—people find it really, really helpful. For me to understand their headaches helps them a lot."

In their quest for communication and better treatment, both young women neurologists interviewed also expressed relative comfort in asking patients about related issues that may have been considered "too private" in the past. An example is discussing the possible impairment of sexual functioning from antidepressant use (which no doctor has ever brought up with me), even in women patients. Dr. Paula Mendes, who had studied at the Mayo Clinic, said that she is open to her patients also talking about past abuse or marital troubles, which may affect their overall stress levels and thus their pain. This partnership also includes being open to alternative medicine, which is what these two doctors were brought up with in medical school. Dr. Mendes even had a rotation in acupuncture during her residency, to make alternative medicine truly "complementary" (instead of adversarial) to her practice.

Twenty-five years ago, when I wrote my first comprehensive report about pain in America, I learned a lot of useful information. As I wrote on page 13 of the conclusion of my sixth-grade report, "If anybody I know when I get older is struck with chronic pain, then I could advise them on what alternatives are available, or if I am struck with pain, I'll know that there are ways to help me."

Today, I hope to retain my natural optimism about the future, despite being infinitely more acquainted with the immense challenges of treating and living with chronic pain. I well know that maintaining optimism will not be easy. I have to face the fact that, as it does for many of us, the Headache may get worse—probably because it already has recently, once again.

One night in the beginning of 2003, my life was again jolted by a simple slapsticklike scene, something you would expect from a Three Stooges short, just before the thing with the two fingers in the eyes and just after the buzz saw to the head. It happened as I walked into my apartment and pulled the string of the overhead light to turn it on. At once, the heavy glass globe light fixture, big enough to house a large salad, fell to bump me on the head and then shatter across the floor. I had replaced it a month earlier and apparently hadn't adequately tightened the two screws holding it in place, and the string had loosened the screws every time I had pulled it. As much as I had resisted this possibility for years, now I had to face the fact that I had literally been waylaid by a few loose screws.

I wasn't upset about the added head pain resulting from that incident that night, but I became depressed about the element of it that still has never gone away. To this day, more than a year later, my head feels as if that accident had just happened. Now, more than a year later, my overall level of pain is about double what it was before January 2003, with the top of my head burning almost constantly, to different degrees, joining the stabbing behind both eyes and temples.

And adding to the confusion, some of the old schemes and signposts of understanding the Headache, which I had cobbled together through the years from both superstition and science, now don't often work anymore. The Headache has taken a new form, newly immune to logic. Last week, I woke up every day feeling this added pain and heaviness, blaming it on what I assumed was a rainy day outside, as I had cannily in the past. However, after I opened the thick shades, I saw only pure, clear sunlight streaming in. Now, I could no longer use the weather as a sign of especially severe pain. Now, the pain didn't have any such "reasonable" explanation.

Again, I involuntarily revisited Elisabeth Kübler-Ross's stages to cope with a new reality. Denial and isolation, anger, depression, acceptance, and hope. They continued to repeat themselves over the months with new intensity. During these times, even more than normally, taking my own advice of acceptance and proper pain management, imparted in the previous chapter, was very difficult. At times while working on this book, I tried as hard as I could to remember inspiring passages in the chronic pain meditation book *Living with It Daily* about what spirituality had to offer me, but I came up blank. To be honest, I didn't care at all what wisdom Louisa May Alcott and Helen Keller had to say. I tried to remember that one Buddhist quote from long ago: "There is no way to enlightenment . . . Hmm. How did it go?" The depression, now overtaking the effect of the 20 mg of Prozac, just blocked all such coping thoughts.

And many of the people who had helped me in the past were no longer available. I thought a few times of talking to my neighbor, Carol, and then I remembered that she was now gone.

Her front door was now plain, like the others in our building, without the mezuzah on her doorpost. I realized that the only trace of her ever being there were little hot-pink wildflowers that grew in a horseshoe pattern in the sidewalk cracks surrounding her third-floor back porch, which had formerly housed a formidable garden.

I could now only hope that she had found happiness and peace in a better place: Florida, where she had retired in 2003.

Before she had left, I remember her wanting to help me but feeling frustrated. "I always thought that when people were ready to leave pain," she had said, "they would be able to leave it. This just doesn't make any sense."

Actually, this freak accident with the light fixture has had one positive use. It did corroborate the current neurological model of chronic daily headache: The nerves do become more and more sensitive over time and then dysfunctionally carve out new neural pathways for pain that the brain begins to recognize as normal. It's like someone walking through a field and tramping down a new path, which then gets more and more established the more it is traveled. Now I have one more path up there in my head, and unfortunately, no one knows how to reverse it.

Furthermore, this new neurological trail forged across the top of my head also illustrates that chronic pain can be a progressive disease. I got the Headache first behind the left eye, and then behind both eyes, and now also on the top of the head.

Unfortunately, and I have learned the hard way (as I usually end up learning everything), real life is not like the cartoons or soap operas, where when someone gets hit on the head, a brain problem is corrected (some people have jokingly suggested this to me through the years as a headache cure). True, I did read that first lady Mary Lincoln had her terrible headaches cured for the rest of her life after a horse-drawn buggy accident in 1863, but I assume that story is apocryphal.

Like all other chronic pain patients, with or without such neurological knowledge, I worry a lot about the future, about my vulnerability. The pain got worse so easily, after one simple accident, so why won't it happen again? Will I end up in life like the triumphant and enviable Ortho Tri-Cyclen pixie woman, or more like defeated Charlie at the end of *Flowers for Algernon* stupidly and superstitiously clutching his rabbit's foot? What happens if some nimrod bonks me on the head, and then I won't be able even to write anymore? Will I end my days as a drug addict—and even worse, as a drug addict still in pain? If I became totally incapacitated and even able to get disability, would I be able to live on $585 a month (the amount I would now receive from the state of Illinois)? Would I have to stop my six channels of HBO, not to mention STARZ and ENCORE? Does Whole Foods accept food stamps for its eight-dollar chipotle chicken breast with a tamarind glaze?

I can only hope that some day, in my lifetime, coming to my rescue will be my real higher power: Big Pharma. Perhaps, bolstered by wider academic research, it will find an answer, even a partial one, in a test tube, and I will find a doctor compassionate and patient enough to lead me through its dispensation.

With this hope in mind, I continue to stand by the final line of my 1979 report conclusion, which is now eerily relevant to my life: "I would also like to know if scientists ever make a nonaddictive endorphin drug."

One of my greatest hopes is indeed that Big Pharma will do for chronic daily headache what it has done for many of those with depression (with Prozac and other SSRIs) or episodic migraines (with Imitrex and other triptans). But I still know not to expect wonders. I now know and recognize that progress in medicine is usually made slowly, in small increments; any improved drug I may be fortunate enough to try will probably give me a degree of relief, not a total cure. I'm now aware, and wary, of rampant overpromising by both the pharmaceutical industry and doctors—as well as the seemingly more "progressive" mind-over-matter folks. Armed with this new realistic attitude, I still have no choice but to continue my journey, with the continuing guidance of handfuls of newspaper clippings, random advice from those I meet at parties, and my own "healthy witness."

Meanwhile, as another constant, I also continue to find absolutely no meaning in the pain itself. (I find the Headache to be as profound as a malfunctioning car alarm that just won't shut off, which is probably the best metaphor I've heard for chronic pain.)[12] Instead, I'm striving to follow my more natural instincts to find meaning in life beyond the pain. I'm talking about meaning that is more piercing, more pulsating, more blazing, and more bracing than any headache.

In this daily struggle, one added comfort will be that I am not alone with all these fears—and these hopes. Most of the Tired Girls, those fellow "neurosomatics" whom I have met along the way, would agree that no matter how bad the storms of doubt (and guilt and shock and anger and denial) become this thing of hope always follows. It somehow just shows up, however briefly at times, making every weight, and every wait, easier to bear.

NOTES

○ ○ ○ ○ ○ ○ ○ ○ ○

Chapter One

1. This is a common experience of those with chronic migraines, with 71 percent of respondents to an online survey of the National Headache Foundation reporting that they visit the ER as many as three times in the course of a year. *NHF Head Lines*, March–April 2004, p. 11.

2. Actually, antidepressants are used for many other types of pain conditions, including postherpetic neuralgia (pain after shingles), diabetic neuropathy (nerve damage), pain following a stroke (rooted in the central nervous system), fibromyalgia, vulvodynia, irritable bowel syndrome, and rheumatoid arthritis.

3. See Levin 2004; Manzoni and Torelli 2003.

4. See Silberstein, Lipton, and Goadsby 2002, p. 6.

5. Hofmann 1979, p. 15.

6. Information from Bove 1970; Edmeads 1991; Rapoport and Edmeads 2000; Sacks 1992, 239–248; Young and Silberstein 2004, p. 100.

7. I have made a decision to change all names of doctors in this book partly for reasons of consistency. I don't want to give the actual names of some and not of others. I also view individual doctors criticized here as not unique in their behavior. They represent attitudes endemic in the medical system—and headache treatment—as a whole (although some institutions like the "Chicago Headache Clinic" exercise more power and influence than others, especially with nonstop uncritical media coverage). However, in journalistic fashion, I have stayed true to the facts when reporting about my experiences with doctors.

Chapter Two

1. Rist 2000.

2. Nardil specifically is the MAOI of choice for headaches. It is the only one highlighted in the U.S. Headache Consortium Guidelines, despite, as with the other off-label chronic-headache preventives, an "absence of relevant randomized placebo-controlled trials," reports the October 2003 newsletter of the National Headache

Foundation, p. 12. For a more detailed history of antidepressants, see Solomon 2001, p. 331.

3. Lampl et al. 2003, p. 878.

Chapter Three

1. Migraine is an additional risk factor for stroke, with the greatest risk for those over thirty-five and with migraine with aura. See Tietjen and Brey 2004, pp. 136–137.

2. Corman, Leung, and Guberman 1997, pp. 240–244.

3. National Migraine Association 1999.

Chapter Four

1. Prince et al. 2004. Also see Mire 2003.

2. Jamison, Anderson, and Slater 1995.

3. Nielsen 1994, November 13 entry.

4. I made this up, but her real name was even more old-school-marmish.

5. Scher, Lipton, and Stewart 2002. Also see Stewart et al. 2003, p. 2449.

6. See Silberstein, Lipton, and Goadsby 2002, p. 24.

Chapter Six

1. See Goldstein 2001; Evans and Pascual 2000.

2. See Ambler et al. 2001. Note: The survey also reported that 85 percent were taking drugs "that might enhance interest in sex."

3. See example of mention by Goldstein 2001.

4. For a critique, see Schlesinger 1996.

5. See Stewart et al. 1992.

6. Cited in Showalter 1985, p. 144.

Chapter Seven

1. See "How Is Your Doctor Treating You?" *Consumer Reports* 1995, p. 82.

2. See Hoffman and Tarzian 2001.

3. Welch, Aurora, and Gelman 2001. Reported by Jauhar 2003.

4. Srikiatkhachorn 2002.

Chapter Eight

1. For analysis, see Kryst 1996, p. 249.

2. Quoted in Penzien 1998.

3. Showalter 1985, p. 28.

4. Weir Mitchell 1887, p. 126.

5. For a more complete history, see Meldrum 2003.

6. Quoted in Kiester 1987, p. 182.

Chapter Nine

1. According to the April 2004 "Americans Living with Pain Survey" (ALPS), sponsored by the American Chronic Pain Association.

2. See Fontanarosa 2000, p. 11.

3. Marchand 2003.

4. Marchand and Arsenault 2002b.

5. Marchand et al. 1993.

6. Marchand and Arsenault 2002a.

7. See Elias 2004, describing a presentation to be made at the 2004 American Psychosomatic Society meeting in Orlando.

8. See Vickers et al. 2004.

9. Actually, the wisdom that Dr. Chung imparted went beyond Chinese medicine. Much of the advice about discipline, exercise, and balance has been commonsense knowledge for migraine sufferers through the ages and promoted by all types of doctors. In fact, Aretaeus, writing in the second century, advised, "Promenades long, straight, without tortuousities, in a well-ventilated place, under trees of myrtle and laurel. . . . It is a good thing to take journeys. . . . Exercises should be sharper, so as to induce sweat and heat. . . . Cultivate a keen temper, without irascibility." Quoted in Sacks 1970, p. 232.

10. Fontanarosa 2000, p. 10.

11. Quoted in Edmeads 1991, p. 7.

Chapter Twelve

1. See Haspel 2004.

2. See Bigal et al. 2002.

3. See Low and Merikangas 2003.

4. Now out of business.

Chapter Thirteen

1. See Peres et al. 2002, quoting Spierings and van Hoof, 1997.

2. See Peres, "Fibromyalgia is Common in Patients with Transformed Migraine," 2001.

3. Kenney 2003.

4. Marcus 2002, p. 22.

5. Robinson, Riley, and Myers 2000, quoted in Fillingim 2000, p. 41.

6. Statistics about nonmigraine disorders are from a presentation by Dr. Roger Fillingim of the University of Florida, "Sex, Gender and Pain: Clinical and Experimental Findings," at the 2003 meeting of the American Pain Society. He compiled this data from several sources, including Crombie et al. 1999 and Merskey and Bogduk 1994. Also see Unruh 1996 for more detail.

7. See Faucett 1997.

8. Hoffman and Tarzian 2001, p. 16.

9. See Pringsheim and Gooeren 2004.

10. Marcus 2002, p. 20.

11. Bigal, Lipton, and Stewart, 2004, p. 100.

12. Loder and Marcus 2003, p. 2.

13. Fillingim and Maixner 1995.

14. See Robbins 1994.

15. See Robinson et al. 2000 and Tietjen 2004 for recent studies.

16. See Silberstein, Lipton, and Goadsby 2002, p. 137.

Chapter Fourteen

1. Marchand and Arsenault 2002a.

2. Stamets 2002.

3. The first article in a mainstream medical journal to critique naturopathic medicine is Atwood 2003.

4. Sacks 1970, p. 305, quoting *De Anima Brutorum*.

5. I cribbed this joke partially from a story in *The Onion*.

6. Morris quotes from Price's 1994 novel that recounts his battle with spinal cancer, and the resulting pain from surgery to remove an "eel-sized" tumor from his spinal cord. Of course, in relating Price's story, Morris was just quoting accurately from his memoir. But the way this story of "mind over matter" is presented, as a definitive medical case study, is misleading. Also, on its own, it may be harmless, but then it also joins countless other anecdotal stories without long-term follow-up circulating in the media that overall portray a picture that everyone (but you) is transcending pain for good with his or her mind.

Chapter Fifteen

1. Perrin 1998, p. 414.

Chapter Sixteen

1. Silberstein, Lipton, and Goadsby 2002.

2. Gobel, Isler and Hasenfraz 1995, Silberstein, Lipton, and Goadsby 2002.

3. Sacks 1992, pp. 299, 301.

4. Report by Eric Eross of the Mayo Clinic in Scottsdale, Arizona, presented at the 2004 Forty-sixth Annual Scientific Meeting of the American Headache Society.

5. Robbins 2000, p. 7.)

6. Conis 2003.

7. Colino 2004.

8. Of course, I should state here that sometimes, in some people, these problems, and not genetic neurological defects, actually are at the root of the headache.

9. For a rare realistic view of surgery used to treat pain, specifically back pain, see Kolata 2004.

10. I did not attend his particular session but did have a tape of it transcribed for study.

11. Willis 1685, p. 380.

12. Meldrum 2003, p. 2472.

13. An example is the recent coverage of supraorbital nerve stimulation (SOS), in which electrodes are implanted in the patient's head. When stimulated, they are thought to operate as a kind of gate that blocks pain signals from reaching the brain, or that activates pain-relieving endorphins. In a March 9, 2004, story about new pain options, the *Chicago Tribune* profiled a Milwaukee woman who had allegedly been cured by the surgery at Northwestern Memorial Hospital's pain management clinic. But the article said nothing about side effects or about people for whom the surgery may have been useless. A similar feature about this process, on the local Chicago ABC-WLS TV newscast on January 23, 2003, portrayed another successful case with a similar surgery at another medical center.

Chapter Seventeen

1. Rapoport and Edmeads 2000; Silberstein, Stiles, et al. 2000; Edmeads 1991; Kiester 1987.

2. Dallek 2002, p. 50.

Chapter Eighteen

1. Gray et al. 1999, p. 41.

2. Boyles 2004.

3. Adams and Young 2003.

4. American Chronic Pain Association 2003, pp. 6–7.

5. He cited Safer 2002.

6. In a landmark case, Pfizer, the maker of Neurontin, was fined $430 million on May 13, 2004 for marketing the drug for unapproved uses. These include for pain, headaches, bipolar disorder and other psychiatric illnesses. On December 13, 2003, the *New York Times* reported that federal officials had subpoenaed Johnson & Johnson, the makers of Topamax, approved for treating epilepsy in 1996, for documents on the sales and marketing of their drugs. According to a September 22, 2003 *Los Angeles Times* report, "The Food and Drug Administration repeatedly has chastised Allergan for advertisements that it says suggest the drug Botox is effective for unapproved uses and has criticized the company for minimizing the drug's side effects." See Piccalo 2003.

7. Piccalo 2003.

Chapter Nineteen

1. Ehrenreich and English 1978, p. 281; Hoffmann and Tarzian 2001, p. 17.

2. Metzl 2003, p. 147.

3. Chino and Davis 2000, p. 150.

4. Kot 2004.

Chapter Twenty

1. Actually, this possibility is not as remote as I thought. More recently, I met another former patient of the "Chicago Headache Clinic" whose doctor there had prescribed her Viagra after antidepressants taken for headache control had squelched her ability to have an orgasm. The Viagra didn't work.

Chapter Twenty-One

1. Oliver 2002.
2. See Welch, Michael, and Goadsby 2002.
3. Isler 1986.
4. In a summary in the May 2003 issue of the journal *Headache*, Dr. Lawrence Robbins described the lack of proven *long-term* effectiveness of many standard preventives in 646 "moderate or severe chronic daily headache" patients: "Only 46 percent of patients obtained long-term relief from preventive medications. . . . This study suggests that over the long term many patients do discontinue the daily preventatives; short-term studies may overestimate the value of the current preventive medications" (573). The medications studied were antidepressants, both the newer SSRIs (such as Prozac) and the older tricyclics (such as Elavil), Depakote (antiepileptic), and beta blockers (hypertensives).
5. In a 1999 report for the federal government, Rebecca N. Gray and her colleagues at Duke University comprehensively reveal these gaps in drugs tested for migraine prevention in particular. In fact, although many types of antidepressants are widely used for headache prevention, the one antidepressant that the group found with "reasonably consistent evidence supporting the efficacy" for this purpose, amitriptyline (Elavil), had been the subject of only three placebo-controlled studies. The calcium blocker verapamil (brand names: Calan, Isoptin, Verelan), also widely used for this purpose, was the subject of only two convincing small placebo-controlled studies, with high dropout rates. "Our best estimate of the efficacy of this agent therefore carries substantial uncertainty," wrote the authors (7). Of these studies of verapamil, the largest placebo-controlled trial included thirty participants.

"Several specific agents have been shown to be efficacious for the prevention of migraine; however, there are few data to guide the choice among agents, and poor tolerability and lack of availability in the US limit the usefulness of many of the drugs reviewed," these authors stated in the report (1).

Typically, only a small number of placebo-controlled studies with relatively small sample groups, often of fewer than a hundred patients, exist for each off-label drug use for migraine control. This standard of being "placebo-controlled" means that a drug is shown not just to act as a placebo, which actually has the well-known effectiveness rate of 30 percent. And a known flaw in studies for headache prevention is that subjects often do not have what qualifies as chronic daily headache, but instead have the less common episodic migraine. See Matchar, McCrory, and Gray 2000.

Chapter Twenty-Two

1. This odd reasoning, that a patient automatically forfeits her right to have her pain treated if she has mental problems, goes way back. It also oddly continues right to the present. I was alarmed to read the following explanation of the pain of psychiatric patients in Dr. Frank Vertosick's highly regarded 2000 book *Why We Hurt*: "Their pain derives from their faulty interface with the outside world and that includes a distorted perception of their own bodies. It's a psychological pain, almost a kind of metaphysical pain, that does not answer to real-world entities like morphine or aspirin. The solution to this type of pain lies in the realm of psychiatry, not pain medicine" (232).

2. Max 2003.

3. Related to this concept, but on a higher educational level, is the Chronic Illness Initiative established at DePaul University's School for New Learning (designed for returning students) in Chicago. This allows such people to get college degrees, at their own pace, with fewer requirements to be on campus, flexible time requirements (a greatly reduced schedule), and assistance with a special advisor.

4. Kot 2004.

5. Clark, www.hopkins-arthritis.som.jhmi.edu/mngmnt/depression.html.

6. Stewart et al. 2003.

7. See Levin 2004, quoting Scher 1998, Castillo 1999, and Lu 2001. Scher, Castillo.

8. By the Joint Commission on Accreditation of Healthcare Organizations; see http://www.jcaho.org.

9. Ruppert 2003; Jauhar 2003; Irvine 2003.

10. Later she went back to Michigan to have an experimental pulsed radiofrequency procedure, that is, having nerves in her head cauterized, which actually helped about 40 percent, despite causing increased neck pain. She is now waiting for FDA approval of a microchip implant to block pain signals to the brain.

11. Reported at the Forty-sixth Annual Scientific Meeting of the American Headache Society in 2004, by Dr. Jonathan Gladstone of the Mayo Clinic branch in Scottsdale, Arizona.

12. I use this description with the caveat that we should all take any metaphor used for a disease with a grain of salt, as metaphors can limit our perception of the real complexities involved.

BIBLIOGRAPHY

o o o o o o o o o

Adams, Chris, and Alison Young. "Drug-Makers' Promotions Boost Off-Label Use by Doctors," *Miami Herald*, November 3, 2003.

Ambler, Nicholas, et al. "Sexual Difficulties of Chronic Pain Patients," *Clinical Journal of Pain* 17, no. 2 (June 2001): 138–145.

American Chronic Pain Association. *Medications and Chronic Pain: Supplement 2003*. Rocklin, Calif. See http:www.theacpa.org.

"Americans Living with Pain Survey," conducted by Roper Public Affairs and Media, on behalf of the American Chronic Pain Association, April 2004. See http://www.theacpa.org.

Armstrong, Karen. "The Loneliness of the Intellectual Woman," *New Statesman*, June 5, 2000.

Ashton, C. Heather. *Benzodiazepines: How They Work and How to Withdraw: Medical Research Information from a Benzodiazepine Withdrawal Clinic*, rev. August 2002 (booklet prepared by author). Order at http://www.benzo.org.uk/manual/index.htm.

Atwood, I. V., and C. Kimball. "Naturopathy: A Critical Appraisal," *Medscape General Medicine* 5, no. 4, posted December 30, 2003, at http://www.medscape.com.

Aurora, Sheena K. "Imaging Chronic Daily Headache," *Current Pain and Headache Reports* 7 (2001): 209–211.

Beinfield, Harriet, and Efrem Korngold. *Between Heaven and Earth: A Guide to Chinese Medicine*. New York: Ballantine, 1991.

Bernardi, Andria. "Half-Cranium," *River Oak Review* (Oak Park, Ill.), Spring-Summer 2003, 67–75.

Bigal, M. E., et al. "Chronic Daily Headache: Identification of Factors Associated with Induction and Transformation," *Headache* 42, no. 7 (July-August 2002): 575–581.

Bigal, Marcelo E., et al. "Chronic Daily Headache: Correlation Between the 2004 and the 1988 International Headache Society Diagnostic Criteria," *Headache* 44, no. 7 (2004): 684–691.

Bigal, M., R. Lipton, and W. Stewart. "The Epidemiology and Impact of Migraine," *Curr. Neurol. Neurosci. Rep.* 4, no. 2 (March 2004): 98–104.

Bove, F. J. *The Story of Ergot*. New York: Karger, 1970.

Boyles, Salynn. "Epilepsy Drug May Reduce Daily Headaches: But Experts Say

Neurontin Is Not a Top Choice," Web-MD, January 6, 2004. http://www.webmd.com.

Breiling, Brian. *Light Years Ahead*. Berkeley, Calif.: Celestial Arts, 1996.

Breuer, Joseph, and Sigmund Freud. *Studies in Hysteria*, 1895. Reprinted with authorized translation and introduction by A. A. Brill. New York: Coolidge Foundation, 1937.

Buchholz, David. *Heal Your Headache: The 1–2–3 Program*. New York: Workman, 2002.

Burns, Bill, Cathy Busby, and Kim Sawchuk, eds. *When Pain Strikes*. Minneapolis: University of Minnesota Press, 1999.

Burstein, R., M. F. Cutrer, and D. Yarnitsky. "The Development of Cutaneous Allodynia During a Migraine Attack: Clinical Evidence for the Sequential Recruitment of Spinal and Supraspinal Nociceptive Neurons in Migraine," *Brain* 123, pt. 8 (2000): 1703–1709.

Carroll, Lewis. *Alice's Adventures in Wonderland* [1865] and *Through the Looking-Glass* [1872]. Edited with an introduction and notes by Hugh Haughton. New York: Penguin Classics, 1998.

Chesler, Phyllis. *Women and Madness*. New York: Doubleday, 1972.

Chino, Alan F., and Corrine D. Davis. *Validate Your Pain! Exposing the Chronic Pain Cover-Up*. Sanford, Fla.: Health Access Press, 2000.

Clark, Michael. "Chronic Pain, Depression and Antidepressants: Issues and Relationships," accessed August 28, 2004, at http://www.hopkins-arthritis.som.jhmi.edu/mngmnt/depression.html.

Cleveland, Martha. *Chronic Illness and the Twelve Steps: A Practical Approach to Spiritual Resilience*. Center City, Minn.: Hazelden, 1988.

Colino, Stacey. "Why You've Got That Headache," *Redbook*, February 2004, pp. 46, 48, 54.

Conis, Elena. "That Raging Headache May Be Anger-Based," *Los Angeles Times*, July 14, 2003.

Corman C. L., N. M. Leung, and A. H. Guberman. "Weight Gain in Epileptic Patients During Treatment with Valproic Acid: A Retrospective Study." *Can. J. Neurol. Sci.* 24, no. 3 (August 1997): 240–244.

Couch, J., and C. Bearss. "Relief of Migraine with Sexual Intercourse" [abstract], *Headache* 30 (1990): 302.

Cousins, Norman. *Anatomy of an Illness: As Perceived by the Patient*. New York: W. W. Norton, 1979.

Cowan, Penney. *From Patient to Person: First Steps: A Workbook for People with Chronic Pain*. Rocklin, Calif.: American Chronic Pain Association, 2000.

Crombie, I. K., et al., eds. *Epidemiology of Pain*. Seattle: IASP Press, 1999.

Crook, Joan. "Women with Chronic Pain." In *Chronic Pain: Psychosocial Factors in Rehabilitation*, edited by R. Roy and E. Tunks. Baltimore: Williams & Wilkins, 1982.

Dallek, Robert. "The Medical Ordeals of JFK," *Atlantic Monthly*, December 2002, pp. 49–61.

Davidoff, Robert A. *Migraine: Manifestations, Pathogenesis, and Management*. Oxford University Press, 2002.

Davis, Lennard J., ed. *The Disability Studies Reader*. New York: Routledge, 1997.

De Beauvoir, Simone. *The Second Sex*, 1952. Reprinted. New York: Knopf, 1974.

Descartes, René. *Treatise of Man*, 1662. Translated by Thomas Steele Hall. Cambridge: Harvard University Press, 1972.

Didion, Joan. "In Bed." Reprinted in *The White Album*, edited by Joan Didion. New York: Pocket Books, 1979.

Dreher, Diane. *The Tao of Inner Peace*. New York: Ballantine, 1991.

Edmeads, John. "The Treatment of Headache: A Historical Perspective." In *Drug Therapy for Headache*, edited by R. Michael Gallagher. New York: Marcel Dekker, 1991.

Ehrenreich, Barbara, and Deirdre English. *For Her Own Good: 150 Years of the Experts' Advice to Women*. New York: Anchor Books, 1978.

Elias, Marilyn. "Acupuncture's Secret: Blood Flow to the Brain," *USA Today*, March 3, 2004.

Evans, Randolph W., and Julio Pascual, "Expert Opinion: Orgasmic Headaches: Clinical Features, Diagnosis and Management," *Headache* 40, no. 6 (June 2000): 491.

Evans, Randolph W., and James W. Couch. "Orgasm and Migraine," *Headache* 41, no. 5 (May 2001): 512.

Faucett, Julia. "The Ergonomics of Women's Work." In *Women's Health: Complexities and Differences*, edited by Sheryl Burt Ruzek, Virginia L. Olesen, and Adele E. Clarke. Columbus: Ohio State University Press, 1997.

Fillingim, R. B., and W. Maixner. "Gender Differences and the Responses to Noxious Stimuli," *Pain Forum* 4, no. 4 (1995): 209–221.

Fillingim, Roger B., ed. *Sex, Gender and Pain: Progress in Pain Research and Management*, vol. 17. Seattle: IASP Press, 2000.

————. "Sex Differences in Pain and Analgesia," conference paper presented at the annual meeting of the American Pain Society, March 20, 2003.

Fine, Michelle, and Adrienne Asch, eds. *Women with Disabilities*. Philadelphia: Temple University Press, 1988.

Fishman, Scott, with Lisa Berger. *The War on Pain*. New York: HarperCollins, 2000.

Fontanarosa, Phil B., ed. *Alternative Medicine: An Objective Assessment*. Chicago: American Medical Association, 2000.

Gawande, Atul. *Complications: A Surgeon's Notes on an Imperfect Science*. New York: Metropolitan Books, 2002.

Gerber, Richard. *Vibrational Medicine: New Choices for Healing Ourselves*. Santa Fe, N.M.: Bear, 1988.

Gilman, Charlotte Perkins. "The Yellow Wallpaper," 1892. Reprinted in *Fiction 100*, edited by James H. Pickering. New York: Macmillan, 1985, 426–435.

Gobel H., H. Isler, and H. P. Hasenfraz. "Headache Classification and the Bible: Was St. Paul's Thorn in the Flesh Migraine?" *Cephalalgia* 15 (1995): 182–190.

Goldstein, Jay A. *Tuning the Brain: Principles and Practice of Neurosomatic Medicine*. New York: Haworth Press, 2004.

Goldstein, Jerome. "Sexual Aspects of Headache," *Postgraduate Medicine* 109, no. 1 (January 2001): 81–92. http://www.postgradmed.com/issues/2001/01_01/goldstein.htm (accessed December 1, 2003).

Gray, R. N., et al. "Evidence Report: Drug Treatments for the Prevention of Migraine," *Technical Review* 2, no. 3 (1999). Available at http://www.clinpol.mc.duke.edu.

Hanley, J. J., David Simpson, and Gordon Quinn, producers. "Refrigerator Mothers." Documentary film. Chicago: Kartemquin Films, 2002. Available for order at fanlight.com.

Harden, Holly. "The Fish That Swim in My Head, A Life with Migraine Headaches," *Utne Reader* (September-October 2003): 45–47. Originally published in *Fourth Genre.*

Harrison, Jim. *The Woman Lit by Fireflies.* Boston: Houghton Mifflin, 1990.

Haspel, Tamar. "Do You Have a Food Allergy?" *Fitness*, March 2004, pp. 64–67.

Hatak, Kristine. *A Guided Tour of Hell: Migraine in the Words of Its Victims.* Roseville, Calif.: Dry Bones Press, 1999.

Hillyer, Barbara. *Feminism and Disability.* Norman: University of Oklahoma Press, 1993.

Hoffman, Diane E., and Anita J. Tarzian. "The Girl Who Cried Pain: A Bias Against Women in the Treatment of Pain." *J. Law Med.* Ethics 29 (2001): 13–27.

Hofmann, Albert. *LSD: My Problem Child, Reflections on Sacred Drugs, Mysticism, and Science.* New York: J. P. Tarcher, 1979.

Hogshire, Jim. *Pills-a-Go-Go: A Fiendish Investigation into Pill Marketing, Art, History and Consumption.* Venice, Calif.: Feral House, 1999.

Hornbacher, Marya. *Wasted: A Memoir of Anorexia and Bulimia.* New York: HarperCollins, 1998.

"How Is Your Doctor Treating You?" *Consumer Reports*, February 1995, pp. 81–88.

Hustvedt, Siri. *The Blindfold.* New York: W. W. Norton, 1992.

"The International Classification of Headache," The International Headache Society, *Cephalalgia* 24 (2004): s1–s150. Also see http:www.I-h-s.org.

Irvine, Martha. "Chronic Headaches Often Start in Teen Years" (AP story), *Chicago Sun-Times*, November 23, 2003, p. 42A.

Isler, Hansruedi. "Thomas Willis' Two Chapters on Headache of 1672: A First Attempt to Apply the 'New Sciences' to This Topic," *Headache* 26 (1986): 95–98.

Jackson, Marni. *Pain: The Fifth Vital Sign.* New York: Crown, 2002.

Jamison, Robert N., Karen O. Anderson, and Mark A. Slater. "Weather Changes and Pain: Perceived Influence of Local Climate on Pain in Chronic Pain Patients," *Pain* 61, no. 2 (May 1995): 309–315.

Jauhar, Sandeep. "Over-the-Counter Headache," *New York Times Magazine*, January 12, 2003, section 6, p. 40.

Kabat-Zinn, Jon. *Full Catastrophe Living.* New York: Delta, 1990.

Kaminer, Wendy. *Sleeping with Extraterrestrials.* New York: Vintage, 1999.

Kaysen, Susanna. *Girl, Interrupted.* New York: Turtle Bay Books, 1993.

———. *The Camera My Mother Gave Me.* New York: Knopf, 2001.

Kelman, Leslie. "Women's Issues of Migraine in Tertiary Care," *Headache* 44, no. 1 (2004): 2–7.

Kempner, J. "A Sociologic Perspective in Migraine in Women." In *Migraine in Women*, edited by Elizabeth Loder and Dawn Marcus. Hamilton, Ontario, Canada: Decker, 2003.

Kenney, Kim. "Headaches and CFIDS," *CFIDS Chronicle* 16, no. 4 (Fall 2003): 6.

Kettlewell, Caroline. *Skin Game: A Cutter's Memoir.* New York: St. Martin's Press, 1999.

Keyes, Daniel. *Flowers for Algernon* (novel version). New York: Bantam, 1975.

Kiester, Edwin, Jr. "Doctors Close In on the Mechanisms Behind Headache," *Smithsonian Magazine* 1, no. 9 (December 1987): 175–190.

Knapp, Caroline. *Drinking: A Love Story*. New York: Dell, 1996.

Kolata, Gina. "With Costs Rising, Treating Back Pain Often Seems Futile," *New York Times*, February 9, 2004, pp. A1, A12.

Kot, Greg. "'I Was Begging Them to Institutionalize Me'" (interview with Jeff Tweedy), *Chicago Tribune*, June 6, 2004, section 7, p. 6.

Kruit, Mark C., et al. "Migraine as a Risk Factor for Subclinical Brain Lesions," *Journal of the American Medical Association* 291 (2004): 427–434.

Kryst, Sandra. "Engendering Pain: Discourse on the Experience of Chronic Headache in the United States," Ph.D. dissertation, University of Kentucky, 1996. Abstract in *Dissertation Abstracts International*; publ. no. 1996-95014-069, vol. 57, no. 1-A (July 1996) US: University Microfilms International, 0299.

Kübler-Ross, Elisabeth. *On Death and Dying*. New York: Macmillan, 1969.

Lack, Dorothea Z. "Women and Pain: Another Feminist Issue." *Women and Therapy* 1, no. 1 (1982): 55–64.

Lampl, Christian, et al. "Relationship of Locus of Control in Women with Migraine and Healthy Volunteers," *Headache* 43, no. 8 (2003): 878.

Levin, Morris. "Chronic Daily Headache and the Revised International Headache Society Classification," *Current Pain and Headache Reports* 8 (2004): 59–65.

Lipton, Richard B., and Julie Pan. "Is Migraine a Progressive Brain Disease?" *Journal of the American Medical Association* 291 (2004): 493–494.

Living, Edward. *On Megrim, Sick-Headache, and Some Allied Disorders: A Contribution to the Pathology of Nerve-Storms*, 1873. Nijmegen, The Netherlands: Arts & Boeve, 1997.

Loder, Elizabeth, and Dawn Marcus, eds. *Migraine in Women*. Hamilton, Ontario, Canada: Decker, 2003.

Loeser, John D. "The Decade of Pain Control and Research." Reprint of speech to March 2003 meeting. *American Pain Society Bulletin*, May-June 2003, pp. 1, 4–8.

Low, Nancy C. P., and Kathleen Ries Merikangas. "The Comorbidity of Migraine," *CNS Spectrums* 8, no. 6 (June 2003): 433–444.

Lu, S. R., Fuh J. L., Chen W. T., et al. "Chronic Daily Headache in Taipei, Taiwan: Prevalence, Follow-up and Outcome Predictors." *Cephalalgia* 21 (2001): 980–986.

Manzoni, G. C., and P. Torelli. "International Headache Society Classification: New Proposals About Chronic Daily Headache," *Neurological Sciences* 24 (2003): S86–S89.

Marchand, S. "Neurophysiological Mechanisms of Non Pharmacological Recruitment of Endogenous Pain Modulation systems," conference paper presented at the annual meeting of the American Pain Society, March 20, 2003.

Marchand, S., and P. Arsenault. "Odors Modulate Pain Perception. A Gender-Specific Effect." *Physiol Behav.* 76 (2002a): 251–256.

Marchand, S., and P. Arsenault. "Spatial Summation for Pain Perception: Interaction of Inhibitory and Excitatory Mechanisms." *Pain* 95 (2002b): 201–206.

Marchand, S., J. Charest, J. Li, J. R. Chenard, B. Lavignole, and L. Laurencelle. "Is

TENS Purely a Placebo Effect? A Controlled Study on Low Back Pain." *Pain* 54 (1993): 99–106

Marcus, Dawn. "Central Sensitization: A New Theory of Migraine," *Headache* 13, no. 3. *Newsletter of American Council on Headache Education*, Mt. Royal, N.J. (Fall 2002): 5. See http://www.achenet.org.

_____. "Central Sensitization: An Important Factor in the Pathogenesis of Chronic Headache," *Headache and Pain*, April 2003, p. 22.

Matchar, David B., Douglas C. McCrory, and Rebecca N. Gray. "Toward Evidence-Based Management of Migraine," *Journal of the American Medical Association* 284 (2000): 2640–2641.

Max, Mitchell B. "How to Move Pain and Symptom Research from the Margin to the Mainstream," *Journal of Pain* 4, no. 7 (September 2003): 355–360.

Maxwell, Harold. *Migraine: Background and Treatment*. Bristol: John Wright, 1966.

McEwan, Ian. *Atonement*. New York: Random House, 2001.

Meldrum, Marcia L. "A Capsule History of Pain Management," *Journal of the American Medical Association* 290, no. 18 (November 12, 2003): 2470–2475.

Merskey, H., and N. Bogduk. *Classification of Chronic Pain*. Seattle: IASP Press, 1994.

Merskey, Harold. "History of Psychoanalytic Ideas Concerning Pain." In *Personality Characteristics of Patients with Pain*, edited by Robert J. Gatchel and James N. Weisberg. Washington, D.C.: American Psychological Association, 2000, 25–35.

Metzl, Jonathan Michel. *Prozac on the Couch: Prescribing Gender in the Era of Wonder Drugs*. Durham, N.C.: Duke University Press. 2003.

Mire, Lucas J. "Weather May Be a Headache for Migraine Sufferers," and "Aches and Pains 101," July 11, 2003, at http://weather.com.

Morris, David B. *The Culture of Pain*. Berkeley: University of California Press, 1991.

_____. *Illness and Culture in the Postmodern Age*. Berkeley: University of California Press, 1998.

Munson, Peggy. *Stricken: Voices from the Hidden Epidemic of Chronic Fatigue Syndrome*. Binghamton, N.Y.: Haworth Press, 2000.

National Institute of Neurological Disorders and Stroke of the National Institutes of Health. "21st Century Prevention and Management of Migraine Headaches," *Clinician* 19, no. 11 (December 2001).

National Migraine Association (MAGNUM). "Elvis Presley's Private Struggle with Intractable Migraines Revealed," April 19, 1999, press release on www.migraines.org/new/news9904/htm.

Nielsen, Patricia D. *Living with It Daily: Meditations for People with Chronic Pain*. New York: Dell, 1994.

Olesen, J., T. J. Steiner, and R. B. Lipton. *Reducing the Burden of Headache*. Oxford: Oxford University Press, 2003.

Oliver, Joan Duncan. "At Home in Our Bodies," *Tricycle Magazine,* Winter 2002.

Packard, Russell C. "Woman with Nearly Continuous Headaches for Whom 'Nothing Has Worked,'" *Headache and Pain* (September 2003): 111–113.

Penzien, Donald B. "Headache and Personality." Excerpted from article in *Headache* 9, no. 3 (Fall 1998). On web site of American Council for Headache Education, http://www.achenet.org.

Peres, M. P., et al. "Fibromyalgia Is Common in Patients with Transformed Migraine," *Neurology* 57, no. 7 (October 9, 2001): 1326–1328.

Peres, M. F. P., et al. "Fatigue in Chronic Migraine Patients," *Cephalalgia* 22, no. 9 (November 2002): 720.

Perrin, Dennis. *Mr. Mike: The Life and Work of Michael O'Donoghue.* New York: Avon Books, 1998.

Piccalo, Gina. "Taking Aim at Botox," *Los Angeles Times.* September 22, 2003.

Prince, Patricia B., et al. "The Effect of Weather on Headache," *Headache* 44, no. 6 (2004): 596–602.

Pringsheim, Tamara, and Louis Gooeren. "Migraine Prevalence in Male to Female Transsexuals on Hormone Therapy." *Neurology* 63, no. 3 (August 10, 2004): 593–594.

Rapoport, Alan M., and John Edmeads. "Migraine: The Evolution of Our Knowledge," *Archives of Neurology* 57, no. 8 (August 2000): 1121–1123.

Reese, Hazel Lucretia. *I Will Not Complain! My Life with Chronic Illness.* Baltimore: Publish America, 2004.

Register, Cheri. *The Chronic Illness Experience.* (Originally titled *Living with Chronic Illness: Days of Patience and Passion.* New York: Free Press, 1987.) Center City, Minn.: Hazelden, 1999.

Rist, Curtis. "The Pain Is in the Brain." *Discover,* March 2000. Found excerpted at http://britannica.com.

Robbins, Lawrence. "Headache and the Immune System," *National Headache Foundation Newsletter,* Chicago (Winter 1994): 3.

_____. *Management of Headache and Headache Medications.* New York: Springer-Verlag, 2000.

_____. "Practical Headache Pearls," *Practical Pain Management,* July/August 2002. From reprinted flyer.

_____. "Long-Term Efficacy of Preventive Medications for Chronic Daily Headache" [abstract], *Headache* 43, no. 5 (May 2003): 573.

Robbins, Lawrence, and Susan S. Lang. *Headache Help: A Complete Guide to Understanding Headaches and the Medicines That Relieve Them.* New York: Houghton Mifflin, 1995.

Robinson, Michael E., Joseph L. Riley III, and Cynthia D. Myers. "Psychosocial Contributions to Sex-Related Differences in Pain Responses." In *Sex, Gender and Pain: Progress in Pain Research and Management,* vol. 17, edited by Roger Fillingim. Seattle: IASP Press, 2000, 41–68.

Ruppert, Susanne. "Living with Pain." *O Magazine,* September 2003, p. 177.

Ruzek, Sheryl Burt, Virginia L. Olesen, and Adele E. Clarke. *Women's Health: Complexities and Differences.* Columbus: Ohio State University Press, 1997.

Sacks, Oliver. *Migraine,* 1970. Reprint. Berkeley, Calif.: University of California Press, 1992.

Safer, D. J. "Design and Reporting Modifications in Industry-Sponsored Comparative Psychopharmacology Trials," *Journal of Nervous and Mental Disease* 190 (2002): 583–592.

Scarry, Elaine. *The Body in Pain: The Making and Unmaking of the World.* Oxford University Press, 1985.

Scher, A. I., R. B. Lipton, and W. Stewart. "Risk Factors for Chronic Daily

Headache," *Current Pain and Headache Reports* 6, no. 6 (2002): 486–491.

Schlesigner, Lynn. "Chronic Pain, Intimacy and Sexuality: A Qualitative Study of Women Who Live with Pain," *Journal of Sex Research* 33, no. 3 (1996): 249.

Seaman, Barbara. *The Doctors' Case Against the Pill*, 25th anniversary edition. Alameda, Calif.: Hunter House, 1995.

Seuss, Dr. *Oh, the Places You'll Go!* New York: Random House, 1990.

Shealy, C. Norman, and Caroline M. Myss. *The Creation of Health: The Emotional, Psychological, and Spiritual Responses That Promote Health and Healing.* Walpole, N.H.: Stillpoint, 1988.

Shorter, Edward. *From Paralysis to Fatigue: A History of Psychosomatic Illness in the Modern Era.* New York: Free Press, 1992.

Showalter, Elaine. *The Female Malady: Women, Madness and English Culture, 1830–1980.* New York: Pantheon, 1985.

_____. *Hystories: Hysterical Epidemics and the Modern Media.* New York: Columbia University Press, 1987.

Silberstein, Stephen, et al. *An Atlas of Headache.* New York: Parthenon, 2002.

Silberstein, Stephen, Richard B. Lipton, and Peter J. Goadsby. *Headache in Clinical Practice.* London: Martin Dunitz, 2002.

Simon, Lizzie. *Detour: My Bipolar Road Trip in 4-D.* New York: Atria Books, 2002.

Slater, Lauren. *Prozac Diary.* New York: Penguin, 1998.

Solomon, Andrew. *The Noonday Demon: An Atlas of Depression.* New York: Simon & Schuster, 2001.

Sontag, Susan. *Illness as Metaphor.* New York: Anchor Books, 1978.

Spierings, E. L., and M. J. van Hoof. "Fatigue and Sleep in Chronic Headache Sufferers: An Age- and Sex-Controlled Questionnaire Study," *Headache* 37 (1997): 549–552.

Srikiatkhachorn, A. "Chronic Daily Headache: A Scientist's Perspective," *Headache* 42, no. 6 (June 2002): 532–537.

Stamets, Bill. "Lecture Notes: Dr. Mesmer's Cure for Pain," *Chicago Reader*, May 3, 2002, p. 35.

Stewart, W. F., et al. "Prevalence of Migraine Headache in the United States: Relationship to Age, Income, Race and Other Sociodemographic Factors," *Journal of the American Medical Association* 267 (1992): 64–69.

Stewart, Walter F., et al. "Lost Productive Time and Cost Due to Common Pain Conditions in the US Workforce," *Journal of the American Medical Association* 290, no. 18 (November 12, 2003): 2443–2454.

Stukin, Stacie. "Freedom from Addiction," *Yoga Journal*, May-June 2002.

Talvi, Sijla. "Women on the Edge," *In These Times*, August 15, 2003.

Teitelbaum, Jacob. *From Fatigued to Fantastic: A Manual for Moving Beyond Chronic Fatigue and Fibromyalgia.* Garden City Park, N.Y.: Avery, 1996.

Tepper, Stewart J. *Understanding Migraine and Other Headaches.* Jackson: University Press of Mississippi, 2004.

Thernstrom, Melanie. "Pain, the Disease," *New York Times Magazine*, December 16, 2001, pp. 66–71.

Tietjen, Gretchen E. "Abuse and Headache," *Headache* 15, no. 1. *Newsletter of American Council on Headache Education*, Mt. Royal, N.J. (Spring 2004): 5. See http://www.achenet.org.

Tietjen, Gretchen E., and Robin L. Brey. "Contraception, Estrogen Replacement Therapy, Migraine, and Stroke." In *Migraine in Women*, edited by Elizabeth Loder and Dawn Marcus, Hamilton, Ontario, Canada: Decker, 2003, 134–143.

Turner, Kristina. *The Self-Healing Cookbook*. Vashon Island, Wash.: Earthtones Press, 1987.

Tzu, Lao. *Tao Te Ching*. Translated and with an introduction by D. C. Lau. New York: Penguin Books, 1963.

Unruh, Anita M. "Gender Variations in Clinical Pain Experience," *Pain* 65 (1996): 123–167.

"US Subpoenas 2 Drug Makers," *New York Times*, December 13, 2003.

Vertosick, Frank T. *Why We Hurt: The Natural History of Pain*. New York: Harcourt, 2000.

Vickers, Andrew J., et al. "Acupuncture for Chronic Headache in Primary Care: Large, Pragmatic, Randomised Trial." *BMJ* 328 (March 15, 2004): 744.

Weil, Andrew. *Spontaneous Healing*. New York: Knopf, 1995.

Weiller, C., et al. "Brain Stem Activation in Spontaneous Human Migraine Attacks," *Nat. Medicine* 1, no. 7 (1995): 658–660.

Weir Mitchell, Silas. *Fat and Blood: and How to Make Them*. Philadelphia: Lippincott, 1877.

———. *Doctor and Patient*. Philadelphia: Lippincott, 1887.

Welch, K., A. Michael, and Peter J. Goadsby. "Chronic Daily Headache: Nosology and Pathopsychology," *Current Opinion in Neurology* 15, no. 3 (June 2002): 287–295.

Welch K. M., et al. "Periaqueductal Gray Matter Dysfunction in Migraine: Cause or the Burden of Illness?" *Headache* 412, no. 7 (July-August 2001): 629–637.

Wendell, Susan. *The Rejected Body*. New York: Routledge, 1996.

Willis, Thomas. *De Anima Brutorum . . . (Two Discourses on the Soul of Brutes Which Is the Vital and Sensitive Soul of Man)*, Oxonii: e Theatro Sheldoniano, 1672. On microfilm. Ann Arbor, Mich.: University Microfilms International, 1979. 1 microfilm reel; 35 mm. (Early English books, 1641–1700; 969:27).

———. *London Practice of Physick*. Printed for T. Dring, C. Harper, and J. Leigh. London: Thos. Basset & Wm. Crooke, 1685. On microfilm. Ann Arbor, Mich.: University Microfilms International, 1983. 1 microfilm reel; 35 mm. (Early English books, 1641–1700; 1371:2).

Wolf, Stuart, and Helen Goodell. *Harold G. Wolff's Stress and Disease*. Springfield, Ill.: Charles C. Thomas, 1953.

Woolf, Virginia. *On Being Ill*, 1st ed. London: Hogarth Press, 1930. Reprinted. Ashfield, Mass.: Paris Press, 2002.

Wurtzel, Elizabeth. *Prozac Nation*. New York: Riverhead Books, 1994.

Young, William B., and Stephen D. Silberstein. *Migraine and Other Headaches*. New York: Demos Medical, 2004.

Young-Bruehl, Elisabeth. *Freud on Women: A Reader*. New York: W. W. Norton, 1990.

P A T I E N T
R E S O U R C E S

○ ○ ○ ○ ○ ○ ○ ○ ○

For Coping with Chronic Pain (Mentally and Emotionally)

From the American Chronic Pain Association (http://theacpa.org):

- *From Patient to Person: First Steps*, by Penney Cowan (workbook). The videotape version is also recommended.
- *Pathways Through Pain* series (videotapes). The first one, *Accepting the Pain*, is especially recommended.

Cleveland, Martha. *Chronic Illness and the Twelve Steps: A Practical Approach to Spiritual Resilience*. Center City, Minn.: Hazelden, 1988.

Kabat-Zinn, Jon. *Full Catastrophe Living*. New York: Delta, 1990. (On meditation)

Nielsen, Patricia D. *Living with It Daily: Meditations for People with Chronic Pain*. New York: Dell, 1994.

Register, Cheri. *The Chronic Illness Experience*. Originally titled *Living with Chronic Illness: Days of Patience and Passion*. New York: Free Press, 1987. Reprinted. Center City, Minn.: Hazelden, 1999.

For Coping with Head Pain (Physically)

Robbins, Lawrence, and Susan S. Lang. *Headache Help: A Complete Guide to Understanding Headaches and the Medicines That Relieve Them*. New York: Houghton Mifflin, 1995.

Tepper, Stewart J. *Understanding Migraine and Other Headaches*. Jackson: University Press of Mississippi, 2004.

Young, William B., and Stephen D. Silberstein. *Migraine and Other Headaches*. New York: Demos Medical, 2004.

First-Person Accounts

Memoirs

Hatak, Kristine. *A Guided Tour of Hell: Migraine in the Words of Its Victims.* Roseville, Calif.: Dry Bones Press, 1999.

Levy, Carol Jay. *A Pained Life: A Chronic Pain Journey.* CITY, 2003. (Trigeminal neuralgia)

Reese, Hazel Lucretia. *I Will Not Complain! My Life with Chronic Illness.* Baltimore: Publish America, 2004. (Chronic daily headache)

Essays

Bernardi, Andria. "Half-Cranium," *River Oak Review* (Oak Park, Ill.), Spring-Summer 2003, pp. 67–75.

Cahn, Susan K. "Come Out, Come Out Whatever You've Got! Or, Still Crazy After All These Years," *Feminist Studies* 29, no. 1 (Spring 2003): 7; 12 pages. (Chronic fatigue syndrome)

Didion, Joan. "In Bed." Reprinted in *The White Album*, edited by Joan Didion. New York: Pocket Books, 1979.

Harden, Holly. 2003. "The Fish That Swim in My Head, A Life with Migraine Headaches," *Utne Reader* (September–October 2003): 45–47. Originally published in *Fourth Genre*.

Fiction

Harrison, Jim. *The Woman Lit By Fireflies.* Boston: Houghton Mifflin, 1990.

Hustvedt, Siri. *The Blindfold.* New York: W. W. Norton, 1992.

Web Sites with Patient Dialogues

http://ww.headaches.about.com
http://www.migrainepage.com
http://www.painaid.org

Nonprofit Organizations

American Chronic Pain Association
    Offers support group referral. http://www.theacpa.org

American Council on Headache Education (ACHE)
    Offers newsletter, *Headache*, with latest medical information; support group; and doctor referral. http://www.achenet.org

American Pain Foundation
    Offers electronic and paper newsletters, among many other patient resources. http://www.painfoundation.org

MAGNUM: National Migraine Association (Migraine Understanding Group: A National Understanding for Migraineurs) http://www.migraines.org/

Migraine Action Association (Great Britain)
http://www.migraine.org.uk/
National Headache Foundation
Offers newsletter, *Head Lines*, with latest medical information; support group
referral. http://www.headaches.org
World Headache Alliance
http://www.w-h-a.org

On Women and Pain (Academic Books)

Fillingim, Roger B., ed. *Sex, Gender and Pain: Progress in Pain Research and
Management*, vol. 17. Seattle: IASP Press, 2000.
Loder, Elizabeth, and Dawn Marcus, eds. *Migraine in Women*. Hamilton, Ontario,
Canada: Decker, 2003.
Wendell, Susan. *The Rejected Body.* New York: Routledge, 1996.
Wilson, Elizabeth A. *Psychosomatic: Feminism and the Neurological Body*. Durham,
N.C.: Duke University Press, 2004.

Medical Journals and Resources
(Clear Summaries at Start of Articles)

Cephalalgia (published on behalf of the International Headache Society);
http://www.blackwellpublishing.com/journal.asp?ref=0333–1024
Current Pain and Headache Reports; http://www.current-
reports.com/home_journal.cfm?JournalID=PA
Headache: The Journal of Head and Face Pain (published on behalf of American
Headache Society); http://www.ahsnet.org/journal/
For the latest diagnostic classifications of headaches, see the web page of the
International Headache Society: http://www.I-h-s.org.

A C K N O W L E D G M E N T S

○ ○ ○ ○ ○ ○ ○ ○ ○

Thanks to those who made this book possible:

- My family, especially my parents
- All patients and doctors interviewed for this book
- Agent Daniel Greenberg
- Editor Marnie Cochran at Da Capo Press

And to those who also really helped:

- Medical consultants: Dr. Megan Shanks (Chicago) and Dr. Elizabeth Loder (Boston)
- Research support: Gender Studies Program of Northwestern University, Galter Health Sciences Library at the Feinberg School of Medicine (reference and interlibrary loan desks), and Dr. Jack Kamen
- Helpful editorial support: Tamara Dean, Kyra Auslander, and Bridget Brown
- Transcription and transcript analysis: GinaMaria Scoleri
- Special support: Heather Barrow, Paul Creamer, Anna Minkov, Wendy Bower, Rivka Solomon, Beth Schulman, Felicia Kornbluh, Clare Sullivan, and Dick Detzner and Sasha Rubel.
- And last but not least: Ingrid Finstuen, Erin Sprague, and Lissa Warren at Da Capo; Laura Micham and the Sallie Bingham Center for Women's History and Culture at Duke University; National Writers Union; Ragdale Foundation; American Pain Society; American Headache Society, Julie Semancek; Teri Robert of headaches.about.com; Susan Barron of the National Headache Foundation in Chicago, and the participants in her support group; Elizabeth Hart, Barbara Seaman, lawyer Eldon Hamm and

Jeffrey Rabin, Mitch Newman, Steve Rhodes, Iris Chang, Beth Austin, Steve Rhodes, Josh Kilroy, Ken and Becky Kurson, Linda Michaels, Mike Ramsey, Joanna Kempner, Estelle Carol and Bob Simpson, Neal Pollack, Adam Langer, Stephany Creamer, Sandi Wisenberg, Amy Keller, Ellen Frank, Dr. Sandra Bartky, Evan Winer, Paul Moulton, Thousand Waves Spa and Janet, Dragon's Life Chinese Medicine, my doctors, Suzen Alvord, and the staff and clients of Transcription Professionals.

INDEX

○ ○ ○ ○ ○ ○ ○ ○ ○